July 2017

Dear Auntie Noreen,

Hope you enjoy – if anything
it will help you sleep!!

Lots of love,

Fairy xxx.

DR Teresa Kennedy
Lydon.
husband DR Senbad
Dr of Science.

GW00669786

Advances in Experimental Medicine and Biology

Series editors
Irun R. Cohen
Department of Cell Bio
The Weizmann Institute of Science
Rehovot, Israel

Abel Lajtha
N.S.Kline Institute for Psychiatric Rrch
Orangeburg, New York, USA

John D. Lambris
Pathology and Lab Med, 401 Stellar Chance
University of Pennsylvania
Philadelphia, Pennsylvania, USA

Rodolfo Paoletti
University of Milan
Milan, Italy

Advances in Experimental Medicine and Biology presents multidisciplinary and dynamic findings in the broad fields of experimental medicine and biology. The wide variety in topics it presents offers readers multiple perspectives on a variety of disciplines including neuroscience, microbiology, immunology, biochemistry, biomedical engineering and cancer research. Advances in Experimental Medicine and Biology has been publishing exceptional works in the field for over 30 years and is indexed in Medline, Scopus, EMBASE, BIOSIS, Biological Abstracts, CSA, Biological Sciences and Living Resources (ASFA-1), and Biological Sciences. The series also provides scientists with up to date information on emerging topics and techniques. 2015 Impact Factor: 1.953

More information about this series at http://www.springer.com/series/5584

Susanne Sattler • Teresa Kennedy-Lydon
Editors

The Immunology
of Cardiovascular Homeostasis
and Pathology

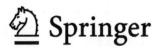 Springer

Editors
Susanne Sattler
Hammersmith Campus
Imperial College London National Heart
and Lung Institute
London, UK

Teresa Kennedy-Lydon
Hammersmith Campus
Imperial College London National Heart
and Lung Institute
London, UK

ISSN 0065-2598   ISSN 2214-8019   (electronic)
Advances in Experimental Medicine and Biology
ISBN 978-3-319-57611-4   ISBN 978-3-319-57613-8   (eBook)
DOI 10.1007/978-3-319-57613-8

Printed on acid-free paper

This Springer imprint is published by Springer Nature
The registered company is Springer International Publishing AG
The registered company address is: Gewerbestrasse 11, 6330 Cham, Switzerland

Preface

Cardiovascular immunology is a newly emerging research area based on the increasingly evident existence of several layers of crosstalk between the cardiovascular and the immune system. Nevertheless, there is still little overlap between research into cardiovascular biology and immunology. However, emerging knowledge is challenging this paradox and forcing communication between the two fields. As a result, we are now approaching a time where the immune system is rapidly being appreciated for its role other than fighting infections, particularly in the cardiovascular sciences.

For this book, we have sought to bring together experts on various aspects of cardiovascular immunology, with the aim of providing an overview of the crosstalk between the cardiovascular and the immune system under homeostasis and during disease. First, we discuss our changing understanding of the immune system and its various roles in physiological processes other than host defence. We then describe the immunological capacities and functions of the most important cardiovascular cell types, including cardiomyocytes, fibroblasts, endothelial cells, pericytes as well as resident macrophages, the most prominent cardiac immune cell population. This is followed by an exploration of areas, in which disturbance of immune regulation and aberrant activation of the immune system is causative in the development of cardiovascular disease including atherosclerosis and cardiac and cardiovascular autoimmunity. We conclude with two chapters on the crucial role of the endogenous innate and adaptive immune system in heart repair and regeneration after tissue damage.

With this comprehensive coverage of state-of-the-art knowledge on the mutual and interdependent link between the cardiovascular and the immune system, we hope to provide a valuable resource for readers with either immunology or cardiovascular background.

London, UK   Susanne Sattler
London, UK   Teresa Kennedy-Lydon

Introduction

Most textbooks still describe the immune system largely in the light of infectious disease. However, we now know that defence against invaders is only one of several roles of the immune system aiming for the maintenance or restoration of tissue integrity. Non-self-recognition and defence against infectious microorganisms even seem to be an evolutionary younger addition to the ancient mechanism of phagocytosis, which is the crucial basis for fundamental physiological processes during development and homeostasis.

As such the immune system cannot be separated from the rest of the body but is an integral part of any organ system or physiological process. To name just a few striking examples, ovulation, mammary gland development, the establishment of a successful pregnancy through fetomaternal tolerance, embryonic development through developmental apoptosis, angiogenesis, bone and brain development and of course wound healing and regeneration of adult tissues are all dependent on a variety of immune effector cells or molecules.

A crucial role of the immune system beyond the control of infectious diseases has also become evident in the cardiovascular system. Immune cells and molecules play critical roles as effectors in cardiovascular health and disease. The heart itself contains a diverse population of tissue-resident immune cells, which are crucial in the continuous maintenance of tissue integrity. Moreover, the vasculature is in intimate contact with immune effectors in the blood and thus particularly susceptible to inflammatory changes. Conversely, parenchymal and stromal cells of the heart and vasculature have a wide range of crucial immunological functions and are active players in shaping immune responses.

Although the field of cardiovascular immunology is still in its infancy, it's becoming increasingly evident that a tightly controlled interplay between the two systems is essential to maintain cardiovascular health. Taking into account the effects on both systems will have potential to significantly improve future therapeutic strategies.

Contents

Contributors

Alexander R. Pinto Australian Regenerative Medicine Institute, Monash University, Melbourne, VIC, Australia

The Jackson Laboratory, Bar Harbor, ME, USA

Anastasia Bougea, MD, PhD Department of Neurology, University of Athens Medical School, Aeginition Hospital, Athens, Greece

William Bracamonte-Baran Department of Pathology, Division of Immunology, Johns Hopkins University School of Medicine, Baltimore, MD, USA

Daniela Čihákova Department of Pathology, Division of Immunology, Johns Hopkins University School of Medicine, Baltimore, MD, USA

W. Harry Feinstone Department of Molecular Microbiology and Immunology, Johns Hopkins University Bloomberg School of Public Health, Baltimore, MD, USA

Marco Folci Allergy, Clinical Immunology and Rheumatology Unit, IRCCS Istituto Auxologico Italiano, Milan, Italy

Stefan Frantz Department of Internal Medicine III, University Clinic Halle, Halle, Germany

Milena B. Furtado The Jackson Laboratory, Bar Harbor, ME, USA

Australian Regenerative Medicine Institute, Monash University, Melbourne, VIC, Australia

Elena Generali Rheumatology and Clinical Immunology, Humanitas Research Hospital, Rozzano, Milan, Italy

Rebecca Gentek Centre d'Immunologie de Marseille-Luminy (CIML), Aix-Marseille Université, Centre National de la Recherche Scientifique (CNRS), Institut National de la Santé et de la Recherche Médicale (INSERM), Marseille, France

Muneer Hasham The Jackson Laboratory, Bar Harbor, ME, USA

Guillaume Hoeffel Centre d'Immunologie de Marseille-Luminy (CIML), Aix-Marseille Université, Centre National de la Recherche Scientifique (CNRS), Institut National de la Santé et de la Recherche Médicale (INSERM), Marseille, France

Alexei Ilinykh Australian Regenerative Medicine Institute, Monash University, Melbourne, VIC, Australia

Teresa Kennedy-Lydon Heart Science, NHLI, Imperial College London, London, UK

Anne A. Knowlton Molecular and Cellular Cardiology, Cardiovascular Division, Department of Medicine, University of California, Davis, Davis, CA, USA

Department of Pharmacology, University of California, Davis, CA, USA

The Department of Veteran's Affairs, Northern California VA, Sacramento, CA, USA

Vânia Nunes-Silva Instituto Gulbenkian de Ciência, Oeiras, Portugal

Mohammed Shamim Rahman Division of Immunology and Inflammation, Department of Medicine, Imperial College London, London, UK

Gustavo Campos Ramos Department of Internal Medicine III, University Clinic Halle, Halle, Germany

Martin-Luther-Universität Halle-Wittenberg Universitätsklinik und Poliklinik für Innere Medizin III, Halle, Germany

Piersandro Riboldi Allergy, Clinical Immunology and Rheumatology Unit, IRCCS Istituto Auxologico Italiano, Milan, Italy

Susanne Sattler National Heart and Lung Institute, Imperial College London, London, UK

Carlo Selmi Rheumatology and Clinical Immunology, Humanitas Research Hospital, Rozzano, Milan, Italy

BIOMETRA Department, University of Milan, Milan, Italy

Nikolaos Spantideas, PhD Department of Neurology, University of Athens Medical School, Aeginition Hospital, Athens, Greece

Caterina Sturtzel, PhD Innovative Cancer Models, Children's Cancer Research Institute, St. Anna Kinderkrebsforschung e.V, Vienna, Austria

Kevin Woollard Division of Immunology and Inflammation, Department of Medicine, Imperial College London, London, UK

Part I
The Immune System in Tissue and Organ Homeostasis

Chapter 1
The Role of the Immune System Beyond the Fight Against Infection

Susanne Sattler

1.1 Introduction: Our Changing Understanding of the Immune System

Our current understanding of the immune system varies drastically from the view that prevailed just over 20 years ago. Early observations during infectious diseases lead to a major focus on the immune system's ability to discriminate between self and non-self and defence against pathogenic microorganisms. In its classical definition, the immune system comprises of humoral factors such as complement proteins, as well as immune cells and their products including antibodies, cytokines/chemokines and growth factors. This system of humoral and cellular factors is considered responsible for defending the host from invading pathogens.

However, the roles of immune cells and factors are not limited to host defence, but extend to development, tissue homeostasis and repair (Fig. 1.1). In addition, there are crucial immunological functions played by stromal and mesenchymal cells, which are not commonly considered part of the immune system, such as fibroblasts and endothelial cells. On top of that, it is now also appreciated that the inflammatory status of the environment is important in defining the type of response to any antigen and that the immune system is in fact crucial for the maintenance and restoration of tissue homeostasis in both sterile and infectious situations.

S. Sattler
National Heart and Lung Institute, Imperial College London,
Hammersmith Campus, Du Cane Road, London W12 0NN, UK
e-mail: s.sattler@imperial.ac.uk

© Springer International Publishing AG 2017
S. Sattler, T. Kennedy-Lydon (eds.), *The Immunology of Cardiovascular Homeostasis and Pathology*, Advances in Experimental Medicine and Biology 1003, DOI 10.1007/978-3-319-57613-8_1

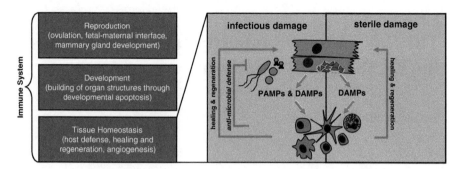

Fig. 1.1 The fundamental roles of the immune system beyond host defence: The immune system is essential for reproduction, development and homeostasis. Sterile tissue damage such as physical trauma or ischemia/reperfusion injury (e.g. myocardial infarct) induces an inflammatory reaction to initiate wound healing and/or regenerative mechanisms. The same basic immunological mechanisms will eliminate microbes if they are present due to injury at a barrier sites (e.g. skin) or primary infectious tissue damage (e.g. viral myocarditis). Necrotic cells in damaged tissue release damage/danger-associated molecular patterns (DAMPs) such as HMGB1, IL-33, ATP, heat-shock proteins, nucleic acids and ECM degradation products. Microbes are recognised by the immune system through their expression of pathogen-associated molecular patterns (PAMPs) such as LPS, flagellin, dsRNA and unmethylated CpG motifs in DNA. *ATP* adenosine triphosphate, *HMGB1* high mobility group box 1, *ECM* extracellular matrix

1.2   A Brief Historical Perspective

What is believed to be the first record of an immunological observation dates from 430 BC. During a plague outbreak in Athens, the Greek historian and general Thucydides noted that people that were lucky enough to recover from the plague did not catch the disease for a second time [1]. The beginnings of modern-day immunology are usually attributed to Louis Pasteur and Robert Koch. Pasteur, in contrast to common belief at the time, suggested that disease was caused by germs [2], and Robert Koch confirmed this concept in 1891 with his postulates and proofs, for which he received the Nobel Prize in Physiology or Medicine in 1905 [3, 4]. These very early observations were fundamental for the first identification and early characterisation of the immune system but also skewed all subsequent definitions towards a defence machinery against invading microorganisms.

1.2.1   The Traditional View of Immunity: Evolution to Protect from Infectious Microorganisms

The immune system has long been considered to have evolved primarily because it provided host protection from infectious microorganisms and correspondingly a survival advantage. Genes of the immune system have been suggested to be under particularly high evolutionary pressure due to the need to prevent pathogenic microorganisms from harming the host. Hosts are therefore under selective pressure to resist pathogens, whereas pathogens are selected to overcome increasing host defences [5]. This process of a stepwise increase in resistance by the host and subsequent mechanisms for evasion by the pathogen is the basis for a well-established co-evolutionary dynamics, the 'host–pathogen arms race' [6].

In 1989, Charles Janeway proposed his 'Pattern Recognition Theory' [7], which still provides the conceptual framework for our current understanding of innate immune recognition and its role in the activation of adaptive immunity. Janeway proposed the existence of an evolutionary conserved first line of defence consisting of antigen-presenting cells equipped with pattern recognition receptors (PRR) which recognise common patterns found on microorganisms, which are different and thus distinguishable from those of host cells. These innate immune cells take up foreign antigens, present them to adaptive immune cells and thus determine the following adaptive immune response. Janeway's model also suggested that the innate immune system evolved to discriminate infectious non-self from non-infectious self as microbial patterns were not present on host tissues [8]. A few years later, the first family of pattern recognition receptors, the Toll-like receptors (TLRs), were indeed discovered [9]. Notably, Toll-like receptors (TLRs) are also one of several striking examples of convergent evolution in the immune system [10]. TLRs are used for innate immune recognition in both insects and vertebrates. The ancient common ancestor, a receptor gene with function during developmental patterning, subsequently evolved a secondary function in host defence. This happened independently in insects and vertebrates after the vertebrate and invertebrate lineage had separated [11].

All this seemed to strongly support the concept that the primary role of the immune system is to defend against potentially infectious microorganisms.

1.2.2   The Danger View of Immunity: Evolution to Protect from Endogenous Danger

Charles Janeway's model is still considered largely correct today, although too simplistic as it fails to explain certain aspects of immunity including sterile immune responses in the absence of infectious agents as well as the unresponsiveness to a variety of non-self-stimuli such as dietary antigens and commensal microorganisms. In 1994, Polly Matzinger proposed the 'Danger Hypothesis' [12]. Her model, again on purely theoretical grounds, suggested that the primary driving force of the immune system is the need to detect and protect against danger as equivalent to tissue injury. Importantly, in the same year, a group of scientists working on kidney transplantation discussed the possibility that in addition to its foreignness, it was the injury to an allograft which ultimately caused an immune response and rejection [13]. Activation of innate immune events by injury-induced exposure of normally hidden endogenous molecules has since been demonstrated countless times [14, 15]. Examples for such endogenous molecules include nucleic acids [16], heat-shock proteins [17], cytoskeletal proteins [18], HMBG-1 [19], SAP130 [20], IL-33 [21] and IL-1a [22]. In addition to proteins that are normally hidden from detection by the immune system, there are small molecules released as a result of endogenous stress including high glucose [23], cholesterol [24] and ATP [25]. All these agents have been shown to contribute to sterile inflammatory responses and have been termed damage/danger-associated molecular patterns (DAMPs).

Thus, an inflammatory environment caused by tissue injury (danger hypothesis) alerts the immune system and is the prerequisite to an adaptive immune response (self versus non-self pattern recognition hypothesis).

1.2.3 The Integrative View of Immunity: Evolution as a System to Establish and Maintain Tissue Homeostasis

Considering the crucial importance of the innate immune response to tissue injury to initiate tissue repair processes and mount an effective adaptive response, the question arises if the early evolution of the immune system may have been driven by the need to maintain tissue homeostasis and the ability to deal with tissue injury rather than infection. Strikingly, the Russian developmental zoologist Ilya Metchnikoff discovered phagocytosis in echinoderms at the end of the nineteenth century and proposed the phagocyte and innate immunity as the centre of the immune response. Metchnikoff's already developed a concept of immunity as a summary of all those activities that defined organismal identity and which regarded host defence mechanisms as only subordinate to this primary function [26]. The evolutionary development of the process of phagocytosis provides a very strong argument for the immune system being more than just a defence mechanism. Evolutionary old organisms, such as amoeba, already use this ancient mechanism, albeit mainly for feeding [27, 28]. In multicellular organisms, phagocytosis is first used during embryogenesis for the removal of dying cells and the recycling of their molecules. In adults, phagocytosis continues to play a crucial role during tissue remodelling [29, 30]. Only the evolutionary appearance of the major histocompatibility complex (MHC) locus in jawed fish seems to have allowed the phagosomes to play a role in the establishment of adaptive immunity [31].

Decades of research using ever more sophisticated technologies allow the conclusion that defence against 'non-self' is only one of many layers of how the immune system protects us from disease. This is most evident in the evolutionary ancient mechanism of phagocytosis, which is still the most fundamental basis for tissue development, homeostasis and repair.

1.3   Functions of Immune Cells Beyond Host Defence

In this section, examples of non-defence functions of classical immune cells during reproduction, embryonic development, angiogenesis and post-injury repair and regeneration will be discussed.

1.3.1   *Reproduction*

The immune system plays a crucial role in reproduction both before and during pregnancy, and leucocytes are found in male and female reproductive tissues [32–34]. Several classical inflammatory mediators participate in the process of ovulation. Granulocytes, macrophages and T lymphocytes migrate to the ovulation site and are activated locally, suggesting an active role of leucocytes in the tissue remodelling which occurs during ovulation [35]. Mice deficient of the major macrophage growth factor, colony-stimulating factor-1 (CSF-1), show severe fertility defects, as CSF-1 is involved in feto-maternal interactions during pregnancy and has a crucial role in the development of the mammary gland [36–39]. Eotaxin, a major chemokine for local recruitment of eosinophils into tissue, also contributes to mammary gland development [40, 41].

Establishment and maintenance of feto-maternal tolerance during pregnancy has intrigued immunologists for a long time, and to date a set of anatomical, cellular and molecular regulatory mechanisms that protect the fetus from immune-mediated rejection has been uncovered [42]. The feto-maternal interface is an immunologically highly dynamic site rich in cytokines and hormones [43, 44]. During the first few weeks after fertilisation, interstitial and endovascular infiltration of trophoblast cells leads to the recruitment of maternal immune cells and the production of pro-inflammatory cytokines [45]. Maternal immune responses have been proposed to protect from trophoblast over-invasion while allowing for the acceptance of the semi-allogeneic fetal–placental unit. 40% of cells in the decidua during the first trimester are CD45$^+$ leucocytes. 50–60% of decidual leucocytes are a unique type of natural killer (NK) cells which is not present outside the context of pregnancy and has crucial trophic function by helping to remodel the spiral arterioles of the uterus that supply the placenta with blood [46]. Failure to sufficiently remodel these vessels leads to inadequate placental perfusion, intrauterine growth restriction and pre-eclampsia, two important obstetric complications [47]. The remaining leucocytic infiltrates are roughly 10% T lymphocytes, 1–2% dendritic cells (DCs) and 20–25% decidual macrophages [48]. The decidual macrophage population are subdivided into a CD11c^{high} and CD11c^{low} population, which are responsible for antigen processing and presentation. Depending on the macrophage subset, antigen presentation leads to either an induction of maternal immune cell tolerance to fetal antigens (CD11c^{high}) or homeostatic functions including the clearance of apoptotic cells during placental construction (CD11c^{low}) [49, 50]. Thus, besides being a potential threat to the developing fetus due to allorecognition of foetal antigens, decidual leucocytes play a crucial role in the development of the fetal–placental unit [51].

1.3.2   Development

Macrophages both initiate and respond to developmental apoptosis [52, 53]. Notably however, and a major sign of the fundamental role of the phagocytic process, non-immune cells are able to take over phagocytosis if necessary. In mice lacking macrophages due to a deficiency for the hemopoietic-lineage-specific transcription factor PU.1, the task of developmental phagocytosis is taken over by mesenchymal cells, although they are significantly less efficient than professional macrophages in recognition, engulfment and degradation of apoptotic debris [54]. Comparable roles of macrophages in developmental apoptosis have been reported in evolutionary older vertebrate species and insects. In the frog *Xenopus laevis*, macrophage phagocytosis is involved in programmed cell death of tail and body muscle during metamorphosis [55]. In the *Drosophila* embryo, the development of the tracheal system is created through migration, rearrangement and elimination of cells, which are engulfed and removed by macrophages [56].

Bone Development   Bone osteoclasts are multinucleated cells that resorb bone material during development and form by fusion of mononuclear precursors of the monocyte/macrophage lineage. CSF-1 is an important factor involved in osteoclast differentiation [57]. The toothless (tl) mutation in the rat is a naturally occurring, autosomal recessive mutation in the *Csf1* gene and causes severely reduced numbers of macrophages and a profound deficiency of bone-resorbing osteoclasts and peritoneal macrophages. This results in severe osteopetrosis, with a highly sclerotic skeleton, lack of marrow spaces and failure of tooth eruption [58]. Administration of CSF-1 can correct these defects demonstrating the crucial importance of macrophages in bone development [59].

Brain Development   Brain microglia are highly motile phagocytic cells that infiltrate and take up residence in the developing brain, where they are thought to provide surveillance and scavenging function [60]. They assist during embryonic development by mediating induced cell death of neurons [61]. Both CSF-1 and its receptor are expressed in the developing mouse brain, and CSF-1 deficiency induces neurological abnormalities [62]. During postnatal brain development, microglia actively engulf synaptic material and play a major role in synaptic pruning [63]. They can remove entire dendritic structures after depletion of appropriate inputs, a process termed synaptic stripping. They accumulate, through signalling mediated by the chemokine receptor CXCR3, at the lesion site, and dendritic structures are removed within a few days [64, 65]. Microglia cells may also be a source of other brain cells, as isolated microglia cells in culture have the potential to generate neurons, astrocytes and oligodendrocytes [66, 67]. Microglia also release factors that influence adult neurogenesis and glial development [68, 69]. They secrete neurotrophins of the nerve growth factor (NGF) family, suggesting that they promote development and normal function of neurons and glia [70] and have autocrine function on microglial proliferation and phagocytic activity in vitro [71].

1.3.3   Angiogenesis

The formation of blood vessels is essential for tissue development and tissue homeostasis in all vertebrates. Monocytes and macrophages are known to be involved in the formation of new blood vessels and are involved in all phases of the angiogenic process. They are capable of secreting a vast repertoire of angiogenic effector molecules, including matrix-remodelling proteases, pro-angiogenic growth factors (VEGF/VPF, bFGF, GM-CSF, TGF-α, IGF-I, PDGF, TGF-β) and cytokines (IL-1, IL-6, IL-8, TNF-α, substance P, prostaglandins, interferons, thrombospondin 1) [72]. The expansion of the blood vessel network during angiogenesis starts with sprouting and is followed by anastomosis. Vessel sprouting is induced by a chemotactic gradient of the vascular endothelial growth factor (VEGF), which stimulates tip cell protrusion to initiate vessel growth [73]. Macrophages are crucial for the fusion of tip cells to add new circuits to the existing vessel network by physically bridging and guiding neighbouring tip cells until they are fused [74].

1.3.4   Tissue Homeostasis, Regeneration and Repair

The immune system is crucial in wound healing and regeneration after tissue damage. There is a wealth of information available about the involvement of immune cells in the repair of all major organs including the skin [75, 76], skeletal and heart muscle [77–82], kidney [83, 84], liver [85], brain [86, 87] and gut [88]. If damage to blood vessels is involved, the activated coagulation system initiates the first stages of healing with the release of chemical mediators that promote vascular permeability and leucocyte adhesion and recruitment. Coagulation activates platelets which produce growth factors such as transforming growth factor-β (TGF-β) and platelet-derived growth factor (PDGF), which activate fibroblasts and act as chemoattractants for leucocytes [89]. However, even without activation of the coagulation cascade, alarmins released from necrotic cells recruit leucocytes. Infiltrating neutrophils and macrophages remove dead cells and secrete chemokines and cytokines, including tumour necrosis factor (TNF) and interleukin-1 (IL-1), which further upregulate leucocyte adhesion molecules to increase immune cell recruitment and induce the production of additional growth factors and proteases such as matrix metalloproteases. Matrix metalloproteases degrade the extracellular matrix which allows for tissue remodelling. Fibroblast growth factor (FGF), PDGF, prostaglandins and thrombospondin-1 promote new blood vessel growth, fibroblast proliferation and collagen deposition. Tissue remodelling is accompanied by parenchymal regeneration or regrowth of the epithelial cell layer with resolution of the healing process [90].

Recently, several innate-type lymphoid cell (iLC) subsets have been identified and characterised that seem to play a particularly important role in sterile inflammatory settings. These cell types include lymphoid tissue-inducer cells (LTi), innate type 2 helper cells and $\gamma\delta$ T lymphocytes [91]. They rapidly express effector cytokines that are commonly associated with adaptive T-helper lymphocyte responses such as IL-17, IL-13, IL-4 and IL-22 production [92, 93]. Their role in wound healing and regeneration is strongly mediated by the cytokines they produce. LTi cells play a central role in promoting appropriate thymic regeneration in sterile inflammatory settings, an effect which is mediated largely through the cytokine IL-22 which promotes epithelial repair and tissue regeneration [94]. Further, the endogenous alarmin IL-33 has profound effects on innate type 2 helper cells and thereby plays a central role in driving type 2 immunity under sterile and infectious settings [95, 96]. Tissue repair processes following injury are dominated by type 2 immune cells producing cytokines such as IL-4, IL-5, IL-10 and IL-13. Many type 2 processes promote the 'walling off' of large invaders through granuloma formation and matrix deposition, which are the same mechanisms employed to close open wounds [97]. Shifting the inflammatory type 1 response towards a type 2 response is beneficial for quick wound healing, which likely was the evolutionary most cost-effective approach to deal with large parasites or insect bites, although this may come at the cost of fibrotic repair and long-term loss of tissue functionality [80, 98]. Intense research efforts in the field of regenerative medicine are trying to find the right balance between pro-inflammatory and reparative immune responses to prevent scarring and fibrotic repair and boost regenerative healing instead.

1.4   Concluding Remarks

Both evolutionary development and functional variety in current day organisms strongly support a notion of the immune system as an all-encompassing machinery to ensure system integrity. Protection from disease caused by invading pathogenic microorganisms is, although the most easily observed, only one manifestation of the workings of this machinery. Instead, the immune system is essential for development, surveillance, protection and regulation to maintain or if necessary re-establish homeostasis.

References

1. Retief FP, Cilliers L. The epidemic of Athens, 430-426 BC. S Afr Med J. 1998;88(1):50–3.
2. Plotkin SA. Vaccines: past, present and future. Nat Med. 2005;11(4 Suppl):S5–11.
3. King LS. Dr. Koch's postulates. J Hist Med Allied Sci. 1952;7(4):350–61.
4. The Nobel Prize in Physiology or Medicine 1905: Nobel Media; 2013 Available from: http://www.nobelprize.org/nobel_prizes/medicine/laureates/1905/.
5. Woolhouse ME, Webster JP, Domingo E, Charlesworth B, Levin BR. Biological and biomedical implications of the co-evolution of pathogens and their hosts. Nat Genet. 2002;32(4):569–77.
6. Decaestecker E, Gaba S, Raeymaekers JA, Stoks R, Van Kerckhoven L, Ebert D, et al. Host-parasite 'Red Queen' dynamics archived in pond sediment. Nature. 2007;450(7171):870–3.
7. Janeway CA Jr. Approaching the asymptote? Evolution and revolution in immunology. Cold Spring Harb Symp Quant Biol. 1989;54(Pt 1):1–13.
8. Janeway CA Jr. The immune system evolved to discriminate infectious nonself from noninfectious self. Immunol Today. 1992;13(1):11–6.

9. Takeda K, Kaisho T, Akira S. Toll-like receptors. Annu Rev Immunol. 2003;21:335–76.

10. Bailey M. Evolution of the immune system at geological and local scales. Curr Opin HIV AIDS. 2012;7(3):214–20.

11. Leulier F, Lemaitre B. Toll-like receptors--taking an evolutionary approach. Nat Rev Genet. 2008;9(3):165–78.

12. Matzinger P. Tolerance, danger, and the extended family. Annu Rev Immunol. 1994;12:991–1045.

13. Land W, Schneeberger H, Schleibner S, Illner WD, Abendroth D, Rutili G, et al. The beneficial effect of human recombinant superoxide dismutase on acute and chronic rejection events in recipients of cadaveric renal transplants. Transplantation. 1994;57(2):211–7.

14. Manson J, Thiemermann C, Brohi K. Trauma alarmins as activators of damage-induced inflammation. Br J Surg. 2012;99(Suppl 1):12–20.

15. Chan JK, Roth J, Oppenheim JJ, Tracey KJ, Vogl T, Feldmann M, et al. Alarmins: awaiting a clinical response. J Clin Invest. 2012;122(8):2711–9.

16. Barrat FJ, Meeker T, Gregorio J, Chan JH, Uematsu S, Akira S, et al. Nucleic acids of mammalian origin can act as endogenous ligands for Toll-like receptors and may promote systemic lupus erythematosus. J Exp Med. 2005;202(8):1131–9.

17. Basu S, Binder RJ, Ramalingam T, Srivastava PK. CD91 is a common receptor for heat shock proteins gp96, hsp90, hsp70, and calreticulin. Immunity. 2001;14(3):303–13.

18. Ahrens S, Zelenay S, Sancho D, Hanc P, Kjaer S, Feest C, et al. F-actin is an evolutionarily conserved damage-associated molecular pattern recognized by DNGR-1, a receptor for dead cells. Immunity. 2012;36(4):635–45.

19. Scaffidi P, Misteli T, Bianchi ME. Release of chromatin protein HMGB1 by necrotic cells triggers inflammation. Nature. 2002;418(6894):191–5.

20. Yamasaki S, Ishikawa E, Sakuma M, Hara H, Ogata K, Saito T. Mincle is an ITAM-coupled activating receptor that senses damaged cells. Nat Immunol. 2008;9(10):1179–88.

21. Moussion C, Ortega N, Girard JP. The IL-1-like cytokine IL-33 is constitutively expressed in the nucleus of endothelial cells and epithelial cells in vivo: a novel 'alarmin'? PLoS One. 2008;3(10):e3331.

22. Eigenbrod T, Park JH, Harder J, Iwakura Y, Nunez G. Cutting edge: critical role for mesothelial cells in necrosis-induced inflammation through the recognition of IL-1 alpha released from dying cells. J Immunol. 2008;181(12):8194–8.

23. Zhou R, Tardivel A, Thorens B, Choi I, Tschopp J. Thioredoxin-interacting protein links oxidative stress to inflammasome activation. Nat Immunol. 2010;11(2):136–40.

24. Duewell P, Kono H, Rayner KJ, Sirois CM, Vladimer G, Bauernfeind FG, et al. NLRP3 inflammasomes are required for atherogenesis and activated by cholesterol crystals. Nature. 2010;464(7293):1357–61.

25. Mariathasan S, Weiss DS, Newton K, McBride J, O'Rourke K, Roose-Girma M, et al. Cryopyrin activates the inflammasome in response to toxins and ATP. Nature. 2006;440(7081):228–32.

26. Tauber AI. The birth of immunology. III. The fate of the phagocytosis theory. Cell Immunol. 1992;139(2):505–30.

27. Desjardins M, Houde M, Gagnon E. Phagocytosis: the convoluted way from nutrition to adaptive immunity. Immunol Rev. 2005;207:158–65.

28. Solomon JM, Rupper A, Cardelli JA, Isberg RR. Intracellular growth of Legionella pneumophila in Dictyostelium discoideum, a system for genetic analysis of host-pathogen interactions. Infect Immun. 2000;68(5):2939–47.

29. Lichanska AM, Hume DA. Origins and functions of phagocytes in the embryo. Exp Hematol. 2000;28(6):601–11.

30. Aderem A, Underhill DM. Mechanisms of phagocytosis in macrophages. Annu Rev Immunol. 1999;17:593–623.

31. Pfeifer JD, Wick MJ, Roberts RL, Findlay K, Normark SJ, Harding CV. Phagocytic processing of bacterial antigens for class I MHC presentation to T cells. Nature. 1993;361(6410):359–62.

32. Oakley OR, Frazer ML, Ko C. Pituitary-ovary-spleen axis in ovulation. Trends Endocrinol Metab. 2011;22(9):345–52.

33. Care AS, Diener KR, Jasper MJ, Brown HM, Ingman WV, Robertson SA. Macrophages regulate corpus luteum development during embryo implantation in mice. J Clin Invest. 2013;123(8):3472–87.
34. Carlock CI, Wu J, Zhou C, Tatum K, Adams HP, Tan F, et al. Unique temporal and spatial expression patterns of IL-33 in ovaries during ovulation and estrous cycle are associated with ovarian tissue homeostasis. J Immunol. 2014;193(1):161–9.
35. Brannstrom M, Mayrhofer G, Robertson SA. Localization of leukocyte subsets in the rat ovary during the periovulatory period. Biol Reprod. 1993;48(2):277–86.
36. Cohen PE, Nishimura K, Zhu L, Pollard JW. Macrophages: important accessory cells for reproductive function. J Leukoc Biol. 1999;66(5):765–72.
37. Pollard JW, Hennighausen L. Colony stimulating factor 1 is required for mammary gland development during pregnancy. Proc Natl Acad Sci U S A. 1994;91(20):9312–6.
38. Van Nguyen A, Pollard JW. Colony stimulating factor-1 is required to recruit macrophages into the mammary gland to facilitate mammary ductal outgrowth. Dev Biol. 2002;247(1):11–25.
39. Ingman WV, Wyckoff J, Gouon-Evans V, Condeelis J, Pollard JW. Macrophages promote collagen fibrillogenesis around terminal end buds of the developing mammary gland. Dev Dyn. 2006;235(12):3222–9.
40. Gouon-Evans V, Rothenberg ME, Pollard JW. Postnatal mammary gland development requires macrophages and eosinophils. Development. 2000;127(11):2269–82.
41. Gouon-Evans V, Lin EY, Pollard JW. Requirement of macrophages and eosinophils and their cytokines/chemokines for mammary gland development. Breast Cancer Res. 2002;4(4):155–64.
42. Erlebacher A. Mechanisms of T cell tolerance towards the allogeneic fetus. Nat Rev Immunol. 2013;13(1):23–33.
43. Tayade C, Black GP, Fang Y, Croy BA. Differential gene expression in endometrium, endometrial lymphocytes, and trophoblasts during successful and abortive embryo implantation. J Immunol. 2006;176(1):148–56.
44. Habbeddine M, Verbeke P, Karaz S, Bobe P, Kanellopoulos-Langevin C. Leukocyte population dynamics and detection of IL-9 as a major cytokine at the mouse fetal-maternal interface. PLoS One. 2014;9(9):e107267.
45. von Rango U. Fetal tolerance in human pregnancy--a crucial balance between acceptance and limitation of trophoblast invasion. Immunol Lett. 2008;115(1):21–32.
46. Koopman LA, Kopcow HD, Rybalov B, Boyson JE, Orange JS, Schatz F, et al. Human decidual natural killer cells are a unique NK cell subset with immunomodulatory potential. J Exp Med. 2003;198(8):1201–12.
47. Zhang J, Chen Z, Smith GN, Croy BA. Natural killer cell-triggered vascular transformation: maternal care before birth? Cell Mol Immunol. 2011;8(1):1–11.
48. Trundley A, Gardner L, Northfield J, Chang C, Moffett A. Methods for isolation of cells from the human fetal-maternal interface. Methods Mol Med. 2006;122:109–22.
49. Houser BL. Decidual macrophages and their roles at the maternal-fetal interface. Yale J Biol Med. 2012;85(1):105–18.
50. Abrahams VM, Kim YM, Straszewski SL, Romero R, Mor G. Macrophages and apoptotic cell clearance during pregnancy. Am J Reprod Immunol. 2004;51(4):275–82.
51. Moffett A, Loke C. Immunology of placentation in eutherian mammals. Nat Rev Immunol. 2006;6(8):584–94.
52. Lobov IB, Rao S, Carroll TJ, Vallance JE, Ito M, Ondr JK, et al. WNT7b mediates macrophage-induced programmed cell death in patterning of the vasculature. Nature. 2005;437(7057):417–21.
53. Rao S, Lobov IB, Vallance JE, Tsujikawa K, Shiojima I, Akunuru S, et al. Obligatory participation of macrophages in an angiopoietin 2-mediated cell death switch. Development. 2007;134(24):4449–58.
54. Wood W, Turmaine M, Weber R, Camp V, Maki RA, McKercher SR, et al. Mesenchymal cells engulf and clear apoptotic footplate cells in macrophageless PU.1 null mouse embryos. Development. 2000;127(24):5245–52.
55. Nishikawa A, Murata E, Akita M, Kaneko K, Moriya O, Tomita M, et al. Roles of macrophages in programmed cell death and remodeling of tail and body muscle of *Xenopus laevis* during metamorphosis. Histochem Cell Biol. 1998;109(1):11–7.

56. Baer MM, Bilstein A, Caussinus E, Csiszar A, Affolter M, Leptin M. The role of apoptosis in shaping the tracheal system in the Drosophila embryo. Mech Dev. 2010;127(1–2):28–35.
57. Stanley ER, Chen DM, Lin HS. Induction of macrophage production and proliferation by a purified colony stimulating factor. Nature. 1978;274(5667):168–70.
58. Van Wesenbeeck L, Odgren PR, MacKay CA, D'Angelo M, Safadi FF, Popoff SN, et al. The osteopetrotic mutation toothless (tl) is a loss-of-function frameshift mutation in the rat Csf1 gene: Evidence of a crucial role for CSF-1 in osteoclastogenesis and endochondral ossification. Proc Natl Acad Sci U S A. 2002;99(22):14303–8.
59. Wiktor-Jedrzejczak W, Bartocci A, Ferrante AW Jr, Ahmed-Ansari A, Sell KW, Pollard JW, et al. Total absence of colony-stimulating factor 1 in the macrophage-deficient osteopetrotic (op/op) mouse. Proc Natl Acad Sci U S A. 1990;87(12):4828–32.
60. Reemst K, Noctor SC, Lucassen PJ, Hol EM. The indispensable roles of microglia and astrocytes during brain development. Front Hum Neurosci. 2016;10:566.
61. Marin-Teva JL, Dusart I, Colin C, Gervais A, van Rooijen N, Mallat M. Microglia promote the death of developing Purkinje cells. Neuron. 2004;41(4):535–47.
62. Michaelson MD, Bieri PL, Mehler MF, Xu H, Arezzo JC, Pollard JW, et al. CSF-1 deficiency in mice results in abnormal brain development. Development. 1996;122(9):2661–72.
63. Paolicelli RC, Bolasco G, Pagani F, Maggi L, Scianni M, Panzanelli P, et al. Synaptic pruning by microglia is necessary for normal brain development. Science. 2011;333(6048): 1456–8.
64. Trapp BD, Wujek JR, Criste GA, Jalabi W, Yin X, Kidd GJ, et al. Evidence for synaptic stripping by cortical microglia. Glia. 2007;55(4):360–8.
65. Rappert A, Bechmann I, Pivneva T, Mahlo J, Biber K, Nolte C, et al. CXCR3-dependent microglial recruitment is essential for dendrite loss after brain lesion. J Neurosci. 2004;24(39):8500–9.
66. Yokoyama A, Sakamoto A, Kameda K, Imai Y, Tanaka J. NG2 proteoglycan-expressing microglia as multipotent neural progenitors in normal and pathologic brains. Glia. 2006;53(7): 754–68.
67. Butovsky O, Bukshpan S, Kunis G, Jung S, Schwartz M. Microglia can be induced by IFN-gamma or IL-4 to express neural or dendritic-like markers. Mol Cell Neurosci. 2007;35(3):490–500.
68. Ekdahl CT, Claasen JH, Bonde S, Kokaia Z, Lindvall O. Inflammation is detrimental for neurogenesis in adult brain. Proc Natl Acad Sci U S A. 2003;100(23):13632–7.
69. Monje ML, Toda H, Palmer TD. Inflammatory blockade restores adult hippocampal neurogenesis. Science. 2003;302(5651):1760–5.
70. Mallat M, Houlgatte R, Brachet P, Prochiantz A. Lipopolysaccharide-stimulated rat brain macrophages release NGF in vitro. Dev Biol. 1989;133(1):309–11.
71. Elkabes S, DiCicco-Bloom EM, Black IB. Brain microglia/macrophages express neurotrophins that selectively regulate microglial proliferation and function. J Neurosci. 1996;16(8):2508–21.
72. Sunderkotter C, Steinbrink K, Goebeler M, Bhardwaj R, Sorg C. Macrophages and angiogenesis. J Leukoc Biol. 1994;55(3):410–22.
73. Gerhardt H, Golding M, Fruttiger M, Ruhrberg C, Lundkvist A, Abramsson A, et al. VEGF guides angiogenic sprouting utilizing endothelial tip cell filopodia. J Cell Biol. 2003;161(6):1163–77.
74. Fantin A, Vieira JM, Gestri G, Denti L, Schwarz Q, Prykhozhij S, et al. Tissue macrophages act as cellular chaperones for vascular anastomosis downstream of VEGF-mediated endothelial tip cell induction. Blood. 2010;116(5):829–40.
75. Mirza R, DiPietro LA, Koh TJ. Selective and specific macrophage ablation is detrimental to wound healing in mice. Am J Pathol. 2009;175(6):2454–62.
76. Goren I, Allmann N, Yogev N, Schurmann C, Linke A, Holdener M, et al. A transgenic mouse model of inducible macrophage depletion: effects of diphtheria toxin-driven lysozyme M-specific cell lineage ablation on wound inflammatory, angiogenic, and contractive processes. Am J Pathol. 2009;175(1):132–47.
77. Nahrendorf M, Swirski FK, Aikawa E, Stangenberg L, Wurdinger T, Figueiredo JL, et al. The healing myocardium sequentially mobilizes two monocyte subsets with divergent and complementary functions. J Exp Med. 2007;204(12):3037–47.

78. Arnold L, Henry A, Poron F, Baba-Amer Y, van Rooijen N, Plonquet A, et al. Inflammatory monocytes recruited after skeletal muscle injury switch into antiinflammatory macrophages to support myogenesis. J Exp Med. 2007;204(5):1057–69.
79. Frantz S, Hofmann U, Fraccarollo D, Schafer A, Kranepuhl S, Hagedorn I, et al. Monocytes/macrophages prevent healing defects and left ventricular thrombus formation after myocardial infarction. FASEB J. 2013;27(3):871–81.
80. Sattler S, Rosenthal N. The neonate versus adult mammalian immune system in cardiac repair and regeneration. Biochim Biophys Acta. 2016;1863(7 Pt B):1813–21.
81. Gallego-Colon E, Sampson RD, Sattler S, Schneider MD, Rosenthal N, Tonkin J. Cardiac-restricted IGF-1Ea overexpression reduces the early accumulation of inflammatory myeloid cells and mediates expression of extracellular matrix remodelling genes after myocardial infarction. Mediat Inflamm. 2015;2015:484357.
82. Tonkin J, Temmerman L, Sampson RD, Gallego-Colon E, Barberi L, Bilbao D, et al. Monocyte/macrophage-derived IGF-1 orchestrates murine skeletal muscle regeneration and modulates autocrine polarization. Mol Ther. 2015;23(7):1189–200.
83. Lin SL, Li B, Rao S, Yeo EJ, Hudson TE, Nowlin BT, et al. Macrophage Wnt7b is critical for kidney repair and regeneration. Proc Natl Acad Sci U S A. 2010;107(9):4194–9.
84. Zhang MZ, Yao B, Yang S, Jiang L, Wang S, Fan X, et al. CSF-1 signaling mediates recovery from acute kidney injury. J Clin Invest. 2012;122(12):4519–32.
85. Meijer C, Wiezer MJ, Diehl AM, Schouten HJ, Schouten HJ, Meijer S, et al. Kupffer cell depletion by CI2MDP-liposomes alters hepatic cytokine expression and delays liver regeneration after partial hepatectomy. Liver. 2000;20(1):66–77.
86. Glod J, Kobiler D, Noel M, Koneru R, Lehrer S, Medina D, et al. Monocytes form a vascular barrier and participate in vessel repair after brain injury. Blood. 2006;107(3):940–6.
87. London A, Cohen M, Schwartz M. Microglia and monocyte-derived macrophages: functionally distinct populations that act in concert in CNS plasticity and repair. Front Cell Neurosci. 2013;7:34.
88. Seno H, Miyoshi H, Brown SL, Geske MJ, Colonna M, Stappenbeck TS. Efficient colonic mucosal wound repair requires Trem2 signaling. Proc Natl Acad Sci U S A. 2009;106(1):256–61.
89. Martin P, Leibovich SJ. Inflammatory cells during wound repair: the good, the bad and the ugly. Trends Cell Biol. 2005;15(11):599–607.
90. DiPietro LA. Wound healing: the role of the macrophage and other immune cells. Shock. 1995;4(4):233–40.
91. Russell SE, Walsh PT. Sterile inflammation - do innate lymphoid cell subsets play a role? Front Immunol. 2012;3:246.
92. Cai Y, Shen X, Ding C, Qi C, Li K, Li X, et al. Pivotal role of dermal IL-17-producing gammadelta T cells in skin inflammation. Immunity. 2011;35(4):596–610.
93. Barlow JL, Bellosi A, Hardman CS, Drynan LF, Wong SH, Cruickshank JP, et al. Innate IL-13-producing nuocytes arise during allergic lung inflammation and contribute to airways hyperreactivity. J Allergy Clin Immunol. 2012;129(1):191–8 e1-4.
94. Dudakov JA, Hanash AM, Jenq RR, Young LF, Ghosh A, Singer NV, et al. Interleukin-22 drives endogenous thymic regeneration in mice. Science. 2012;336(6077):91–5.
95. Kim HY, Chang YJ, Subramanian S, Lee HH, Albacker LA, Matangkasombut P, et al. Innate lymphoid cells responding to IL-33 mediate airway hyperreactivity independently of adaptive immunity. J Allergy Clin Immunol. 2012;129(1):216–27 e1-6.
96. Sattler S, Smits HH, Xu D, Huang FP. The evolutionary role of the IL-33/ST2 system in host immune defence. Arch Immunol Ther Exp. 2013;61(2):107–17.
97. Allen JE, Wynn TA. Evolution of Th2 immunity: a rapid repair response to tissue destructive pathogens. PLoS Pathog. 2011;7(5):e1002003.
98. Schneider DS, Ayres JS. Two ways to survive infection: what resistance and tolerance can teach us about treating infectious diseases. Nat Rev Immunol. 2008;8(11):889–95.

Part II
Immune Functions and Properties of Resident Cells in the Heart and Cardiovascular System

Chapter 2
Paying for the Tolls: The High Cost of the Innate Immune System for the Cardiac Myocyte

Anne A. Knowlton

The cardiac myocyte, which continuously contracts and relaxes to deliver blood throughout the body, differs markedly from the specialized cells of the immune system. The adaptive, or acquired, immune system with the production of distinct antibodies in response to specific threats was long considered the mainstay of protection against infection; however, the production of antibodies and the full immune response against a threat takes 4–7 days, a long period for an infectious agent to propagate without response. Janeway hypothesized the existence of a simpler, less specific, but more rapid immune response, which he termed innate immunity [1]. In contrast to the specialized immune system found in advanced organisms, innate immunity is widely expressed and found in both more primitive life forms and in humans. Furthermore, the innate immune response and its receptors are found in cell types and tissues that were long viewed as non-immunologic. The persistence of innate immunity is essential for rapid protection against infections, given the long time needed to produce antibodies, but the flip side is that inadvertent activation of innate immunity by proteins, RNA, and other endogenous ligands can lead to cell and tissue inflammation/damage. Unfortunately a number of essential and otherwise innocuous molecules activate different TLRs leading to an inflammatory response, which can be deleterious leading to myocyte death/injury and to organ dysfunction. Predominantly TLR4 has been shown to have a significant role in cardiac injury, with other TLRs including TLR2, having lesser roles [2–7]. In this chapter we will focus on TLRs and the cardiac myocyte. Subsequent chapters will address other aspects immunity and the heart.

A.A. Knowlton
Cardiovascular Division, Department of Medicine, Molecular and Cellular Cardiology, University of California, Davis, One Shields Avenue, Davis, CA 95616, USA

Department of Pharmacology, University of California, Davis, CA, USA

The Department of Veteran's Affairs, Northern California VA, Sacramento, CA, USA
e-mail: aaknowlton@ucdavis.edu

© Springer International Publishing AG 2017   17
S. Sattler, T. Kennedy-Lydon (eds.), *The Immunology of Cardiovascular Homeostasis and Pathology*, Advances in Experimental Medicine and Biology 1003, DOI 10.1007/978-3-319-57613-8_2

Innate Immunity and TLRs Innate immunity includes epithelial barriers to invading organisms; phagocytic cells, such as macrophages and dendritic cells; the complement system; and the TLRs. The Toll receptor was first identified as an essential receptor for dorsal ventral patterning in the embryonic *Drosophila*, but subsequent work has demonstrated that it has a role in defending against fungal infections in the adult Drosophila [8, 9]. Ten TLRs have been identified in humans and 13 in mice (Table 2.1). TLRs 1–10 are expressed in humans and 1–13 in mice, but TLR10 is inactive in the mouse. TLRs 1, 2, 4, 5, 6, 10, 11, 12, and 13 are expressed on the cell surface, and TLRs 3, 7, 8, and 9 localize to the membranes of intracellular organelles, including endosomes and the endoplasmic reticulum. TLRs recognize pathogen-associated molecular patterns (PAMPs) and alarmins, which are endogenous molecules that signal cell and tissue damage and lead to enhanced injury and self-damage. Lipopolysaccharides (LPS) and flagellin are examples of PAMPS, while alarmins include HMGB1 and heat shock proteins (HSPs), which are an endogenous, protective response. PAMPs and alarmins are both types of DAMPs (damage-associated molecular patterns), which in cardiac myocytes includes proteins released after ischemia/reperfusion injury. Key ligands for the TLRs are summarized in Table 2.1.

Heat Shock Proteins (HSPs) Heat shock proteins are well known as protective proteins that make cells resistant to stress-induced cell damage [35–38]. Among the HSPs, HSP60 is highly conserved intracellular protein that is expressed both constitutively and under stress conditions and that serves as a molecular chaperone to facilitate mitochondrial protein folding [39–41]. Although the HSPs are protective and the endogenous increase in HSPs in response to injury reduces cell damage, they can lead to inflammation and even to apoptosis, in other words, a paradoxical deleterious response [42, 43]. HSP70, which has four isoforms, including the

Table 2.1 TLRs in human and mouse

TLR	Ligand	
TLR1	Triacyl lipopeptides	[10]
TLR2	Lipoprotein, lipopeptides, atypical LPS, HSP70	[11–13]
TLR3	Double-stranded RNA	[14, 15]
TLR4	LPS, HMGB1, HSP60, HSP70?	[2, 11, 16–20]
TLR5	Flagellin	[21]
TLR6	Diacyl lipopeptides, lipoteichoic acid	[22, 23]
TLR7	Single-stranded RNA Imidazoquinoline compounds imiquimod and R-848	[24–26]
TLR8	Single-stranded RNA	[25]
TLR9	CpG DNA	[27]
TLR10	Negative regulator of MYD88-dependent and MYD88-independent signaling	[28, 29]
TLR11	Profilin, flagellin	[30] Mouse, not humans
TLR12	Profilin	[31]
TLR13	Bacterial 23 s ribosomal RNA	[32]

Humans have TLR1–10. Mice have TLR1–9 plus TLR11–13. TLR10 in the mouse is nonfunctional as it is disrupted by retroviral insertions, but the rat has been found to have the complete TLR10 sequence [33, 34]

constitutive (HSC)70, an inducible HSP70 (HSP72) and a mitochondrial HSP70, is the most ubiquitous and protective of the HSPs having many cellular functions including folding proteins, targeting irreversibly denatured proteins for degradation, and binding newly synthesized peptides at the ribosome, so that they do not interact with the abundant proteins in the surrounding cytosol [44]. HSP60 is primarily a mitochondrial protein, where it is critical in combination with HSP10, with which it forms a barrel, for folding of proteins imported into the mitochondria. HSPs have been considered to be intracellular proteins; however, HSPs have been found in blood samples at levels of 1–100 μg/ml, and this is a problem [45–47].

Extracellular Heat Shock Proteins 60 and 72 as Mediators of Injury   Intracellular HSPs are protective proteins with many key functions that maintain cellular functions, remove or refold denatured proteins, and protect the cell when exposed to a wide range of injuries [38, 48–52]. However, when HSP60 and HSP72 are extracellular, they can be injurious with one mechanism being activation of TLR4 and TLR2, respectively (Fig. 2.1), resulting in the activation of NFκB and production of cytokines, including TNFα [16, 53]. Antibodies to HSP60 can pull down TLR4 from isolated the membrane fraction of cardiac myocytes after 30 min of incubation

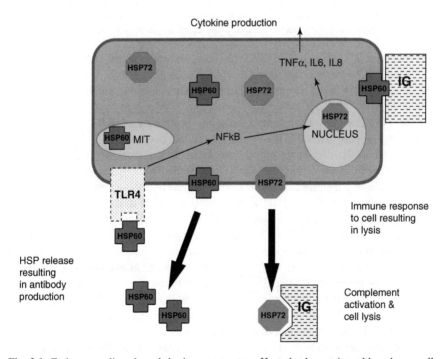

Fig. 2.1 Endogenous ligands and the immune system. Heat shock proteins, although normally protective, can produce injury through several pathways as shown. Both HSP60 and HSP72 have been found in the plasma membrane with injury/stress. Both can be released from the cell, and both have been found in human serum. HSP60 and HSP72 can bind to TLR4/2, respectively, and activate NFκB and cytokine production as shown. Both can elicit antibody response and activation of complement, and both can potentially lead to cell destruction when expressed on cell membrane. Both can also bind to TLRs on monocytes/macrophages leading to a greater inflammatory response

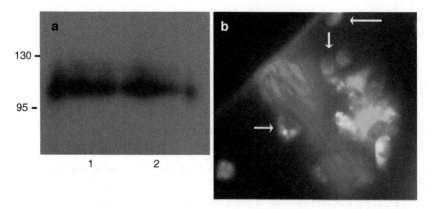

Fig. 2.2 (**a**) Anti-HSP60 immunoprecipitates TLR4 from adult cardiac myocyte plasma membrane fraction. Adult cardiac myocytes were treated with low-endotoxin HSP60 for 30 min at 4 °C, cross-linked, and then fractionated. The plasma membrane fraction was immunoprecipitated with anti-HSP60 and processed for western blotting and developed with anti-TLR4 antibody. Two different immunoprecipitations are shown. (**b**) Monocytes/lymphocytes isolated from the blood were labeled with FITC and added to adult rat cardiac myocytes, labeled with Texas *Red*, and treated with fibronectin. The right pointing *arrow* at the *bottom* left points to a monocyte and the two *arrows* at the *top* identify two lymphocytes based on nuclei characteristics. The monocytes are far smaller than the cardiac myocyte, and any attempt to ingest the larger myocyte can lead to the release of pro-inflammatory factors

with HSP60 at 4 °C (Fig. 2.2a). HSP72 has been reported to bind TLR4, but we have not found this to be the case in cardiac myocytes [2, 54, 55]. Both HSP60 and HSP72 are present in the serum and plasma of humans, even though both are intracellular proteins, and neither are known to be secreted nor to have an extracellular function [45]. HSP60 was present in the serum of diabetics at 6.9 ± 1.9 ng/ml, and similar levels were found in the serum of trauma patients [56, 57]. In contrast, plasma levels of HSP60 were 1 µg/ml or more in 26% of diabetics and 10 µg/ml or more in 7% of diabetics [58]. Similarly 20% of British civil servants had HSP60 plasma levels of 1 µg/ml or more [45]. Anti-HSP60 antibodies were present in the serum of diabetics at titers of 1:100 and 1:250 in 76.5% and 58.8%, respectively [56]. We have reported HSP60 and HSP72 are released in exosomes by cardiac myocytes in the absence of necrosis, and these exosomes are quite stable, not releasing HSP60 under pathophysiologic or physiologic conditions [59, 60]. Whether HSP60 in serum and plasma samples is always present in exosomes is not clear. Many studies of serum/plasma HSPs have used blood samples, which have been stored at -80 °C before analyzing. Freeze/thaw will rupture lipid bilayers, and this would be expected to occur with exosomes. If safely encased in exosomes, then HSP60 and 70 would be unable to bind TLR4 and TLR2.

There are other mechanisms by which the HSPs can activate the immune system. Antibodies to HSPs have been found in human serum, most often to HSP60, but antibodies for HSP72, HSP90, and other HSPs have been reported [61, 62]. 34.4% of patients with *Helicobacter* (*H.*) pylori had antibodies to HSP60 at a 1:1000 titer compared to 0% in *H. pylori*-negative controls ($p < 0.001$), and the same difference was seen for anti-HSP72 antibodies in these patients ($p < 0.001$) [61]. HSP72 alone can activate complement, another component of the innate immune system (Fig. 2.1), and HSP60 complexed with antibody can do the same [63, 64].

Complement activating anti-HSP60 antibodies are associated with increased familial risk of coronary disease [63]. If HSPs are present of the surface of cardiac myocytes, as we have found for HSP60 in ischemic heart failure, antibodies binding to HSP60 will elicit an immune response potentially leading to cell lysis and/or release of inflammatory mediators as macrophages attempt to engulf the much larger myocytes. Adult rat cardiac myocytes were treated with fibronectin, a ligand of TLR4, and monocytes and lymphocytes were added to the culture. As shown in Fig. 2.2b, the monocytes (purified from the blood, they become macrophages when they enter tissues), which are quite small compared to the cardiac myocyte, attempted to engulf portions of the cardiac myocyte, labeled with Texas Red, with some success as evidenced by the change in cell color. It is unknown how the intracellular HSP60 and HSP72 end up in the serum and plasma outside of exosomes, but the potential downstream effects are not benign.

The etiology of the anti-HSP antibodies remains unresolved, although cross-reactivity with bacterial HSPs is one possible mechanism [63, 65]. Overall, the significance of these anti-HSP antibodies remains to be fully elucidated, but studies indicate a role in disease progression including atherosclerosis and potentially heart failure [62, 66]. The presence of both antibody and antigen in the plasma sets the stage for activation of several different aspects of the immune system, as summarized in Fig. 2.1.

Extracellular HSPs and Adaptive Immunity HSPs, particularly HSP60 and HSP72, can present antigens to APCs (antigen-presenting cells, which activate immune system) [46]. HSPs can promote an antibody response to tumors, and this can occur through tumor peptides bound to HSP60 or 72, and can be recreated through fusion proteins containing a combination of HSP72 and tumor antigen [67]. Furthermore T cells reactive to HSPs have been found under certain settings [68–70]. Thus, both elements of innate immunity (TLR activation and complement) and adaptive immunity (T cells, production of antibodies) can be activated by the HSPs, with HSP60 having the most conspicuous effect. Significantly, HSP60 has been found in the plasma of healthy individuals with 25% of them having levels similar or higher to the concentrations used in the current study [45]. We have also found HSP60 in the plasma of rats, although levels were much lower than those reported in British civil servants [71]. Thus, extracellular HSP60 and HSP72 have the potential to activate several different facets of the immune system, and this can lead to inflammation and disease.

Endotoxin/LPS An important caveat for studying HSPs and other molecule effects on the TLRs in culture is that endotoxin is a known ligand of TLR4. There was some controversy as to whether observed effects with other proteins activating TLR-4 occur directly or represent contamination with LPS [72]. However, this issue has been resolved and experimental controls have become more rigorous. Direct comparison of the effects of HSP60 vs. endotoxin in eliciting apoptosis of adult cardiac myocytes demonstrated that endotoxin-free HSP60 induced far more apoptosis than endotoxin [2]. HSPs produced by bacteria transfected with recombinant human HSP can be contaminated with endotoxin, unless measures are taken to remove it either by purchasing verified low-endotoxin HSP or by removing endotoxin with polymyxin. As polymyxin can be toxic to cells, it is best to treat any preparation with polymyxin bound to beads, which is commercially available and easily done.

2.1   TLRs and Cardiac Myocytes

The presence of TLR2 and TLR4 in the membranes of adult cardiac myocytes was first demonstrated in two papers and has been confirmed by others [73–75]. mRNA for many of the TLRs has been shown to be present in mouse heart tissue and rat cardiac myocytes [5, 73]. More recently neonatal rat cardiac myocytes have been shown convincingly to have a functional TLR7, but no analysis of the protein by western or flow cytometry was done [76]. mRNA for TLR2, TLR3, TLR4, TLR5, TLR7, and TLR9 has been shown to be present in mouse heart tissue and HL-1 cells [4]. The investigators also transfected the HL-1 cells with an NFκB luciferase reporter and observed NFκB activation in response to ligands for TLR2, TLR4, and TLR5. Similarly, mRNA for all ten human TLRs has been found in heart tissue, but it has not been shown definitively that all of the TLR proteins are present in human cardiac myocytes. Thus, there is a gap with regard to how many functional TLR receptors are actually expressed in the heart and in cardiac myocytes.

The TLRs are type 1 transmembrane proteins with a leucine-rich repeat (LRR) ectodomain, which is key for ligand recognition, a single transmembrane domain, and a cytoplasmic domain, which is similar to that of the IL-1 receptor. This domain is referred to as the Toll/IL-1 receptor domain or TIR. With activation the TLRs dimerize and mobilize specific adaptor proteins containing TLRs including MyD88, TRIF, and TRAM. These adaptor proteins selectively direct the two activation pathways of the different TLRs. The MyD88 pathway is activated by all TLRs, except for TLR3, and results in NFκB activation and the expression and release of inflammatory cytokines. TLR3 and TLR4 activate the Trif-dependent pathway, which induces activation of interferon regulatory factor or IRF3 as well as NFκB. This leads to both the production of inflammatory cytokines and also to activation of interferon I.

2.2   Heat Shock Proteins, Ischemic Heart Failure, and Innate Immunity

HSP60 in Heart Failure   The heat shock response is lost in ischemic heart failure (IHF), likely in response to repetitive stimulation, except for an unexpected increase in HSP60 and HSP27 [77]. This increase in HSP60 is driven by NFκB, which is chronically activated in IHF [78–80]. The HSP60 gene in both rats and humans contains NFκB binding domains, which are not present in the HSP72 gene, and ChIP assay demonstrated that in IHF, p65 was bound to these sites [80]. Cell fractionation studies demonstrated that in IHF, HSP60 was present as expected in the mitochondria, but 20–25% was present in the cardiac myocyte cytosol, and a small percent was found in the plasma membrane fraction in both rats and humans, as well as in human nonischemic, dilated cardiomyopathy [71]. Flow cytometry studies of fixed cardiac myocytes isolated from the IHF heart demonstrated that HSP60 was on the surface of cardiac myocytes in IHF, and this correlated with apoptosis (Fig. 2.3) [71]. Analysis of plasma samples showed that at a 1:10,000 dilution, control rat plasma was negative for anti-HSP60 antibody, but 20% of 9-week CHF rats and 55% of 12-week CHF rats were positive (Fig. 2.4).

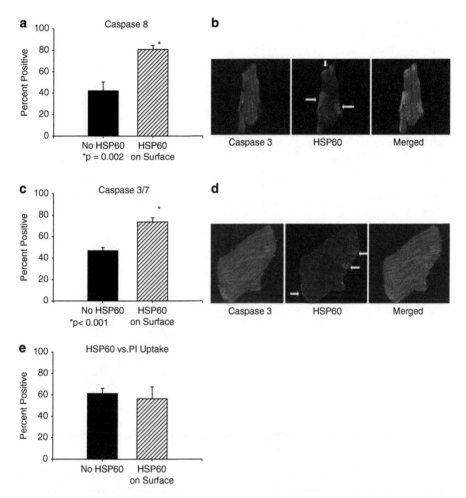

Fig. 2.3 (**a**) Graph summarizes flow cytometry experiments showing that surface localization of HSP60 by flow correlates with activation of caspase-8. In normal myocytes immediately after isolation, 20–25% are positive for caspase-8 activation. For the failing heart cardiac myocytes, overall $56.7 \pm 5.6\%$ were positive for caspase-8 activation (*$p < 0.002$). (**b**) Confocal image of cardiac myocyte stained for activated caspase-8 (*green*, FITC, showing diffuse staining throughout cell) and for HSP60 (*red*). Merged image is shown at the right. (**c**) Graph summarizes flow cytometry experiments showing increased activation of caspase-3/7 when HSP60 is present on the cell surface (*$p < 0.001$). Overall, for the failing heart cardiac myocytes, $59.3 \pm 3.6\%$ were positive for caspase-3/7 activation. (**d**) Confocal image of cardiac myocyte stained for activated caspase-3/7 (*green*) and for HSP60 localization to cell surface (*red*). Caspase-3/7 localized throughout the cell. HSP60 is shown as a fine *red* rim at the edge of the cell. Merged image is shown at right. In **a**–**d**, $n = 6$ experiments/group. (**e**) The uptake of propidium iodide (PI) after isolation. No correlation was present between HSP60 on the surface and PI uptake ($n = 10$/group). Reprinted from the American Journal of Physiology [71]

Fig. 2.4 (**a**) Graph shows percent of heart failure vs. sham control rats with plasma anti-HSP60 antibody at 1:10,000 dilutions. (**b**) Example of a slot blot. Only samples with a band lining up with HSP60 marker (shown on *left*) were scored as positive. $N = 11–15$/group. * $p = 0.004$ vs. 9 weeks. Reprinted from the American Journal of Physiology [71]

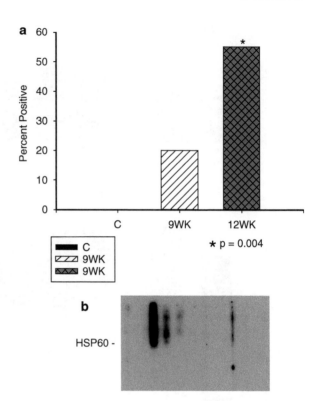

2.3   HSP60, TLR4, Cardiac Myocyte Apoptosis, and Necrosis

We hypothesized that surface HSP60 seen with IHF cardiac myocytes activated TLR4, as it had been reported that HSP60 was a ligand for TLR4 [16, 81]. In a series of experiments in isolated adult rat cardiac myocytes, we investigated whether low-endotoxin, extracellular (ex) recombinant human HSP60 activated TLR4 and what were the downstream signaling events [2]. We found that treatment with exHSP60 led to activation of NFκB, caspase-3/7 activation, and DNA fragmentation (Fig. 2.5). NFκB activation resulted in increased TNFα and IL-1β expression by the cardiac myocytes. Both heat inactivation and anti-HSP60 antibodies blocked this sequence of events, as did a blocking antibody to TLR4, but not to TLR2. TNFα neutralizing antibodies prevented the HSP60-induced apoptosis, while neutralizing antibodies to IL-1β had no effect [2]. Thus, HSP60 is a ligand for TLR4, and extracellular HSP60 causes cardiac myocyte apoptosis in part through increased expression and release of TNFα [2]. Studies with TLR4 mutant (Hej) mice cardiac myocytes provide further insight into the mechanisms of TLR-mediated injury in response to extracellular HSP60 [75]. Investigation of cardiac myocyte injury after treatment with HSP60 in Hej mouse cardiac myocytes and their wild-type controls revealed that not only did exHSP60 increase apoptosis in WT mouse cardiac myocytes, but it also increased necrosis, and anti-HSP60 antibody

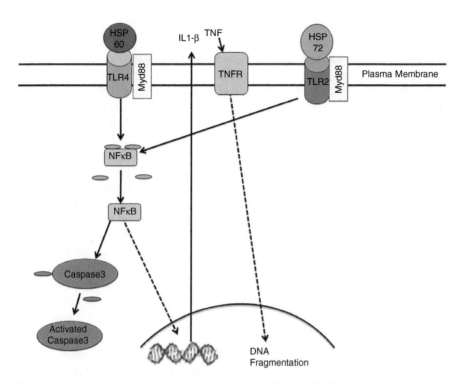

Fig. 2.5 Diagram summarizes key signaling pathways for TLR2 and TLR4. Both TLR2 and TLR4 signal through MD88 leading to inflammatory cytokine expression via both IRF5 and the activation of NFκB. TLR4 also activates the TRAM/TRIF pathway, which leads to further cytokine production, but also to expression of interferon type 1. Figure based on Kim et al. [2]

treatment markedly decreased LDH release after hypoxia/reoxygenation [75]. In contrast the Hej mutant mouse cardiac myocytes had no change in media LDH levels after hypoxia/reoxygenation. TLR2 and TLR4 blocking antibodies each significantly reduced LDH release in WT mouse cardiac myocytes after hypoxia/reoxygenation, but the effect was less than that seen with anti-HSP60 antibodies. Similarly, knockdown of TLR4 with siRNA in mouse cardiac myocytes reduced markers of both necrosis and apoptosis [6]. Sparstolonin B, which is derived from a Chinese herb used to treat tumors, is a TLR2/TLR4 antagonist. Sparstolonin B treatment prevented increased expression of TLR2/4 in H9C2 cells after hypoxia/reoxygenation as well as decreasing the post H/R inflammatory response, including blocking the increase in MSP-1, as well as inhibiting activation of ERK 1/2 and JNK [82]. However, sparstolonin B has also been reported to inhibit angiogenesis and block cell cycle progression in endothelial cells, which would be a drawback for treatment of cardiovascular disease [83].

TLR2/4, Protein Kinase C (PKC)α, Nox2, and Necrosis NADPH oxidase (Nox)2 is one of the seven known Nox family proteins. Nox2 and Nox4 are the most abundant Nox proteins in the heart. Nox2 is associated with the plasma membrane, and Nox4 is predominantly intracellular and associated with organelle membranes. Nox2 and Nox4 have been shown to be important and equal contributors of ROS in myocardial ischemia/reperfusion [84]. LPS is commonly used to model sepsis, and researchers have found that TLR4 has a role in LPS-mediated increased ROS and cell death [85, 86]. TLR4 has been reported to mediate activation of Nox2 and Nox4 in human umbilical vein endothelial cells (HUVECS) [85]. In HUVECS cell death from necrosis after LPS treatment occurred prior to any increase in cytokine expression [85]. Similarly Nox1, which was expressed at low levels in the heart, and Nox2 expression increased in the heart after treatment with endotoxin [86]. Modeling this in H9c2 cells demonstrated that siRNA to knockdown TLR4 prevented the LPS-induced increase in Nox1 mRNA [86]. In macrophages, TLR4-mediated activation of Nox2 by minimally oxidized (mm) LDL [87]. In isolated, adult mouse cardiac myocytes, PKCα was rapidly activated by phosphorylation via TLR2 and TLR4 after hypoxia/reoxygenation, and this activation was gone within an hour. PKCα activation was followed by an increase in Nox2 protein levels. Inhibiting this response reduced necrosis [75]. Thus, with hypoxia/reoxygenation and with in vivo ischemia, TLR2 and TLR4 activation will lead to both apoptosis and necrosis. Findings in vivo by the Lin laboratory demonstrate that HSP60-released myocardial ischemia further exacerbates cardiac injury [5]. A mutant, nonfunctional TLR-4 receptor was associated with smaller infarct size, but this reduced infarct size did not translate into preservation of function [7, 88–90].

TLR2, TLR4, and Their Ligands There have been some conflicting results regarding the ligands for TLR2 and TLR4 for cardiac myocytes, as well as other cell types. The importance of HSP60 activation of TLR4, but not TLR2, as a mechanism of cardiac injury in vivo has been demonstrated by Tian and colleagues [5]. In C9C2 cells, isolated adult rat cardiac myocytes, and in the studies of in vivo cardiac ischemia in a rat model, HSP60 was shown to activate TLR4 with MyD88, but not Trif, leading to activation of p38 and JNK. Neither in vitro nor in vivo was TLR2 activated by HSP60. Activation of TLR4 by HSP60 in the setting of ischemia led to increased expression of both TLR2 and TLR4, via TLR4-mediated activation of JNK/NFκB, as well as increased TNFα and IL-1β expression through HSP60 activation TLR4/MyD88-p38/NFκB. Li and colleagues reported both in vivo and in vitro with isolated cardiac myocytes that ischemia/simulated ischemia-related injury was mediated in part by HSP60 and TLR4 [17]. These findings are consistent with our own results showing that exHSP60 activated TLR4, but not TLR2 in adult rat cardiac myocytes [2]. In cardiac myocytes, HSP70 is a ligand for TLR2 [91]. However, studies in other cell types differ with regard to HSPs as ligands for the TLRs. Vascular smooth muscle cell (VSMC) proliferation was stimulated by treatment with HSP60 in a dose-dependent manner, and blocking antibodies to TLR2 and TLR4 each inhibited the response, with the greatest inhibition observed when the TLR2 and TLR4 blocking antibodies were given in combination [92]. Work on the immune response demonstrated that HSP60 acting via TLR2, but not TLR4, stimulated Tregs [93]. Both of these studies support that in other cell types, HSP60 stimulates TLR2, and both studies used low-endotoxin HSP60. The cause of this difference in TLR2/4 ligand between cardiac myocytes and other cell types is not readily apparent at this point.

Other TLRs Cardiac myocytes also have been found to express TLR7, which is activated by RNA [76]. Cardiac RNA when added to neonatal rat cardiac myocytes in culture induced expression of MIP-2, and this response was stronger when the RNA was complexed with Lipofectamine (Life Technologies). NFκB was activated by treatment with RNA, and both IL1-β and MIP-2 were increased at the mRNA level after the treatment with cardiac RNA. This inflammatory response was inhibited by pretreatment with RNase or by the specific TLR7 inhibitor IRS661. TLR7 knockout, but not TLR9 knockout, markedly attenuated the inflammatory response to RNA in bone-derived macrophages. These experiments provide convincing evidence of TLR7 being present in cardiac myocytes and the importance of TLR7, but not TLR9, for the inflammatory response to RNA. TLR9 has been reported to mediate protection of cardiac myocytes and neurons by modulating cell metabolism [94].

2.4 Beyond Toll-Like Receptors: Other Aspects of Innate Immunity Impacting the Heart

The innate immune system and the Toll-like receptors have been studied extensively in immune cells; however, work addressing the function of the Toll-like receptors outside the immune system is nascent [46]. As discussed, HSP60 and HSP72 have been found in the plasma of many individuals. Furthermore, many individuals make antibodies to heat shock proteins, possibly secondary to conservation of sequence during evolution or from exposure to HSPs during vaccinations. These circulating HSPs and antibodies have the potential to activate the immune system. The role of these chronic extracellular HSPs in disease processes has yet to be definitively identified, although there is work associating circulating HSPs with early atherosclerosis in young individuals [95]. The level of circulating HSP60 was highly consistent over 5 years and correlated with circulating anti-HSP60 antibodies. Work in the atherosclerotic ApoE3 mouse demonstrating that TLR-4 has a role in atherosclerosis and in outward arterial remodeling supports these findings [96, 97]. In older individuals because of the many confounding factors contributing to atherosclerosis and the high prevalence of atherosclerosis, the effect of HSP6O and anti-HSP60 antibodies would be difficult to discern. More work is needed to elucidate the role of extracellular HSPs and their antibodies in human disease.

As our understanding of the Toll-like receptors increases, it has become apparent that these receptors have pleiotropic effects, with both protective and destructive events triggered by their activation. In the immune system, TLR-2 and TLR-4 have been implicated in signaling leading to apoptosis. TLR-4, as well as TLR-2, has been described in macrophages as causing apoptosis, as well as the induction of the innate immune response [98]. In microglial cells, TLR-4-mediated activation induced cell death, which is a mechanism by which activated immune cells are eliminated [98]. In the immune system, this would have an advantage, as self-destruction of an activated macrophage turns off the inflammatory response, preventing indefinite propagation.

TLRs and Extracellular Proteins as Ligands: Experimental Caveats—The potential effects of extracellular HSP60 and other proteins have generated significant interest, particularly with regard to inflammation and as a source of increased injury after myocardial infarction, which results in the release of cellular contents into the bloodstream as a result of necrotic cell death. Endotoxin contamination is an important issue in working with purified proteins and other molecules. As endotoxin is a ligand for TLR4, it is essential that work in this area be conducted with low-endotoxin material and controls to avoid misinterpretation of results.

2.5 Conclusions

In the last 10–15 years, the role of endogenous proteins as potential ligands for some of the Toll-like receptors has provided another mechanism for autoimmune-mediated inflammation and tissue/cell damage. In particular heat shock proteins, as well as other proteins, such as HMGB1, have been identified as binding TLR2 and TLR4 when extracellular, and it has become clear that the intracellular HSPs are extracellular. The immune system now must be recognized as a potential foe, not just in established autoimmune diseases, such a lupus, but also in cardiovascular disease where both the innate immune system and the adaptive immune system can contribute to cardiac myocyte injury and death. Extension of our understanding of the role of innate immunity activation has not led to application in the clinical setting, even though numerous basic research studies have shown that inhibition of TLR4 can limit infarct size. The availability of specific TLR inhibitors makes this feasible, and for reducing infarct size, only temporary inhibition of TLR4 is necessary. Ischemic heart failure with increased HSP60 and HSP60 on the cardiac myocyte surface is another potential target, and we are currently writing a manuscript on TLR4 inhibition and its effect on the progression of ventricular dysfunction in a rat model.

In disease states the HSPs can be increased in response to cell and tissue injury, and this can potentially contribute to disease progression, rather than to protection. In particular, extracellular HSPs can be pro-inflammatory, activating innate and also adaptive immunity, depending on the setting. In cardiac myocytes, extracellular HSP60 appears to have a more damaging effect than HSP72, but both are clearly injurious. Research from our laboratory and others supports a detrimental role for extracellular HSP60 in heart failure and other cardiovascular diseases [99, 100]. Others have demonstrated a tripling of plasma HSP60 with menopause and that exHSP60 induced apoptosis in human bone marrow stromal cells via TLR2 [101]. In contrast, HSP60 inhibited apoptosis via MyD88 in B cells [102]. Thus, the role of exHSP60 in cell injury is complex and at times exHSP60 is clearly beneficial. Further investigation will be needed to understand the role of extracellular HSPs, their antibodies, and the TLRs in disease.

Acknowledgments This work was supported by a RO1 HL079071 and a Merit Award (5101BX000839) from the US Department of Veterans' Affairs, Office of Research and Development, Biomedical Laboratory Research Program.

References

1. Janeway CA Jr. Approaching the asymptote? Evolution and revolution in immunology. Cold Spring Harb Symp Quant Biol. 1989;54(Pt 1):1–13.
2. Kim SC, Stice JP, Chen L, Jung JS, Gupta S, Wang Y, et al. Extracellular heat shock protein 60, cardiac myocytes and apoptosis. Circ Res. 2009;105(12):1186–95.
3. Kaczorowski DJ, Nakao A, Mollen KP, Vallabhaneni R, Sugimoto R, Kohmoto J, et al. Toll-like receptor 4 mediates the early inflammatory response after cold ischemia/reperfusion. Transplantation. 2007;84(10):1279–87.
4. Boyd JH, Mathur S, Wang Y, Bateman RM, Walley KR. Toll-like receptor stimulation in cardiomyocytes decreases contractility and initiates an NF-kB dependent inflammatory response. Cardiovasc Res. 2006;72:384–93.
5. Tian J, Guo X, Liu XM, Liu L, Weng QF, Dong SJ, et al. Extracellular HSP60 induces inflammation through activating and up-regulating TLRs in cardiomyocytes. Cardiovasc Res. 2013;98(3):391–401.
6. Avlas O, Srara S, Shainberg A, Aravot D, Hochhauser E. Silencing cardiomyocyte TLR4 reduces injury following hypoxia. Exp Cell Res. 2016;348(2):115–22.
7. Timmers L, Sluijter JPG, van Keulen JK, Hoefer IE, Nederhoff MGJ, Goumans MJ, et al. Toll-like receptor 4 mediates maladaptive left ventricular remodeling and impairs cardiac function after myocardial infarction. Circ Res. 2008;102(2):257–64.
8. Anderson KV, Jürgens G, Nüsslein-Volhard C. Establishment of dorsal-ventral polarity in the drosophila embryo: genetic studies on the role of the toll gene product. Cell. 1985;42(3):779–89.
9. Imler JL, Hoffmann JA. Toll receptors in innate immunity. Trends Cell Biol. 2001;11(7):304–11.
10. Takeuchi O, Sato S, Horiuchi T, Hoshino K, Takeda K, Dong Z, et al. Cutting edge: role of toll-like receptor 1 in mediating immune response to microbial lipoproteins. J Immunol. 2002;169(1):10–4.
11. Asea A, Rehli M, Kabingu E, Boch JA, Bar, O, Auron PE, et al. Novel signal transduction pathway utilized by extracellular HSP70: role of toll-like receptor (TLR) 2 and TLR4. J Biol Chem. 2002;277:15028–34.
12. Chavakis E, Hain A, Vinci M, Carmona G, Bianchi ME, Vajkoczy P, et al. High-mobility group box 1 activates integrin-dependent homing of endothelial progenitor cells. Circ Res. 2007;100(2):204–12.
13. Yu M, Wang H, Ding A, Golenbock DT, Latz E, Czura CJ, et al. HMGB1 signals through toll-like receptor (TLR) 4 and TLR2. Shock. 2006;26:174–9.
14. Alexopoulou L, Holt AC, Medzhitov R, Flavell RA. Recognition of double-stranded RNA and activation of NF-[kappa]B by toll-like receptor 3. Nature. 2001;413(6857):732–8.
15. Cole JE, Navin TJ, Cross AJ, Goddard ME, Alexopoulou L, Mitra AT, et al. Unexpected protective role for toll-like receptor 3 in the arterial wall. Proc Natl Acad Sci U S A. 2011;108(6):2372–7.
16. Ohashi K, Burkart V, Flohe S, Kolb H. Cutting edge: heat shock protein 60 is a putative endogenous ligand of the toll-like receptor-4 complex. J Immunol. 2000;164:558–61.
17. Li Y, Si R, Feng Y, Chen HH, Zou L, Wang E, et al. Myocardial ischemia activates an injurious innate immune signaling via cardiac heat shock protein 60 and toll-like receptor 4. J Biol Chem. 2011;286(36):31308–19.

18. Bulut Y, Faure E, Thomas L, Karahashi H, Michelsen KS, Equils O, et al. Chlamydial heat shock protein 60 activates macrophages and endothelial cells through toll-like receptor 4 and MD2 in a MyD88-dependent pathway. J Immunol. 2002;168(3):1435–40.

19. Rhee SH, Hwang D. Murine TOLL-like receptor 4 confers lipopolysaccharide responsiveness as determined by activation of NF kappa B and expression of the inducible cyclooxygenase. J Biol Chem. 2000;275(44):34035–40.

20. Sasu S, LaVerda D, Qureshi N, Golenbock DT, Beasley D. Chlamydia pneumoniae and chlamydial heat shock protein 60 stimulate proliferation of human vascular smooth muscle cells via toll-like receptor 4 and p44/p42 mitogen-activated protein kinase activation. Circ Res. 2001;89:244–50.

21. Hayashi F, Smith KD, Ozinsky A, Hawn TR, Yi EC, Goodlett DR, et al. The innate immune response to bacterial flagellin is mediated by toll-like receptor 5. Nature. 2001;410(6832):1099–103.

22. Takeuchi O, Kawai T, Mühlradt PF, Morr M, Radolf JD, Zychlinsky A, et al. Discrimination of bacterial lipoproteins by toll-like receptor 6. Int Immunol. 2001;13(7):933–40.

23. Ozinsky A, Underhill DM, Fontenot JD, Hajjar AM, Smith KD, Wilson CB, et al. The repertoire for pattern recognition of pathogens by the innate immune system is defined by cooperation between toll-like receptors. Proc Natl Acad Sci U S A. 2000;97(25):13766–71.

24. Hemmi H, Kaisho T, Takeuchi O, Sato S, Sanjo H, Hoshino K, et al. Small anti-viral compounds activate immune cells via the TLR7 MyD88-dependent signaling pathway. Nat Immunol. 2002;3(2):196–200.

25. Heil F, Hemmi H, Hochrein H, Ampenberger F, Kirschning C, Akira S, et al. Species-specific recognition of single-stranded RNA via toll-like receptor 7 and 8. Science. 2004;303(5663):1526.

26. Diebold SS, Kaisho T, Hemmi H, Akira S, Reis e Sousa C. Innate antiviral responses by means of TLR7-mediated recognition of single-stranded RNA. Science. 2004;303(5663):1529.

27. Hemmi H, Takeuchi O, Kawai T, Kaisho T, Sato S, Sanjo H, et al. A toll-like receptor recognizes bacterial DNA. Nature. 2000;408(6813):740–5.

28. Jiang S, Li X, Hess NJ, Guan Y, Tapping RI. TLR10 is a negative regulator of both MyD88-dependent and -independent TLR signaling. J Immunol. 2016;196(9):3834–41.

29. Oosting M, Cheng SC, Bolscher JM, Vestering-Stenger R, Plantinga TS, Verschueren IC, et al. Human TLR10 is an anti-inflammatory pattern-recognition receptor. Proc Natl Acad Sci U S A. 2014;111(42):E4478–84.

30. Plattner F, Yarovinsky F, Romero S, Didry D, Carlier MF, Sher A, et al. Toxoplasma profilin is essential for host cell invasion and TLR11-dependent induction of an interleukin-12 response. Cell Host Microbe. 2008;3(2):77–87.

31. Koblansky AA, Jankovic D, Oh H, Hieny S, Sungnak W, Mathur R, et al. Recognition of profilin by toll-like receptor 12 is critical for host resistance to toxoplasma gondii. Immunity. 2013;38(1):119–30.

32. Oldenburg M, Krüger A, Ferstl R, Kaufmann A, Nees G, Sigmund A, et al. TLR13 recognizes bacterial 23S rRNA devoid of erythromycin resistance-forming modification. Science. 2012;337(6098):1111.

33. Akira S, Takeda K. Toll-like receptor signaling. Nat Rev Immunol. 2004;4(7):499–511.

34. Hasan U, Chaffois C, Gaillard C, Saulnier V, Merck E, Tancredi S, et al. Human TLR10 is a functional receptor, expressed by B cells and plasmacytoid dendritic cells, which activates gene transcription through MyD88. J Immunol. 2005;174(5):2942–50.

35. Benjamin IJ, McMillan DR. Stress (heat shock) proteins: molecular chaperones in cardiovascular biology and disease. Circ Res. 1998;83:117–32.

36. Nollen EAA, Morimoto RI. Chaperoning signaling pathways: molecular chaperones as stress-sensing 'heat shock' proteins. J Cell Sci. 2002;115(14):2809–16.

37. Knowlton AA. The role of heat shock proteins in the heart. J Mol Cell Cardiol. 1995;27:121–31.

38. Nakano M, Mann DL, Knowlton AA. Blocking the endogenous increase in HSP72 increases susceptibility to hypoxia and reoxygenation in isolated adult feline cardiocytes. Circulation. 1997;95(6):1523–31.
39. Neupert W, Herrmann JM. Translocation of proteins into mitochondria. Annu Rev Biochem. 2007;76(1):723–49.
40. Young JC, Agashe VR, Siegers K, Hartl FU. Pathways of chaperone-mediated protein folding in the cytosol. Nat Rev Mol Cell Biol. 2004;5(10):781–91.
41. Fink AL. Chaperone-mediated protein folding. Physiol Rev. 1999;79(2):425–49.
42. Knowlton AA, Srivatsa U. Heat-shock protein 60 and cardiovascular disease: a paradoxical role. Futur Cardiol. 2008;4:151–61.
43. Kobba S, Kim SC, Chen L, Kim E, Tran AL, Knuefermann P, et al. The heat shock paradox and cardiac myocytes: role of heat shock factor. Shock. 2011;35(5):478–84.
44. Beckmann RP, Mizzen LA, Welch WJ. Interaction of HSP 70 with newly synthesized proteins: implications for protein folding and assembly. Science. 1990;248:850–4.
45. Lewthwaite J, Owen N, Coates A, Henderson B, Steptoe A. Circulating human heat shock protein 60 in the plasma of British civil servants: relationship to physiological and psychosocial stress. Circulation. 2002;106(2):196–201.
46. Srivastava P. Interaction of heat shock proteins with peptides and antigen presenting cells: chaperoning of the innate and adaptive immune response. Annu Rev Immunol. 2002;20:395–425.
47. Xu Q, Schett G, Perschinka H, Mayr M, Egger G, Oberhollenser F, et al. Serum soluble heat shock protein 60 is elevated in subjects with atherosclerosis in a general population. Circulation. 2000;102:14–20.
48. Knowlton AA, Brecher P, Apstein CS. Rapid expression of heat shock protein in the rabbit after brief cardiac ischemia. J Clin Investig. 1991;87:139–47.
49. Hollander JM, Martin JL, Belke DD, Scott BT, Swanson E, Krishnamoorthy V, et al. Overexpression of wild-type heat shock protein 27 and a nonphosphorylatable heat shock protein 27 mutant protects against ischemia/reperfusion injury in a transgenic mouse model. Circulation. 2004;29:01.
50. Ooie T, Takahashi N, Saikawa T, Nawata T, Arikawa M, Yamanaka K, et al. Single oral dose of geranylgeranylacetone induces heat-shock protein 72 and renders protection against ischemia/reperfusion injury in rat heart. Circulation. 2001;104(15):1837–43.
51. Okubo S, Wildner O, Shah MR, Chelliah JC, Hess ML, Kukreja RC. Gene transfer of heat-shock protein 70 reduces infarct size in vivo after ischemia/reperfusion in the rabbit heart. Circulation. 2001;103(6):877–81.
52. Radford NB, Fina M, Benjamin IJ, Moreadith RW, Graves KH, Zhao P, et al. Cardioprotective effects of 70-kDa heat shock protein in transgenic mice. Proc Natil Acad Sci U S A. 1996;93:2339–42.
53. Chen W, Syldath U, Bellmann K, Burkart V, Kolb H. Human 60-kDa heat-shock protein: a danger signal to the innate immune system. J Immunol. 1999;162:3212–9.
54. Vabulas RM, Ahmad-Nejad P, Ghose S, Kirschning CJ, Issels RD, Wagner H. HSP70 as endogenous stimulus of the toll/interleukin-1 receptor signal pathway. J Biol Chem. 2002;277(17):15107–12.
55. Dybdahl B, Wahba A, Lien E, Flo TH, Waage A, Qureshi N, et al. Inflammatory response after open heart surgery: release of heat-shock protein 70 and signaling through toll-like receptor-4. Circulation. 2002;105(6):685–90.
56. Blasi C, Kim E, Knowlton AA. Improved metabolic control in diabetes, HSP60, and proinflammatory mediators. Autoimmune Dis. 2012;2012:346501.
57. Pespeni M, Mackersie RC, Lee H, Morabito D, Hodnett M, Howard M, et al. Serum levels of Hsp60 correlate with the development of acute lung injury after trauma. J Surg Res. 2005;126(1):41–7.

58. Shamaei-Tousi A, Stephens JW, Bin R, Cooper JA, Steptoe A, Coates ARM, et al. Association between plasma levels of heat shock protein 60 and cardiovascular disease in patients with diabetes mellitus. Eur Heart J. 2006;27(13):1565–70.
59. Gupta S, Knowlton AA. HSP60 trafficking in adult cardiac myocytes: role of the exosomal pathway. Am J Physiol Heart Circ Physiol. 2007;292:H3052–6.
60. Malik ZA, Kott KS, Poe AJ, Kuo T, Chen L, Ferrara KW, et al. Cardiac myocyte exosomes: stability, HSP60, and proteomics. Am J Physiol Heart Circ Physiol. 2013;304(7):H954–65.
61. Go MF, Knowlton AA. Heat shock proteins (HSPs) in H-pylori associated disease. Gut. 2000;47:A39–40.
62. Portig I, Pankuweit S, Maisch B. Antibodies against stress proteins in sera of patients with dilated cardiomyopathy. J Mol Cell Cardiol. 1997;29:2245–51.
63. Veres A, Szamosi T, Ablonczy M, Szamosi JT, Singh M, Karadi I, et al. Complement activating antibodies against the human 60 kDa heat shock protein as an independent family risk factor of coronary heart disease. Eur J Clin Investig. 2002;32:405–10.
64. Prohászka Z, Singh M, Nagy K, Kiss E, Lakos G, Duba J, et al. Heat shock protein 70 is a potent activator of the human complement system. Cell Stress Chaperones. 2002;7:17–22.
65. Zhu J, Quyyumi AA, Rott D, Csako G, Wu H, Halcox J, et al. Antibodies to human heat-shock protein 60 are associated with the presence and severity of coronary artery disease: evidence for an autoimmune component of atherogenesis. Circulation. 2001;103(8):1071–5.
66. Mayr M, Kiechl S, Willeit J, Wick G, Xu Q. Infections, immunity, and atherosclerosis: associations of antibodies to chlamydia pneumoniae, helicobacter pylori, and cytomegalovirus with immune reactions to heat-shock protein 60 and carotid or femoral atherosclerosis. Circulation. 2000;102(8):833–9.
67. Feng H, Zeng Y, Whitesell L, Katsanis E. Stressed apoptotic tumor cells express heat shock proteins and elicit tumor-specific immunity. Blood. 2001;97:3505–12.
68. Mor SH, Breloer M, von Bonin A. Eukaryotic heat shock proteins as molecular links in innate and adaptive immune responses: HSP60-mediated activation of cytotoxic T cells. Int Immunol. 2001;13:1121–7.
69. Heng MK, Heng MCY. Heat-shock protein 65 and activated g/d; T cells in injured arteries. Lancet. 1994;344(8927):921–3.
70. Zanin-Zhorov A, Nussbaum G, Franitza S, Cohen IR, Lider O. T cells respond to heat shock protein 60 via TLR2: activation of adhesion and inhibition of chemokine receptors. FASEB J. 2003;17(11):1567–9.
71. Lin L, Kim SC, Wang Y, Gupta S, Davis B, Simon S, et al. HSP60 in heart failure: abnormal distribution and role in cardiac myocyte apoptosis. Am J Physiol. 2007;293:H2238–47.
72. Gao B, Tsan MF. Endotoxin contamination in recombinant human heat shock protein 70 (Hsp70) preparation is responsible for the induction of tumor necrosis factor alpha release by murine macrophages. J Biol Chem. 2003;278(1):174–9.
73. Frantz S, Kelly RA, Bourcier T. Role of TLR-2 in the activation of nuclear factor kB by oxidative stress in cardiac myocytes. J Biol Chem. 2001;276:5197–203.
74. Frantz S, Kobzik L, Kim YD, Fukazawa R, Medzhitov R, Lee RT, et al. Toll4 (TLR4) expression in cardiac myocytes in normal and failing myocardium. J Clin Investig. 1999;104:271–80.
75. Heiserman JP, Chen L, Kim BS, Kim SC, Tran AL, Siebenborn N, et al. TLR4 mutation and HSP60-induced cell death in adult mouse cardiac myocytes. Cell Stress Chaperones. 2015;20(3):527–35.
76. Feng Y, Chen H, Cai J, Zou L, Yan D, Xu G, et al. Cardiac RNA induces inflammatory responses in cardiomyocytes and immune cells via toll-like receptor 7 signaling. J Biol Chem. 2015;290(44):26688–98.
77. Knowlton AA, Kapadia S, Torre-Amione G, Durand JB, Bies R, Young J, et al. Differential expression of heat shock proteins in normal and failing human hearts. J Mol Cell Cardiol. 1998;30:811–8.

78. Wong SCY, Fukuchi M, Melnyk P, Rodger I, Giaid A. Induction of cyclooxygenase-2 and activation of nuclear factor-{kappa}B in myocardium of patients with congestive heart failure. Circulation. 1998;98(2):100–3.
79. Frantz S, Fraccarollo D, Wagner H, Behr TM, Jung P, Angermann CE, et al. Sustained activation of nuclear factor kappa B and activator protein 1 in chronic heart failure. Cardiovasc Res. 2003;57(3):749–56.
80. Wang Y, Chen L, Hagiwara N, Knowlton AA. Regulation of heat shock protein 60 and 72 expression in the failing heart. J Mol Cell Cardiol. 2010;48(2):360–6.
81. Habich C, Baumgart K, Kolb H, Burkart V. The receptor for heat shock protein 60 on macrophages is saturable, specific, and distinct from receptors for other heat shock proteins. J Immunol. 2002;168(2):569–76.
82. Liu Q, Wang J, Liang Q, Wang D, Luo Y, Li J, et al. Sparstolonin B attenuates hypoxia-reoxygenation-induced cardiomyocyte inflammation. Exp Biol Med. 2014;239(3):376–84.
83. Bateman HR, Liang Q, Fan D, Rodriguez V, Lessner SM. Sparstolonin B inhibits pro-angiogenic functions and blocks cell cycle progression in endothelial cells. PLoS One. 2013;8(8):e70500.
84. Matsushima S, Tsutsui H, Sadoshima J. Physiological and pathological functions of NADPH oxidases during myocardial ischemia/reperfusion. Trends Cardiovasc Med. 2014;24(5):202–5.
85. Simon F, Fernandez R. Early lipopolysaccharide-induced reactive oxygen species production evokes necrotic cell death in human umbilical vein endothelial cells. J Hypertens. 2009;27(6):1202–16.
86. Matsuno K, Iwata K, Matsumoto M, Katsuyama M, Cui W, Murata A, et al. NOX1/NADPH oxidase is involved in endotoxin-induced cardiomyocyte apoptosis. Free Radic Biol Med. 2012;53(9):1718–28.
87. Bae YS, Lee JH, Choi SH, Kim S, Almazan F, Witztum JL, et al. Macrophages generate reactive oxygen species in response to minimally oxidized low-density lipoprotein: toll-like receptor 4- and spleen tyrosine kinase-dependent activation of NADPH oxidase 2. Circ Res. 2009;104(2):210–8.
88. Shimamoto A, Chong AJ, Yada M, Shomura S, Takayama H, Fleisig AJ, et al. Inhibition of toll-like receptor 4 with Eritoran attenuates myocardial ischemia-reperfusion injury. Circulation. 2006;114(1_Suppl):I-270.
89. Kim SC, Ghanem A, Stapel H, Tiemann K, Kneufermann P, Hoeft A, et al. Toll-like receptor 4 deficiency: smaller infarcts, but no gain in function. BMC Physiol. 2007;7:5.
90. Zhao Y, McLaughlin D, Robinson E, Harvey AP, Hookham MB, Shah AM, et al. Nox2 NADPH oxidase promotes pathologic cardiac remodeling associated with doxorubicin chemotherapy. Cancer Res. 2010;70(22):9287–97.
91. Mathur S, Walley KR, Wang Y, Indrambarya T, Boyd JH. Extracellular heat shock protein 70 induces cardiomyocyte inflammation and contractile dysfunction via TLR2. Circ J. 2011;75:2445–52.
92. de Graaf R, Kloppenburg G, Kitslaar P, Bruggeman CA, Stassen F. Human heat shock protein 60 stimulates vascular smooth muscle cell proliferation through toll-like receptors 2 and 4. Microbes Infect. 2006;8(7):1859–65.
93. Zanin-Zhorov A, Cahalon L, Tal G, Margalit R, Lider O, Cohen IR. Heat shock protein 60 enhances CD4+ CD25+ regulatory T cell function via innate TLR2 signaling. J Clin Investig. 2006;116(7):2022–32.
94. Shintani Y, Kapoor A, Kaneko M, Smolenski RT, D'Acquisto F, Coppen SR, et al. TLR9 mediates cellular protection by modulating energy metabolism in cardiomyocytes and neurons. Proc Natl Acad Sci U S A. 2013;110(13):5109–14.
95. Xiao Q, Mandal K, Schett G, Mayr M, Wick G, Oberhollenzer F, et al. Association of serum-soluble heat shock protein 60 with carotid atherosclerosis: clinical significance determined in a follow-up study. Stroke. 2005;36(12):2571–6.
96. Hollestelle SCG, de Vries MR, van Keulen JK, Schoneveld AH, Vink A, Strijder CF, et al. Toll-like receptor 4 is involved in outward arterial remodeling. Circulation. 2004;109(3):393–8.

97. Vink A, Schoneveld AH, van der Meer JJ, van Middelaar BJ, Sluijter JPG, Smeets MB, et al. In vivo evidence for a role of toll-like receptor 4 in the development of intimal lesions. Circulation. 2002;106(15):1985–90.

98. Jung DY, Lee H, Jung B, Ock J, Lee M, Lee WH, et al. TLR4, but not TLR2, signals auto-regulatory apoptosis of cultured microglia: a critical role of IFN-b as a decision maker. J Immunol. 2005;174:6467–76.

99. Giannessi D, Colotti C, Maltinti M, Del Rhy S, Prontera C, Turchi S, et al. Circulating heat shock proteins and inflammatory markers in patients with idiopathic left ventricular dysfunction: their relationships with myocardial and microvascular impairment. Cell Stress Chaperones. 2007;12:265–74.

100. Liu L, Wang Y, Cao Z, Wang M-M, Liu XM, Gao T, et al. Up-regulated TLR4 in cardio-myocytes exacerbates heart failure after long-term myocardial infarction. J Cell Mol Med. 2015;19(12):2728–40.

101. Kim YS, Koh JM, Lee YS, Kim BJ, Lee SH, Lee KU, et al. Increased circulating heat shock protein 60 induced by menopause, stimulates apoptosis of osteoblast-lineage cells via up-regulation of toll-like receptors. Bone. 2009;45(1):68–76.

102. Cohen-Sfady M, Pevsner-Fischer M, Margalit R, Cohen IR. Heat shock protein 60, via MyD88 innate signaling, protects B cells from apoptosis, spontaneous and induced. J Immunol. 2009;183(2):890–6.

Chapter 3
Properties and Immune Function of Cardiac Fibroblasts

Milena B. Furtado and Muneer Hasham

Abbreviations

AIM	Absent in melanoma protein
APC	Antigen-presenting cell
BNP	Brain natriuretic peptide
Ccl2	Chemokine ligand 2 or MCP-1
Ccr2	Chemokine receptor 2 or MCP-1 receptor
CD	Cluster of differentiation
CF	Complement factor
Col1a1	Collagen, type I, alpha 1
Cre	Cre recombinase, tyrosine recombinase enzyme derived from the P1 bacteriophage, recognizes specific DNA sequences (LoxP sites) and catalyzes recombination between two recognition LoxP sites, and commonly used in mouse genetic recombineering to remove particular genes of interest
Cxcl1	Chemokine ligand 1 or GROα
Cxcl2	Chemokine ligand 2 or GROβ
Cxcl8	Chemokine ligand 8 or IL-8
DAMPs	Damage-associated molecular patterns
DC	Dendritic cell
ECM	Extracellular matrix

M.B. Furtado (✉)
The Jackson Laboratory, Bar Harbor, ME 04609, USA

Australian Regenerative Medicine Institute, Monash University,
Melbourne, VIC 3800, Australia
e-mail: milena.furtado@jax.org

M. Hasham
The Jackson Laboratory, Bar Harbor, ME 04609, USA

© Springer International Publishing AG 2017
S. Sattler, T. Kennedy-Lydon (eds.), *The Immunology of Cardiovascular Homeostasis and Pathology*, Advances in Experimental Medicine and Biology 1003, DOI 10.1007/978-3-319-57613-8_3

EGF   Epidermal growth factor
EMT   Epithelial to mesenchymal transition
Erk1   Extracellular signal-regulated kinase 1(serine threonine kinase) or MAPK3
Foxp3   Transcription factor forkhead box P3
Gata   Transcription factor GATA-binding protein
GCSF   Granulocyte colony-stimulating factor
GFP   Green fluorescent protein
GMCSF   Granulocyte macrophage colony-stimulating factor
GRO   Growth-regulated protein
H2   Histamine type 2 receptor
Hand   Transcription factor heart and neural crest derivatives expressed
IFN-γ   Interferon gamma
IL   Interleukin
Ltb4   Leukotriene B4
MAPK3   Mitogen-activated protein kinase 3
MBP   Major basic protein
MCP-1   Monocyte chemotactic protein 1 or Ccl2
MCP-3   Monocyte chemotactic protein 3
mEF-SK4   Anti-feeder antibody, clone mEF-SK4
MHC   Major histocompatibility complex
MIP-2α   Macrophage inflammatory protein-2α
MMP   Matrix metalloproteinase
MPO   Myeloperoxidase
NADPH   Nicotinamide adenine dinucleotide phosphate
Nfatc1   Transcription factor nuclear factor of activated T cells, cytoplasmic, calcineurin-dependent 1
NF-κB   Nuclear factor kappa B
NK   Natural killer
NOD   Nucleotide-binding oligomerization domain containing
PAMP   Pathogen-associated molecular pattern
Pdgfra   Platelet-derived growth factor receptor a
PKC   Protein kinase C
PRR   Pattern recognition receptor
RAGE   Receptor for advanced glycosylation end product-specific receptor
RANTES   Regulated on activation, normal T cell expressed and secreted or CCL5
RIG   Retinoic acid-inducible gene or RLR
RLR   Retinoic acid-inducible gene
ROR t   Retinoic acid receptor-related orphan nuclear receptor
SDF-1   Stromal-derived factor 1or Cxcl12
SHIP   SH2 domain-containing inositol 5-phosphatase
SMA   Smooth muscle actin
Tbx   T-box transcription factor
TF   Tissue factor
TGF-β   Transforming growth factor-β
Th   T helper lymphocyte
Thy1   Thymocyte antigen 1 or CD90
Tie2   Tyrosine kinase with Ig and EGF homology domains 2

TIMP	Tissue inhibitor of metalloproteinase
TLR	Toll-like receptor
TNF-α	Tumor necrosis factor alpha
Tnfr	TNF receptor
Treg	T regulatory lymphocyte
Wt-1	Transcription factor Wilms tumor factor 1

3.1 Introduction

It is estimated that fibrosis accounts for about 45% of all deaths in the developed world [1], highlighting the importance of fibroblasts for overall organ pathology. In the heart, fibrosis is a major contributor to heart failure, a chronic debilitating condition for which there is no cure to date. Once a heart reaches this stage, the only solution to this disease is heart transplantation. Heart failure can have a number of different etiologies (Fig. 3.1). The incidence of cardiovascular disease in developed countries is about 30% of the population, therefore posing enormous burden to the

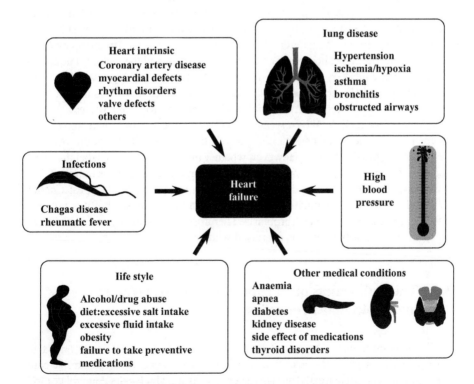

Fig. 3.1 Various etiologies of heart failure. Several heart intrinsic and extrinsic factors can contribute to cardiac pathology, as shown in the diagram. In addition, poor lifestyle choices, such as diet, alcohol, and drug abuse, can also trigger or aggravate heart conditions. Adapted from Cowie et al. [196]

health system [2]. Therefore, a critical understanding of the cardiac fibroblast and how it influences heart function in homeostasis and disease is essential to unravel novel therapeutic approaches to treat heart failure. Important aspects of fibroblast biology will be briefly discussed below, after which immunological properties of these cells will be examined in detail.

3.2   What Is a Cardiac Fibroblast?

The term fibroblast comes from the Latin *fibr* (fiber) and the Greek *blast* (germ, cell, bud) and is reminiscent of the classic but outdated role assigned to this cell type as the main extracellular matrix producer of the body. Modern interpretations of the role of cardiac fibroblasts in the heart include electric isolation and/or conductance in different compartments, cell-cell communication with cardiomyocytes and other cell types, and chemokine/cytokine secretion [3]. In homeostasis, cardiac fibroblasts maintain a symbiotic relationship with other cell types and promote a healthy extracellular matrix balance necessary for proper heart function. In pathogenic circumstances, these cells over-proliferate and differentiate into a myofibroblast phenotype, popularly defined as an "angry" fibroblast, due to its oversecretory and inflammatory-sustaining role. They also express smooth muscle-related molecules, such as smooth muscle actin (SMA) and are able to contract, hence the term *myo*fibroblast [3].

Fibroblasts are seen as a heterogeneous population of cells. Heterogeneity may be due to uncertainties about their embryological origin and the lack of unique protein and genetic markers to separate fibroblasts from other cell types within various organs and body [4]. Particularly for the heart, currently used markers include Thy1 or CD90, vimentin, filamin A, and mEF-SK4 antigen (Miltenyi Biotec). Murine genetic markers include *Wt-1-cre* and *Tbx18-cre* (epicardial-derived fibroblasts), *Nfatc1-cre* and *Tie2-cre* (endocardial-derived fibroblasts), *Periostin-cre*, *Col1a1-GFP*, and *Pdgfra-GFP* [5–8]. However, whether these markers fully label the whole fibroblast fraction and/or are specific to this fraction is arguable. For example, CD90 is expressed by fibroblasts and leukocytes in addition to other cell types; *Col1a1-GFP* and *Pdgfra-GFP* populations fully overlap in flow analysis, but it is not clear if they in fact label all cardiac fibroblasts. Therefore, the use of any of these markers for cardiac fibroblasts should be exercised with caution.

3.3   The Uniqueness of Cardiac Fibroblasts: Origins and Molecular Properties

While many immune cell types can reside in the heart tissue, they do not have their embryological origin in the heart field and therefore are not considered cardiac cells. The heart field is a demarcated area in the embryo from which cells that will contribute to heart formation are specified. The major cell types generated within the heart

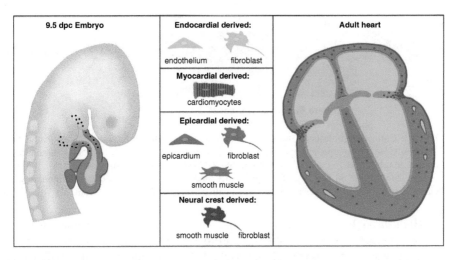

Fig. 3.2 Embryological origin of cardiac fibroblasts and corresponding compartments in the adult heart. *Left panel*—right side view of a 9.5 days post-coitum mouse embryo drawing, depicting the three compartments that contribute cardiac fibroblasts to the heart: pro-epicardial organ (*blue*), endocardium (*green*), and migrating neural crest (*dark gray*). The muscle compartment (cardiomyocytes) is shown in *red*. The *middle panel* shows major cell types contributed by each heart compartment, color-coded to match the *left panel*. The *right panel* shows final contribution of cardiac fibroblasts from various embryological origins to each heart compartment (muscle chambers and valves). Neural crest cells contribute mostly to the outflow tract compartment (aortic root and semilunar valves) and are therefore not depicted here. Reproduced with permission from Furtado et al. [4]

field include endothelial cells, smooth muscle, fibroblasts, and cardiomyocytes. These cell types are produced early in embryonic development (Fig. 3.2) [4]. At 9.5 days post-coitum in murine embryonic development, the heart is composed of only two tissue layers, the muscle (red) and the endocardium (green), which are comprised of cardiomyocytes and endothelial cells, respectively. At this stage, a third layer starts to delaminate from the pro-epicardial organ, which sits under the proper heart. These delaminating cells will cover the heart surface, forming the cardiac epicardium. Epicardial cells also undergo epithelial to mesenchymal transition (EMT) and generate interstitial cells throughout the myocardial space. The two main sources of cardiac fibroblasts are the endocardial and epicardial compartments, both of which undergo EMT early in embryonic development. While the endocardium contributes fibroblasts mostly to the cardiac skeleton, the epicardium will be the major source of interstitial fibroblasts within the muscle compartment. A very small proportion of cardiac fibroblasts are of neural crest cell contribution (Fig. 3.2—dark gray). Many studies describe a fourth source of fibroblasts from the heart as myeloid-derived, named fibrocytes. These cells are capable to produce collagen but retain myeloid cell surface identity (CD45+; CD11b+), and, therefore, whether these cells are actually fibroblasts or a subpopulation of collagen-producing myeloid cells is debatable. Fibrocytes invade injured sites early after insults such as myocardial infarction or pressure overload and seem to participate in injury resolution [4].

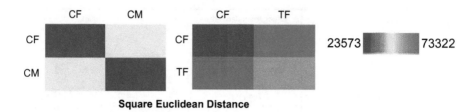

High-throughput molecular profiling of cardiac fibroblasts demonstrated the expression of a broad range of cardiogenic transcription factors, such as T-box factors 2, 5, 20, Hand2, and Gata 4, 5, 6, among others [9, 10]. These transcription factors are normally associated with cardiomyocyte ontogenesis and thought to be specific solely to the muscle compartment. This combination of factors (Gata4, Tbx5, and Hand2) has also been efficiently used to transdifferentiate fibroblasts into cardiomyocytes in vitro and in vivo [11–13], which suggests that cardiomyocytes and fibroblasts show a very similar transcriptional signature. These observations are corroborated by their general transcriptional profile, which shows that cardiac fibroblasts molecularly cluster closer to cardiomyocytes than with an unrelated source of fibroblasts, for example, ones isolated from the mouse tail (Fig. 3.3) [4]. These findings demonstrate that the cardiac fibroblast is a unique cell type, as opposed to a generic body-wide cell, that retains its embryological cardiac identity and is engineered to make part of the cardiac microenvironment. This will be briefly discussed in the next session.

3.4   Cardiac Fibroblasts in Development, Homeostasis, and Disease

Fibroblasts are an integral component of the heart and are commonly used in bioengineering strategies to generate proper heart muscle in vitro [14–17]. In addition, fibroblasts regulate cardiomyocyte proliferation (hyperplasia) or growth in size (hypertrophy) [18] and are surprisingly electrically active, capable of coupling with cardiomyocytes and transmitting electrical impulses [19, 20]. The importance of this cell type for heart formation can be demonstrated by developmental biology studies in the mouse, an important genetic model that allows dissection of mechanistic phenomena, not possible in human subjects. Deletion of genes important for fibroblast biology causes significant malformations in the heart [9, 21–23]. As for adult heart, deletion of fibroblast-specific genes seems to be compatible with a healthy homeostatic balance. However, challenges of heart function have revealed altered pathological remodeling [9, 24]. Fibroblast-specific deletion of the transcription factor *Klf5* using *Periostin-cre* led to reduced cardiac hypertrophy in response to pressure overload but caused severe heart failure under high-overload conditions [24]. Using the same *Periostin-cre*, the cardiogenic transcription factor *Tbx20* has been deleted from murine hearts [9]. Following myocardial infarction, hearts lacking *Tbx20* in fibroblasts showed improved cardiac function and reduced dilation. Combined, these data emphasize the importance of the cardiac fibroblast for the modulation of pathological remodeling of the heart.

3.5 Innate and Adaptive Immune Systems as Modulators of Fibroblast Activity

The adult mammalian heart has very low regenerative capacity, due to the lack of significant cardiomyocyte proliferation after birth. Cardiac repair following an insult requires removal and replacement of dead cells with connective tissue to restore homeostatic balance. Both innate and adaptive immune systems play an important role in this process, which leads to the development of collateral chronic inflammation and fibrosis, normally observed in pathological settings, such as pressure overload or myocardial infarction, and therefore will be discussed in detail in this section.

3.5.1 Innate Immune System, Inflammation, and Fibroblast Activation

The innate immune system and cardiac fibroblasts are intimately associated, sensing environmental cues and communicating with each other to promote adequate response to eliminate insults and restore homeostatic balance. Cardiac injury can be generated by various stimuli, including ischemic, volume, pressure, infection, or allergic reactions. However, most of them converge on induction of fibrosis and pathological remodeling of the heart, which ultimately leads to chronic conditions and heart failure. The innate immune system plays a pivotal role on cardiac fibroblast activation, and sustained inflammation has been linked to the progression of fibrosis (Fig. 3.4).

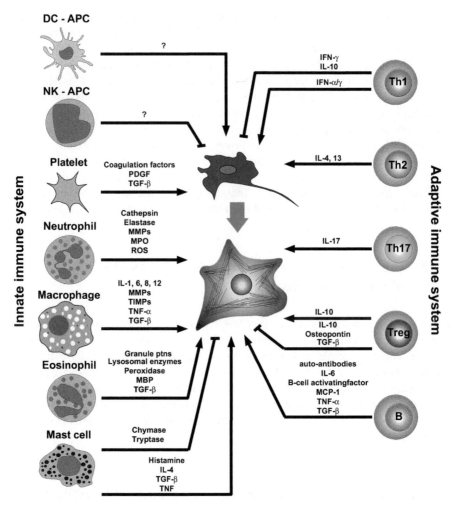

Fig. 3.4 The innate and adaptive immune systems as modulators of fibroblast activity. Various cells of the innate (*left*) or adaptive (*right*) immune system are known to secrete soluble factors that activate (*arrowhead*) or suppress (*bar*) fibroblast activity. Fibroblasts in turn respond to these chemical stimuli and differentiate into myofibroblasts (*center*), highly secretory cells that participate in the fibrotic response. Adapted from Van Linthout et al. [25]

3.5.1.1 Wound Healing Is the Initial Response to Ischemic Events

The coagulation cascade plays an important role in ischemic injuries [25], and platelets are among the first to respond to the injury. Upon endothelial damage, the extrinsic coagulation factor pathway is activated when platelets are exposed to complement factor (CF) III or tissue factor (TF) in the damaged endothelial layer. TF converts CF VII into VIIa (activated VII), which subsequently activates CF X. Activated CF X (Xa) converts prothrombin (CF II) into thrombin (CF IIa), which in turn amplifies the pathway by converting fibrinogen (CF I) into fibrin (CF Ia), culminating in the formation of a fibrin clot or thrombus [26]. In addition to their role in clot formation, CF VII and X exert pro-fibrotic effects in lung fibrosis. CF X is a potent inducer of fibroblast proliferation and myofibroblast differentiation through the activation of TGF-β platelet-derived growth factor (PDGF) signaling using the thrombin PAR1 receptor [27, 28].

3.5.1.2 The Involvement of the Innate Immune System in Fibrosis

The innate response to a heart insult is highly dependent on pattern recognition receptors or PRRs, present in cells of the innate immune system, including platelets. Some of the well-recognized PRRs are the Toll-like receptors or TLRs, nucleotide-binding oligomerization domain (NOD)-like receptors, retinoic acid-inducible gene (RIG)-I-like receptors (also RLRs), absent in melanoma (AIM) 2 receptors, inter-leukin-1 (IL-1) receptors, or the more atypical receptor for advanced glycation end product (RAGE) [29, 30]. PRRs are supposed to recognize conserved pathogen-associated molecular patterns or PAMPs. In the case of sterile inflammation observed in many heart pathological settings, PRRs recognize antigens released from necrotic muscle tissue, named damage-associated molecular patterns or DAMPs [31, 32]. Irrespective of the type of injury, DAMPs released from dying cells, mostly damaged endothelium and cardiomyocytes, are responsible for the activation of inflammation and fibrosis.

Natural killer (NK) cells, neutrophils, dendritic cells, and inflammatory mono-cytes are among the first cells to invade the damaged tissue. NK cells are cytotoxic lymphocytes that are critical for the innate response, as they recognize dead cells and debris in the absence of major histocompatibility complex (MHC) receptors or antibodies, therefore promoting a fast response to clear injury sites of unwanted necrotic tissue. The role of NK cells in cardiac fibroblast activation remains poorly understood. A recent study demonstrated that NK cells exert a beneficial effect in myocardial remodeling, through the c-Kit receptor: c-Kit-deficient mice show impaired production and mobilization of NK cells [33] and have exacerbated patho-logical remodeling following myocardial infarction, with increased dilation and hypertrophy when compared with control hearts. Bone marrow-rescued animals display increased mobilization of NK cells, improved ventricular function and neo-vascularization, and decreased collagen deposition, suggesting an anti-fibrotic role for NK cells [34].

Neutrophils are among the first cells that are chemoattracted to injured sites, due to a cocktail of chemokines and growth factors released from injured cells. They arrive at injured sites within minutes and initiate acute inflammatory response and phagocytose dead cells and debris [25]. Following myocardial infarction, macro-phage inflammatory protein-2α (MIP-2α, Cxcl2, or GROβ), leukotriene B4 (Ltb4), GROα (Cxcl1), IL-8 (Cxcl8), and complement 5a are the main chemokine recruiters of neutrophils [35]. Upon activation, neutrophils release reactive oxygen species, which are mediators of fibrotic response in various disease models, such as pulmonary and hepatic fibrosis, as well as systemic sclerosis [36–38]. Neutrophils have numerous roles in fibroblast recruitment: Reactive oxygen species, generated via nicotinamide adenine dinucleotide phosphate (NADPH) oxidase enzymatic complex, are directly involved in cardiac fibrosis [35, 39, 40]. NADPH oxidases are expressed by various cardiovascular cells, including endothelial, vascular smooth muscle, cardiomyocytes, and fibroblasts [41]. Contrary of the oxidase expressed by neutrophils, enzymatic complex in cardiovascular cells constantly generates low levels of intracellular reactive oxygen species in heart homeostasis. This process is highly enhanced by injury stimuli. However, neutrophil infiltration seems to be a major regulator of fibrosis following injury. Superoxide causes proliferation of fibroblasts and differentiation into myofibroblasts [42, 43]. Although it is difficult to disentangle the role played by neutrophil or resident cell release of reactive oxygen species, it is clear that NADPH oxidases play a fundamental role in the development of cardiovascular fibrosis. Nox2-deficient mice have abolished fibrotic response under pressure overload/hypertrophy stimuli, also measured at the molecular level through reduction of collagens I/III and MMP-2 [44, 45]. In addition, chemical inhibition of NADPH oxidases diminishes myocardial fibrosis [39, 40]. Apart from generating reactive oxygen species, neutrophils also release granules containing about 300 enzymes or other proteins, including myeloperoxidase (MPO), matrix metalloproteinases (MMPs), elastase, and cathepsins, among others. These granules are capable of cleaving connective tissue released by fibroblasts during the fibrotic response [35]. In addition to its secretory role, neutrophils also activate other cells of the innate response, such as inflammatory macrophages, which depending on activation state can be pro-fibrotic, and will be discussed below. Eosinophils are another type of granulocyte implicated in the fibrotic response. Besides secreting TGF-β, their granules contain major basic protein (MBP), peroxidase, and lysosomal hydrolytic enzymes, among others. These factors cause myofibroblast differentiation and are also involved in the induction of EMT, although it is questionable if this event plays a role in cardiac fibroblast-driven pathology in the adult organ [46]. Although the role played by eosinophils in the development of heart failure has not been fully explored, it is clear that hyper-eosinophilia can severely compromise heart function, causing myocarditis and fibrosis, among other pathologies [47]. MBP-1 has been also linked to the development of fibrosis in muscular dystrophy, corroborating a pro-fibrotic role for eosinophils in muscle pathologies [48].

Dendritic cells (DCs) are professional antigen-presenting cells. They express both MHC class I and class II with the processed antigen peptide on their surface to activate the adaptive immune system (B and T lymphocytes) response to inflammation. Similar to Langerhans cells of the skin, resident DCs have also been identified in the vasculature and cardiac valves of healthy individuals and mice [49, 50]. Vascular resident DCs found in mice have an immature phenotype, characterized by low expression of costimulatory molecules such as CD40, CD80, and CD86, which are required to activate the adaptive immune system [51]. However, upon injury, these DCs are promptly activated to present antigens to T lymphocytes [49, 50, 52, 53]. Moreover, DCs play a central role in the recruitment of inflammatory cells, which in turn activate fibroblasts in injury sites, and mounting evidence supports a role for fibroblasts on the recruitment and activation of DCs, discussed in the next section [54–57].

Macrophages occupy center stage in innate immune response, as they are central effectors of both pro- and anti-inflammatory responses. Macrophages secrete a broad range of matrix metalloproteinases (MMPs 1, 7, 8, 9, and 12), which degrade ECM components, as well as tissue inhibitors of MMPs or TIMPs, which promote a balance between degradation versus deposition of ECM in the tissue [58]. MMP-9, in particular, has been associated with the development of fibrosis in various models, including the lung [59], myocarditis and dilated cardiomyopathy [60], myocardial infarction [61], and hypertrophic cardiomyopathy [62]. Despite its regulatory role on ECM homeostasis, MMP-2 has been also implicated in the cleavage of monocyte chemotactic protein 3 (MCP-3), which in turn leads to a reduction of the inflammatory response and consequent fibrosis [63].

Macrophages also secrete substantial amounts of TGF-β, which is among the major pro-fibrotic factors in many organs, including the heart [64–66]. TGF-β induces the expression of ECM components such as collagens, suppresses MMPs, and activates myofibroblasts [65, 67–73]. Inhibition of the TGF-β pathway exerts beneficial anti-fibrotic effects in the heart. Administration of a TGF-β-neutralizing antibody in rats subjected to myocardial injury through pressure overload prevented fibroblast activation, collagen induction, and myocardial fibrosis, as well as reversed diastolic dysfunction [74]. In addition, mice subjected to myocardial infarction that had the same pathway inhibited through gene therapy showed improved survival, reduced fibrosis, reduced ventricular dilation, and improved heart function [75]. It is important to note that TGF-β is a pleiotropic factor with manifold roles in embryological development, homeostasis, and disease; therefore temporal and localized modulation may be important to elicit the desired beneficial effects [76, 77].

Apart from secretion of TGF-β, macrophages are also the major cytokine producers, including the pro-inflammatory IL-1, IL-6, IL-8, IL-12, and tumor necrosis factor alpha (TNF-α). TNF-α seems to exert anti-fibrotic effects through suppression of ECM genes [78] but has an indirect pro-fibrotic effect in fibroblasts through activation of TGF-β [79]. Interestingly, clinical trials in which TNF neutralization was used in heart failure patients failed to show beneficial effects [80]. A possible explanation for the observed effect is due to contrasting activities of TNF-α through its receptors 1 (Tnfr1) and 2 (Tnfr2): Knockout mice lacking *Tnfr1* have attenuated fibrosis and collagen deposition in response to angiotensin II infusion, as well as fewer inflammatory cells [81]. These effects were not observed for *Tnfr2*. In a myocardial infarction model, Tnfr1 activation exacerbates remodeling, hypertrophy, and inflammation, while Tnfr2 ameliorates the same parameters [80]. In summary, macrophages are strongly implicated in the exacerbation of inflammatory cell infiltration through the production of cytokines, chemokines, and growth factors, but they are also potent activators and recruiters of myofibroblasts and therefore play an essential role in the development of fibrosis.

A substantial amount of literature indicates important roles for mast cells in various pathological conditions leading to heart failure. Within a few minutes of reperfusion following ischemic events, resident mast cells are also seen in ischemic sites.

Mast cells degranulate pro-inflammatory and pro-fibrotic mediators such as TNF, TGF-β, histamine, cytokines, and proteases [29, 82], which also interact with the complement cascade, exacerbating histamine release, enhancing edema, increasing endothelium permeability, and further attracting inflammatory cells [83]. Inhibition of histamine activity through blockage of type 2 receptor (H2) reduced pathological hypertrophy in a clinical study, measured functionally and by reduced brain natriuretic peptide (BNP) plasma levels [84]. Another study using ischemia reperfusion in dogs also showed a beneficial effect for H2 inhibition, where hearts had smaller infarcts, although no functional improvement was observed [85].

In volume-overload rat models, proteases such as tryptase and chymase released by mast cells activated MMPs with collagenase, gelatinase, and stromelysin properties, which are directly involved in ECM degradation [86]. However, drug-induced inhibition of mast cell degranulation in the same model led to diminished ventricular hypertrophy and dilation, as well as attenuated pulmonary edema and mortality [86, 87]. In agreement with this, mast cell-deficient rats showed attenuation of myocardial remodeling following volume overload, in which ventricular dilation and collagen degradation were both reduced [88]. In addition, mast cells also activated MMPs through secretion of TNF-α [89–91]. These studies were consistent with pro-fibrotic role for mast cells in cardiac volume overload.

Mast cells have also been implicated in pro-fibrotic remodeling in conditions like myocardial infarction, ischemia reperfusion injury, hypertension, myocarditis, and rejection posttransplantation, among others. In these cases, apart from exacerbating inflammation through recruitment of other immune cells, pathological remodeling has been linked to regulation of myofibroblast activity. Following ischemia or pressure overload, mast cell-deficient mice show hypertrophy, larger infarcts, and ventricular dilation, due to reduced infarct thickness [34, 92–94]. Spontaneously hypertensive rats treated with mast cell-stabilizing drugs showed diminished ventricular fibrosis, despite still showing increased blood pressure and hypertrophy [95]. In addition, treatment of cardiac fibroblasts isolated from hypertensive rats with tryptase, which is normally released by activated mast cells, induced fibroblast proliferation and synthesis of collagen [95]. Interestingly, human mast cells were also found to directly regulate myofibroblast activity *in vitro*, by inducing expression of SMA and causing collagen gel matrix contraction [96]. Moreover, mast cells isolated from myocardial biopsies of patients with end-stage dilated cardiomyopathy caused a 92% increase in collagen production in fibroblasts upon *in vitro* stimulation, measured as 3H-proline incorporation [97].

The presence of mast cells in transplanted hearts has been correlated with development of fibrosis, anaphylaxis, and rejection [98–101]. Activated mast cells were detected in myocardial biopsies of patients post-heart transplantations [100]. In such tissues, the number of mast cells and granules were directly correlated with the volume of fibrosis and severe rejection episodes. In a rat model of heart allograft transplantation, the amount of mast cell infiltration was correlated with the intensity of chronic inflammation but not with acute rejection, suggesting a secondary role for these cells in acute rejection through recruitment of other inflammatory cells, such as macrophages [102]. A second study showed that mast cells in hearts with acute rejection were not cardiac resident mast cells but ones recruited from the host circulation, molecularly differed from resident cells, displaying a "mucosa-like phenotype" [101]. A later study using mast cell-deficient rats concluded that donor heart survival was unexpectedly reduced in rats without mast cells, suggesting a paradoxical protective role after cardiac transplantation [98]. Further studies will be necessary to clarify discrepancies among models, but it is clear that increases in mast cell population are found in transplanted hearts undergoing fibrosis and rejection.

In summary, the many cell components of the innate immune system play an integral role on the initial response to various types of heart insults, which in turn stimulate myofibroblasts, the architects of the fibrotic response seen in adverse heart remodeling.

3.5.2 Adaptive Immune System and Fibrosis

The role of the adaptive immune system in the development of fibrosis is normally underappreciated, but growing body of evidence suggests an important role for acquired immunity in various cardiac pathological conditions, most of which result in fibrosis. This section will review evidence implicating some of the main adaptive immune cells in cardiovascular disease and fibrosis. The presence of T lymphocytes seems to be essential for organ homeostasis; mice deficient in T lymphocytes (SHIP) develop spontaneous intestinal inflammation and fibrosis [103]. T lymphocytes are divided into seven categories: One major category is the T helper (T_h) lymphocytes, which can be further subdivided into T_{h1}, T_{h2}, T_{h3}, T_{h17}, T_{h9}, and T_{fh} subtypes [104]. T_{h1}, T_{h2}, and T_{h17} have been reported to have a part in the development of fibrosis and will be further discussed below. The role, if any, of the other helper subtypes at present is not understood in the context of cardiac fibrosis. T_{h1} lymphocytes normally exert anti-fibrotic but pro-inflammatory effects [105–107] and involve secretion of cytokines IFN-γ, TNF, and IL-2. T_{h2} lymphocytes are characterized by the secretion profile of cytokines like IL-4, IL-5, and IL-13, which exert a pro-fibrotic phenotype [108–111].

Although T_{h1} cytokines can be highly inflammatory, it has been demonstrated that IFN-γ and IL-12 substantially reduced collagen deposition in pulmonary [106] and kidney fibrosis [107]. IFN-γ, however, is a highly controversial cytokine, shown to exert both pro- and anti-fibrotic phenotypes. Both IFN-α and IFN-γ are potent inhibitors of fibroblast-driven collagen synthesis in vitro [112]. In addition, IFN-γ has been found to protect against the development of myocarditis and dilated cardiomyopathy in a mouse model, where pro-fibrotic cytokines TGF-β, IL-1β, and IL-4 were reduced, leading to reduced mast cell degranulation and fibrosis [113]. Other studies have demonstrated pro-fibrotic effects for IFN-γ, which seems to be driven by production of cytokines such as TNF-α [114, 115] and recruitment of macrophages, indirectly leading to further inflammation and fibrosis [116, 117].

In a murine model that uses bleomycin to induce lung fibrosis, IFN-γ-deficient mice showed reduced lung inflammation and fibrosis [118]. Angiotensin II-driven cardiac hypertrophy was also reduced in IFN-γ-deficient mice, which showed decreased infiltration of macrophages and T lymphocytes, as well as attenuated fibrosis [119].

Cytokines produced by T_{h2} lymphocytes are clearly pro-fibrotic in various experimental models, primarily through the induction of ECM remodeling and collagen deposition [120, 121] and secondarily through the recruitment and modulation of macrophage plasticity [122, 123]. IL-13 is among the major cytokines of pro-fibrotic activity [124, 125] and when combined with IL-4 induces myofibroblast differentiation [126]. This cytokine has also been linked to regulation of MMPs in Crohn's disease [127]. In this instance, IL-13 downregulated MMP synthesis, which caused collagen accumulation. Additionally, IL-13 has been found to induce TGF-β secretion by macrophages through the IL-13Rα2, originally thought to be a decoy receptor, in models of colitis and pulmonary fibrosis [122, 128]. The same paradigm was confirmed in a murine model of cardiac transplantation, where treatment of animals with siRNAs for IL-13Rα2 prevented allograft fibrosis [129]. Conversely, signaling through the IL-13Rα1 receptor exerted a protective role in pulmonary injury, where mice deficient in IL-13Rα1 showed increased bleomycin-induced lung fibrosis [130]. Collectively, these data demonstrate that modulation of IL-13 signaling may be a suitable pathway for anti-fibrotic therapeutic intervention.

T helper 17 lymphocytes (T_{h17}) are another distinct subset of pro-inflammatory cells that have been associated with fibrosis in various tissues, including the lung, heart, and liver [131–133]. These cells are defined by the production of IL-17 as their major interleukin, namely, Th17. Among the inflammatory mediators released by Th17 are IL-17a, IL-17f, IL-21, and IL-22 [134]. IL-17a stimulates the release of other pro-inflammatory cytokines, such as IL-1, IL-6, TNF-α, and Cxcl8, granulocyte colony-stimulating factor (GCSF), and granulocyte macrophage colony-stimulating factor (GMCSF). Activation of T_{h17} lymphocytes has been strongly linked to myocarditis [135, 136] and isoproterenol-induced heart failure [131], while the role of this lymphocyte subtype in myocardial infarction has been less explored. In experimental murine autoimmune viral myocarditis, the T_{h17} lymphocytes and their transcription factor retinoic acid receptor-related orphan nuclear receptor (ROR γt) were upregulated 3 weeks after myocarditis induction. Furthermore, ROR γt knockout mice showed resistance to myocarditis [136]. A second study further demonstrated that IL-17 is responsible for the induction of heart fibrosis in this model, through activation of the protein kinase C/extracellular signal-regulated kinase 1/nuclear factor kappa B (PKC/Erk1/NF-κB) pathway [135]. Further support for T_{h17} involvement in heart failure comes from a rat model of isoproterenol-induced heart failure, in which animals were also injected with anti-IL-17 antibodies [131]. This work showed decreased expression of MMP-1 and collagen fibers, counterbalanced by increased expression of TIMPs in IL-17 antibody-injected animals. Blocking of IL-17 also improved myocardial fibrosis, measured by Masson trichrome staining. In a mouse model of myocardial infarction, IL-17 was not upregulated 1 week post-infarct, suggesting that T_{h17} response is not important in acute ischemic heart failure [137]. However, an unpublished study showed IL-17 and T_{h17} increased from 2 weeks after infarction, indicating a role for IL-17 in chronic but not acute infarction [138]. In this case, anti-IL-17 antibodies failed to reduce the fibrotic response in infarcted animals, although ROR γt knockout mice had in fact increased cardiac fibrosis. As this study is yet to be published in a peer-reviewed journal, the jury is still out on the role of T_{h17} in the fibrotic response to myocardial infarction. Taken together, this body of current literature demonstrates a strong pro-fibrotic role for T_{h17} lymphocytes in various pathologies leading to heart failure.

Another major category of T lymphocytes is the regulatory T cells, or T_{regs}, defined by the expression of the transcription factor forkhead box P3 (Foxp3). T_{regs} can exert dual roles on the fibrotic response, depending on stimulatory stimuli. They play an important role in controlling inflammation and consequent promotion [139] or suppression [140] of fibrosis. IL-10 released by T_{regs} has been shown to be a potent anti-fibrotic agent in a mouse myocarditis model, through the inhibition of collagen synthesis by cardiac fibroblasts [141]. Another study engineered monocytes/macrophages that overexpressed IL-10 and showed that this strategy also ameliorated myocarditis [142]. In addition, transfer of T_{regs} to hypertensive mouse hearts also attenuated inflammation and fibrosis, reducing TGF-β1 and the presence of myofibroblasts [140]. Following myocardial infarction, T_{regs} infiltrate the cardiac tissue and participate in injury resolution. Mice depleted of T_{regs} showed reduced heart function and survival, as well as increased dilation after infarction [143, 144]. In agreement with this, increasing the amount of T_{regs} in the heart tissue through cell transfer or agonistic antibodies had beneficial effects on healing [143–149]. This healing activity was probably mediated by IL-10, osteopontin and TGF-β, all found to be produced by infiltrating T_{regs}, and caused a trifold impact on infarct repair through activation of M2-like (anti-inflammatory) macrophages [144], rescue of cardiomyocytes from death [146], and modulation of fibroblast activity [143]. *In vitro*, T_{regs} directly downregulated myofibroblast marker SMA and MMP-3 in cardiac fibroblasts, confirming that T_{regs} exert an anti-fibrotic activity.

Given the important role played by T_{regs} in many heart conditions, many experimental models have successfully established pre-therapeutic assessments for the use of IL-10 to treat various heart pathologies, including ischemia/infarct [150], pressure overload [151], and myocarditis, as previously mentioned. IL-10 has also been linked to cardiac protection in obese animals submitted to exercise [152].

In contradiction with an anti-fibrotic role for IL-10, a recent study showed a detrimental role for targeted release of IL-10 to the posttransplantation heart [153]. This study took advantage of fibronectin, normally overexpressed during chronic heart rejection, to create a vehicle for injection of IL-10 to rats with heterotopic heart transplants undergoing chronic rejection. In this case, IL-10-injected groups showed higher rejection and increased SMA expression, as well as enrichment of inflammatory cells, against the odds. However, the authors suggested a caveat for the observed results, which was that the therapeutic time point used in the study was still in the acute phase of rejection, and proposed a further study to address this issue.

Last, but not least, the role for B lymphocytes in heart fibrosis has only recently raised interest of the scientific community and is so far under-investigated. B lymphocytes are professional antigen-presenting cells (APCs), produce antibodies and secrete cytokines. Similar to T lymphocytes, there are various subsets of B lymphocytes, including a regulatory B lymphocyte population (B_{reg}) [104]. A pro-fibrotic role for B lymphocytes has been demonstrated in liver fibrosis, where B lymphocyte secretion of IL-6-induced myofibroblast differentiation from stellate cells, accompanied of fibroblast proliferation, increased collagen and TIMP synthesis [154, 155]. In systemic sclerosis, autoantibodies produced against fibrillin were shown to directly affect dermal fibroblasts *in vitro*, causing fibrosis through increased ECM expression and induction of TGF-β1 and consequent Smad3 phosphorylation [156]. Another study showed that B lymphocyte-activating factor was a potent inducer of collagen, TIMP1, MMP-9, and SMA in dermal fibroblasts, all pro-fibrotic molecules [157]. Expression of pro-fibrotic/pro-inflammatory cytokines IL-6, Ccl2, and TGF-β was also found in this system.

In the heart, B lymphocytes are involved in the pathology of allograft rejection and autoimmune myocarditis, both of which are intimately linked to fibrosis, as previously mentioned throughout this section. Acute antibody-mediated rejection is one of the main complications following heart transplantation, correlated with poor survival, vasculopathy, and transplant failure [158]. In a mouse model of allograft transplantation, B lymphocytes were found responsible for the generation of atherosclerosis in transplanted tissues [159]. B lymphocyte-deficient recipient mice showed reduced collagen deposition. Furthermore, two other donor-recipient combinations, which had undetectable levels of anti-donor antibodies, presented decreased intimal fibrosis. When these animals were given anti-donor antibodies through passive transfer, the fibrotic lesions reappeared, demonstrating a strong role for B cell-mediated response in allograft rejection. However, it has been recently demonstrated that B lymphocytes exert regulatory roles in transplantation and can mediate chronic allograft heart rejection independently of generation of autoantibodies [160]. Mice deficient in antibody production still experienced vasculopathy, while mice deficient in both antibodies and B lymphocytes were protected. Further data suggested that vasculopathy was dependent on the APC properties of B lymphocytes, which in turn recruited cytotoxic T lymphocytes to transplanted tissue, rather than antibody production. This phenomenon is similar to autoimmune diseases such as Type I diabetes [161].

Myocarditis occurs in three phases; the initial phase involves cardiomyocyte damage through viral/bacterial infections or other agents. The second phase consists of activation of immune cells such as CD4+ T lymphocytes, which leads to the third phase of clonal expansion of B lymphocytes, causing further inflammation and production of circulating autoantibodies directed against the heart tissue [162, 163].

Dilated cardiomyopathy, a progression from persistent myocarditis, has been linked to B lymphocyte epitope spreading in a C-protein-induced myocarditis rat model [164]. Interestingly, patients showing dilated cardiomyopathy associated with myocarditis showed increased numbers of TNF-α secreting B lymphocytes [165]. Moreover, 59% of patient sera also showed increased serum procollagen type III, suggesting this cytokine was involved in the fibrotic response in these patients. In this model, epitope spreading was correlated with aggravation of inflammation and fibrosis. It remains to be fully addressed if B lymphocytes, or subsets of B lymphocytes, play a role in ischemic or pressure overload events, but considering that patients undergoing infarct release structural proteins such as troponin in the blood, the possibility of a humoral response is intriguing and highly plausible. The participation of B lymphocytes in cardiac ischemic injury can be exemplified by a study that showed that antibody mediated or genetic depletion of mature B lymphocytes was beneficial to heart recovery in acute myocardial infarction, in this case through modulation of monocyte mobilization [166].

3.6 Fibroblasts as the Immunomodulatory Hub of the Heart

Most studies place the cardiac fibroblast as a passive cell type in standby for receiving inputs from various immune cells to be activated and promote fibrosis. Indeed, cardiac fibroblasts are receptive to multiple chemical and cellular stimuli, as addressed in the previous section. However, it has become clear that this cell type is highly active in the cardiac tissue milieu and is capable of directly sensing disturbances in homeostatic conditions and reacting to such disturbances appropriately. In a highly active tissue like the heart, which never rests, sustaining homeostasis is no simple task. Besides chemical cues, cardiac fibroblasts are directly connected with cardiomyocytes and other resident cells, through gap junctions, and therefore sense and transmit electrical impulses [3]. Cardiac fibroblasts also respond to mechanical stress and hormonal changes, such as angiotensin II and adrenaline [3]. Although cardiac fibroblasts can sense various types of external stimuli, the goal of this section is to solely focus on immune response cues triggered by the cardiac fibroblast.

Fibroblasts modulate the inflammatory response at various levels, including initial chemotaxis, infiltration, and migration of inflammatory cells, as well as later steps of cell retention, apoptosis, and inflammation resolution or persistence of a chronic condition (Fig. 3.5). Traditionally, endothelial cells have been described as the initiators of vascular inflammation. While that still holds true, it does not necessarily account for the full picture in cardiovascular conditions. Inflammatory cells have been reported to exist within the interstitial myocardium in high quantities, including myeloid and lymphoid cells [7, 167]. Therefore, sensing damage and activating a repair response can also be achieved in a local fashion by interstitial fibroblasts, which trigger endothelial inflammatory response

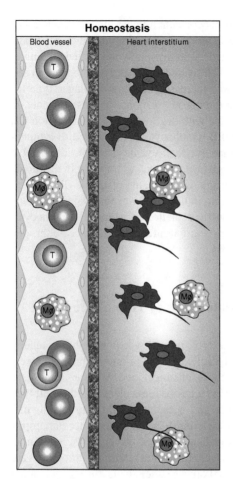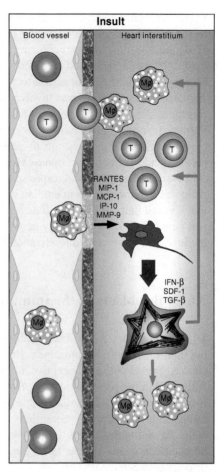

Fig. 3.5 Fibroblasts as the immunomodulatory hub of the heart. Under homeostatic conditions, immune cells and fibroblasts reside in the myocardial interstitium and sense microenvironmental cues (*left panel*). Upon an injury stimulus, such as ischemic or pressure overload events, cardiac fibroblasts cross-talk with various immune cells in the local interstitium and are capable of modulating the activity of both innate and adaptive immune systems. Adapted from Van Linthout et al. [25]

[168]. Indeed, a study using subcutaneous infusion of angiotensin II to induce vascular inflammation in mice showed that inflammation happened predominantly in the tunica adventitia, the most external layer of the aorta closer to the tissue interstitium, and not at the vessel lumen [169]. This was accompanied by production of pro-inflammatory cytokines IL-6 and MCP-1, culminating in macrophage infiltration and aortic dissections (tears). Furthermore, coculture of adventitial fibroblasts with monocytes induced IL-6, MCP-1, and MMP-9 *in vitro*, suggesting a major role for aortic adventitial fibroblasts in the development of local vascular inflammation and dissection. Besides, fibroblasts participating in

the fibrotic response in conditions such as pressure overload and myocardial infarction are solely of a local, cardiac-resident origin [5, 6, 8].

The expression of pattern recognition receptors (PRRs) by cardiac fibroblasts is novel concept [170]. PRRs confer these cells the capability to directly respond to damage-associated molecular patterns (DAMPs) released by damaged myocardium [171–173]. Some of the PRRs found in cardiac fibroblasts include TLRs, NLRs, IL-1R1, and RAGE. Activation of PRRs in turn causes a feed-forward inflammatory response via NF-κB, mitogen-activated protein kinase (MAPK) 8, and p38 stress signaling pathways [174, 175]. Activation of these pathways commonly leads to transcription of pro-inflammatory cytokines. Table 3.1 summarizes DAMPs and PRRs associated with cardiac fibroblast response to damage, as well as the net outcome of triggering their response.

Table 3.1 PRRs and DAMPs involved in regulating fibroblast activity

Damp	Species	Age	Receptor/signaling pathway	Response
S100A1	Rat	Adult	TLR4 MyD88 ERK P38 JNK NF-κB	↓Collagen I ↓CTGF ↓SMA ↑MMP-9 ↑ICAM, IL-10 ↑SDF-1, TSP2
S100A8/9	Mouse	Adult NIH/3T3	RAGE NF-κB	↑Cell migration ←→Cell proliferation ←→Myofibroblast differentiation ↑Cytokines ↑Chemokines ↑Cell proliferation ←→Collagens I, III
IL-1α	Human Mouse	Adult Neonatal NIH/3T3	P38 JNK NF-κB PI3K/AKT IL-1R1	↑Cell migration ↓Myofibroblast differentiation ↓SMA ↑IL-1β, IL-6, TNFα ↑CXCL1, 2, 5, 8 ↑MMP-1, MMP-3, MMP-9, MMP-10 ↑ICAM, VCAM ↑E-selectin ↓ADAMTS1 ↑TNC ↓CTGF ↓Collagen I ↑Collagen III ↑IL-6, MCP-1 ←→Cell proliferation ←→Collagens I, III

(continued)

Table 3.1 (continued)

Damp	Species	Age	Receptor/signaling pathway	Response
HMGB1	Human Rat Mouse	Adult Adult Neonatal Adult Neonatal NIH/3T3	ERK JNK PI3K/AKT TLR4 TLR2 TLR4 PKC-β ERK	↑Cell migration ←→Cell proliferation ←→Myofibroblast differentiation ↑Cytokines ↑Chemokines ↑Growth factors ↓Collagen I ↑Smad7 ↑Cell proliferation ↑Cell migration ↑Collagens I, III ↑TGF-β ↑MMP-2, MMP-9 ↑Collagen I ↓TIMP3 ↑miR-206 ↑Cell proliferation ↑Cell migration ↑Collagens I, II ↑OPN ↑MMP-1, MMP-2 ↑TIMP1 ↑Cell proliferation ↑Collagens I, III
HSP70	Rat	Neonatal	TLR2	↑Cell proliferation ↑Cytokines

Reproduced from Turner [170]

Vascular endothelial cells are known to control leukocyte adhesion to vessels during inflammation [176]. However, interstitial fibroblasts have been shown to also regulate this process in inflamed tissues. Fibroblasts isolated from inflamed synovium, but not normal one, were capable of causing flowing peripheral blood leukocytes to adhere to the endothelial cell line HUVEC *in vitro* [177]. Adhesion was promoted by interaction with integrin VCAM-1, Cxcr4, and its ligand stromal cell-derived factor 1 (SDF-1 or Cxcl12).

Fibroblasts are capable of secreting high levels of MCP-1, MIP-1, RANTES, IP-10, and chemokine receptors, which in turn recruit macrophages and stimulate inflammatory response [25], as well as activate the fibrotic response through an autocrine loop. Chemokine production by fibroblasts seems to be dependent on the NF-κB pathway and the transcription factor RelB. Mice deficient in RelB displayed severe inflammatory syndrome, although the heart looked grossly normal under homeostatic conditions [178]. In normal fibroblasts, incubation with lipopolysaccharide induced transient production of chemokines, and that was correlated with increased RelB expression. Fibroblasts deficient in RelB had exacerbated and persistent (chronic) induction of chemokines, including MIP and RANTES, and this could be reversed using transient transfection of RelB back into fibroblasts.

Murine fibroblasts recovered from kidneys undergoing inflammatory response or cocultured with mononuclear cells were able to produce large quantities of MCP-1, MCP-1 receptor (Ccr2), or MIP-1α [179–181]. Another study showed that MCP-1 induced collagen expression in lung fibroblasts, plausibly through the activation of TGF-β signaling [182]. MCP-1 was also implicated in activating MMP-1 in human fibroblasts [183]. Moreover, a third study found that MCP-1 and IL-6 induced mouse myofibroblast differentiation in an *in vitro* hypoxic model [184]. MCP-1 is a very important cytokine in response to myocardial infarction, controlling inflammatory infiltration and myofibroblast accumulation. While deficiency in MCP-1 caused delayed macrophage recruitment and increased fibrosis in infarcted hearts [185], overexpression of MCP-1 in transgenic hearts led to increased myofibroblast deposition in infarcts [184]; therefore the proposition of a direct role of cardiac fibroblasts for the local regulation of inflammation and fibrosis is of high importance.

In addition to helping the recruitment of leukocytes, cardiac fibroblasts participate in the retention of leukocytes into damaged tissue. This seems to be dependent of the presence of CD40 and costimulatory molecule programmed cell death ligand 1 (B7-H1) on the fibroblast cell surface and the ligands CD40L and CTLA4, respectively, in immune cells [186, 187]. Expression of CD40 in fibroblasts was found to be regulated by IFN-γ and amplified by IL-1α and TNF-α *in vitro* [188]. Interaction with CD40 with its ligand (CD40L) induced expression of intercellular adhesion molecule-1 (ICAM-1) and vascular cell adhesion molecule-1 (VCAM-1) in fibroblasts. Activated fibroblasts also increased proliferation and secretion of IL-6. A second way of retaining leukocytes in the damaged interstitial space involved Cxcr4/SDF-1 signaling. Fibroblasts produced increased quantities of SDF-1 and regulated Cxcr4 expression in immune cells through TGF-β signaling [189, 190]. Taken together, these data demonstrate that fibroblasts can function as APCs and are capable of modulating activity of the adaptive immune system through direct cell-cell contact, in addition to their autocrine role.

Finally, fibroblasts have also been shown to regulate apoptosis of T lymphocytes in inflamed tissues in cell contact-dependent and contact-independent manners [191–193]. Upon stimulation with IFN-γ, fibroblasts express MHC class II, which are normally expressed by hematopoietic cells and participate in antigen presentation. It has been demonstrated that cultured synovial fibroblasts stimulated with IFN-γ not only expressed high levels of MHC II but were also capable of processing soluble protein for presentation to T lymphocytes [194]. This demonstrates that fibroblasts show proper APC function and can also modulate the adaptive immune system.

As for contact-independent regulation of T lymphocytes by fibroblasts, addition of fibroblasts or fibroblast-conditioned media to T lymphocytes *in vitro* resulted in prolonged survival of T lymphocytes in a resting state, absent in proliferation, as opposed to reducing in number after removal of mitogenic cytokine signals. This state was achieved through IFN-β secretion and caused persistence of T lymphocytes in chronic inflammation settings. Administration of IFN-β to T lymphocytes *in vitro* fully mimicked the effect of fibroblast-conditioned media to promote cell survival, while IFN-α did not alter apoptosis [195]. Administration of antibodies against IFN-β reverted cell survival to control levels, corroborating the role of IFN-β secreted by fibroblasts in controlling T lymphocyte survival and expansion. However, it remains to be seen whether cardiac fibroblasts behave in the same manner, as most of the data generated so far used synovial fibroblasts from patients with inflamed joints [192, 195].

Nevertheless, substantial amount of evidence now points to the fibroblast as a major regulator of the immune response or an immunomodulatory hub, as opposed to a passive producer of extracellular matrix. Fibroblasts participate in major steps of the inflammatory response, including induction of leukocyte activation, endothelial adhesion, transendothelial migration, and tissue retention, in addition to their pro-fibrotic role.

3.7   Immunomodulation Therapies that Reduce Fibrosis

Unfortunately, in many pathological scenarios, cardiac fibroblast hyper-activation and myofibroblast differentiation lead to pathological dysfunction and adverse remodeling of the heart, culminating in heart failure. Considering that cardiac fibroblasts are intimately interconnected with various cells and signaling pathways used by the innate and adaptive immune systems, it is not surprising that drugs that affect immunomodulation are also capable of regulating fibrosis. Table 3.2 summarizes some of the validated treatments for fibrosis and shows novel therapeutic targets currently under experimentation or clinical trial. It is important to note that most anti-fibrotic treatments are systemic and not targeted to a particular organ; therefore side effects are commonly seen. Moreover, current therapeutic agents are capable of ameliorating or retarding the pathological process, but no cure has so far been achieved for fibrotic diseases, reinforcing the need for improved therapeutic approaches.

Table 3.2 Current anti-fibrotic therapies used in the clinic and novel experimental drugs

Therapies currently used in the clinic		
Compounds	Targets	Process
AMD3100	Inhibitor of Cxcr4	Immunosuppressant
Captopril, benazepril, enalapril, ramipril, and others	Inhibitors of angiotensin converting enzyme (ACE)	Anti-fibrotic, blood pressure control
Clopidogrel	Inhibitor of platelet aggregation and clot formation	Anti-fibrotic, immunosuppressant
Dasatinib	Inhibitor of BRC-Abl, c-Kit, Src	Anti-fibrotic
Entresto (LCZ696)	Combination of valsartan with sacubitril	See valsartan and sacubitril
Imatinib	Inhibitor of BCR-Abl, c-Kit, PDGFR	Anti-fibrotic
Losartan, valsartan, irbesartan, amlodipine, and others	Angiotensin I and II receptor blockers	Anti-fibrotic, blood pressure control
Metelimumab (CAT-192) and others	Inhibitor of TGFbeta1	Anti-fibrotic, immunosuppressant
Macrolide antibiotics (sirolimus and others)	Inhibitor of mTOR, Fli-1, IL-2 secretion	Anti-inflammatory; immunosuppressant
Nilotinib	Inhibitor of c-Abl, c-Kit, PDGFR	Anti-fibrotic
Nintedanib	Inhibitor of PDGFR, VEGFR, FGFR	Anti-fibrotic
Pirfenidone and others	Inhibitor of TGF-beta, TNF-alpha, and others	Anti-fibrotic, anti-inflammatory, anti-oxidative stress
Sacubitril	Inhibitor of neutral endopeptidases (NEPs) that degrades vasoactive peptides like ANP and BNP	Blood pressure control
Simvastatin, lovastatin, atorvastatin and other statins	Inhibitors of hydroxymethylglutaryl-coenzyme A reductase	Cholesterol lowering; anti-fibrotic
Sorafenib	Inhibitor of PDGFR, VEGFR, and Raf kinases	Anti-fibrotic
Tocilizumab	Inhibitor of interleukin (IL)-6 receptor	Anti-fibrotic, anti-inflammatory

Experimental drugs under clinical trial for various fibrotic diseases			
Compounds	Clinical trial	Targets	Process
Advair	COPD	Agonist for beta-adrenergic receptor	Anti-fibrotic, immunosuppressant

(continued)

Table 3.2 (continued)

Experimental drugs under clinical trial for various fibrotic diseases

Compounds	Clinical trial	Targets	Process
Azaserine, acivicin and others	IPF	Inhibitor of gamma-glutamyl transpeptidase (GTT)	Anti-fibrotic, antioxidant, immunosuppressant
AZD9668	Cystic fibrosis	Inhibitor of neutrophil elastase	Anti-fibrotic, anti-inflammatory
CC-930 (Tanzisertib)	IPF[a]	Inhibitor of the c-Jun N-terminal kinase (JNK)	Anti-fibrotic, anti-inflammatory
Clopidogrel	Myocardial infarction	Inhibitor of platelet aggregation and clot formation	Anti-fibrotic, immunosuppressant
CTX-4430	Cystic fibrosis	Leukotriene A4 hydrolase (LTA4H) inhibitor	Anti-inflammatory
CxCL12 neutralizing antibody	Cystic fibrosis	Inhibitor of chemokine (CXC motif) ligand 12 (CxCl12 or SDF-1)	Immunosuppressant
Doxycycline	Cystic fibrosis	Inhibitor of matrix metalloproteinase (MMP) 9	Anti-bacterial, Immunomodulator, anti-fibrotic
E5564, TAK-242	Sepsis	Inhibitors of Toll-like receptor (TRL)	Anti-inflammatory, antioxidant
Eculizumab	Glomerulonephritis, other kidney pathologies, kidney and heart transplantation	Inhibitor of complement C5	Immunosuppressant
EZ-2053	Lung rejection	Inhibitor of T lymphocytes	Immunosuppressant
Fasudil	Heart failure, atherosclerosis	Inhibitor of Rho kinase (ROCK)	Anti-fibrotic
Fenretinide	Cystic fibrosis	Synthetic retinoic acid agonist	Anti-inflammatory
Fg-3019 and others	Liver/lung/kidney fibrosis, Duchenne muscular dystrophy, glomerulosclerosis	Inhibitor of connective tissue growth factor (CTGF or CCN2)	Anti-fibrotic
Flovent	COPD	Steroid	Immunosuppressant
INT-747 and others (obeticholic acid)	Cirrhosis, hepatitis, cholangitis	Farnesoid X receptor (FXR) agonist	Regulation of glucose and lipid metabolism

(continued)

Table 3.2 (continued)

Experimental drugs under clinical trial for various fibrotic diseases

Compounds	Clinical trial	Targets	Process
Interferon gamma	IPF	Recombinant cytokine	Anti-fibrotic, immunomodulator
Lebrikizumab, QAX576, Tralokinumab	IPF	Inhibitor of interleukin (IL)-13	Anti-fibrotic, anti-inflammatory
MabCampath (alemtuzumab)	Kidney transplantation	Inhibitor of CD52	Immunosuppressant
Prevascar	Scar formation	Inhibitor of TGF-beta signaling (recombinant IL-10)	Anti-fibrotic, Immunosuppressant
Pentoxifylline	Cirrhosis	Inhibitor of phosphodiesterase	Immunosuppressant
Remicade, adalimumab, infliximab, and others	Kidney transplantation, glomerulosclerosis, colitis	Inhibitor tumor necrosis factor (TNF) alpha	Immunosuppressant
Rituximab	IPF, rheumatoid arthritis	Inhibitor of B cells (CD20 antagonist)	Immunosuppressant
Rosiglitazone, fenofibrate, and others	Glomerulosclerosis	peroxisome proliferator-activated receptor gamma (PPAR-gamma) agonist	Anti-fibrotic; regulation of glucose and lipid metabolism
Rilonacept	Systemic sclerosis	Inhibitor of IL-1 (IL-1 modified humanized antibody)	Anti-fibrotic, anti-inflammatory
SB656933	Cystic fibrosis	Inhibitor of neutrophil activation (CXCR2 antagonist)	Anti-fibrotic, immunosuppressant
Tacrolimus (Prograf, Advagraf, Protopic, FK506, and others)	Liver and kidney fibrosis	Inhibitor of IL-2 and T cell activity	Anti-fibrotic, immunosuppressant

Drugs highlighted in bold show both immune and fibrotic properties. Experimental drugs are either under clinical trials for various fibrotic conditions or have only been described in basic research experiments. Sourced at Clinical Trials.gov (May 2016)

COPD chronic obstructive pulmonary disease, *IPF* idiopathic pulmonary fibrosis

[a]Trial terminated due to safety concerns

3.8   Concluding Remarks

We hope the reader has gained a better insight on the cardiac fibroblast as an acceptor and donor of the immune system function. Information described here highlights the complexity of the immune response in cardiovascular homeostasis and disease. This reinforces the difficulty of generating proper anti-inflammatory and anti-fibrotic therapies that are not systemic but organ-specific. Addressing organ-specific properties of cardiac fibroblasts may be an interesting avenue to pursue more stringent therapies. The field of cardiac fibrosis is now booming, as most stem cell therapies have so far failed to reduce cardiovascular pathologies. A bright future is ahead for exploration of the cardiac fibroblast and its immunological properties for the treatment of cardiovascular conditions.

References

1. Wynn TA. Cellular and molecular mechanisms of fibrosis. J Pathol. 2008;214(2):199–210.
2. Mozaffarian D, Benjamin EJ, Go AS, Arnett DK, Blaha MJ, Cushman M, et al. Heart disease and stroke statistics-2016 update: a report from the American Heart Association. Circulation. 2016;133(4):e38–e360.
3. Turner NA, editor. The cardiac fibroblast. 1st ed. Kerala: Research Signpost; 2011.
4. Furtado MB, Nim HT, Boyd SE, Rosenthal NA. View from the heart: cardiac fibroblasts in development, scarring and regeneration. Development. 2016;143(3):387–97.
5. Ali SR, Ranjbarvaziri S, Talkhabi M, Zhao P, Subat A, Hojjat A, et al. Developmental heterogeneity of cardiac fibroblasts does not predict pathological proliferation and activation. Circ Res. 2014;115(7):625–35.
6. Moore-Morris T, Guimaraes-Camboa N, Banerjee I, Zambon AC, Kisseleva T, Velayoudon A, et al. Resident fibroblast lineages mediate pressure overload-induced cardiac fibrosis. J Clin Invest. 2014;124(7):2921–34.
7. Pinto AR, Ilinykh A, Ivey MJ, Kuwabara JT, D'Antoni ML, Debuque R, et al. Revisiting cardiac cellular composition. Circ Res. 2016;118(3):400–9.
8. Ruiz-Villalba A, Simon AM, Pogontke C, Castillo MI, Abizanda G, Pelacho B, et al. Interacting resident epicardium-derived fibroblasts and recruited bone marrow cells form myocardial infarction scar. J Am Coll Cardiol. 2015;65(19):2057–66.
9. Furtado MB, Costa MW, Pranoto EA, Salimova E, Pinto AR, Lam NT, et al. Cardiogenic genes expressed in cardiac fibroblasts contribute to heart development and repair. Circ Res. 2014;114(9):1422–34.
10. Furtado MB, Nim HT, Gould JA, Costa MW, Rosenthal NA, Boyd SE. Microarray profiling to analyse adult cardiac fibroblast identity. Genomics Data. 2014;2:345–50.
11. Ieda M, Fu JD, Delgado-Olguin P, Vedantham V, Hayashi Y, Bruneau BG, et al. Direct reprogramming of fibroblasts into functional cardiomyocytes by defined factors. Cell. 2010;142(3):375–86.
12. Qian L, Huang Y, Spencer CI, Foley A, Vedantham V, Liu L, et al. In vivo reprogramming of murine cardiac fibroblasts into induced cardiomyocytes. Nature. 2012;485(7400):593–8.
13. Song K, Nam YJ, Luo X, Qi X, Tan W, Huang GN, et al. Heart repair by reprogramming non-myocytes with cardiac transcription factors. Nature. 2012;485(7400):599–604.
14. Alavi SH, Kheradvar A. A hybrid tissue-engineered heart valve. Ann Thorac Surg. 2015;99(6):2183–7.
15. Chan V, Neal DM, Uzel SG, Kim H, Bashir R, Asada HH. Fabrication and characterization of optogenetic, multi-strip cardiac muscles. Lab Chip. 2015;15(10):2258–68.
16. Hong H, Dong N, Shi J, Chen S, Guo C, Hu P, et al. Fabrication of a novel hybrid scaffold for tissue engineered heart valve. J Huazhong Univ Sci Technol Med Sci. 2009;29(5):599–603.
17. Noguchi R, Nakayama K, Itoh M, Kamohara K, Furukawa K, Oyama J, et al. Development of a three-dimensional pre-vascularized scaffold-free contractile cardiac patch for treating heart disease. J Heart Lung Transplant. 2016;35(1):137–45.

18. Ieda M, Tsuchihashi T, Ivey KN, Ross RS, Hong TT, Shaw RM, et al. Cardiac fibro-blasts regulate myocardial proliferation through beta1 integrin signaling. Dev Cell. 2009;16(2):233–44.
19. Camelliti P, Borg TK, Kohl P. Structural and functional characterisation of cardiac fibro-blasts. Cardiovasc Res. 2005;65(1):40–51.
20. Kohl P, Camelliti P, Burton FL, Smith GL. Electrical coupling of fibroblasts and myocytes: relevance for cardiac propagation. J Electrocardiol. 2005;38(4 Suppl):45–50.
21. Acharya A, Baek ST, Huang G, Eskiocak B, Goetsch S, Sung CY, et al. The bHLH tran-scription factor Tcf21 is required for lineage-specific EMT of cardiac fibroblast progenitors. Development. 2012;139(12):2139–49.
22. Cai X, Zhang W, Hu J, Zhang L, Sultana N, Wu B, et al. Tbx20 acts upstream of Wnt signal-ing to regulate endocardial cushion formation and valve remodeling during mouse cardiogen-esis. Development. 2013;140(15):3176–87.
23. Moskowitz IP, Wang J, Peterson MA, Pu WT, Mackinnon AC, Oxburgh L, et al. Transcription factor genes Smad4 and Gata4 cooperatively regulate cardiac valve development. [corrected]. Proc Natl Acad Sci U S A. 2011;108(10):4006–11.
24. Takeda N, Manabe I, Uchino Y, Eguchi K, Matsumoto S, Nishimura S, et al. Cardiac fibro-blasts are essential for the adaptive response of the murine heart to pressure overload. J Clin Invest. 2010;120(1):254–65.
25. Van Linthout S, Miteva K, Tschope C. Crosstalk between fibroblasts and inflammatory cells. Cardiovasc Res. 2014;102(2):258–69.
26. Esmon CT. The interactions between inflammation and coagulation. Br J Haematol. 2005;131(4):417–30.
27. Chambers RC. Procoagulant signalling mechanisms in lung inflammation and fibrosis: novel opportunities for pharmacological intervention? Br J Pharmacol. 2008;153(Suppl 1):S367–78.
28. Scotton CJ, Krupiczojc MA, Konigshoff M, Mercer PF, Lee YC, Kaminski N, et al. Increased local expression of coagulation factor X contributes to the fibrotic response in human and murine lung injury. J Clin Invest. 2009;119(9):2550–63.
29. Epelman S, Liu PP, Mann DL. Role of innate and adaptive immune mechanisms in cardiac injury and repair. Nat Rev Immunol. 2015;15(2):117–29.
30. Hartupee J, Mann DL. Role of inflammatory cells in fibroblast activation. J Mol Cell Cardiol. 2015;93:143–8.
31. Rock KL, Latz E, Ontiveros F, Kono H. The sterile inflammatory response. Annu Rev Immunol. 2010;28:321–42.
32. Takeuchi O, Akira S. Pattern recognition receptors and inflammation. Cell. 2010;140(6):805–20.
33. Colucci F, Caligiuri MA, Di Santo JP. What does it take to make a natural killer? Nat Rev Immunol. 2003;3(5):413–25.
34. Ayach BB, Yoshimitsu M, Dawood F, Sun M, Arab S, Chen M, et al. Stem cell factor receptor induces progenitor and natural killer cell-mediated cardiac survival and repair after myocar-dial infarction. Proc Natl Acad Sci U S A. 2006;103(7):2304–9.
35. Ma Y, Yabluchanskiy A, Lindsey ML. Neutrophil roles in left ventricular remodeling follow-ing myocardial infarction. Fibrogenesis Tissue Repair. 2013;6(1):11.
36. Barnes TC, Anderson ME, Edwards SW, Moots RJ. Neutrophil-derived reactive oxygen spe-cies in SSc. Rheumatology (Oxford). 2012;51(7):1166–9.
37. Svegliati-Baroni G, Saccomanno S, van Goor H, Jansen P, Benedetti A, Moshage H. Involvement of reactive oxygen species and nitric oxide radicals in activation and prolif-eration of rat hepatic stellate cells. Liver. 2001;21(1):1–12.
38. Wynn TA. Integrating mechanisms of pulmonary fibrosis. J Exp Med. 2011;208(7):1339–50.
39. Liu XH, Pan LL, Deng HY, Xiong QH, Wu D, Huang GY, et al. Leonurine (SCM-198) attenuates myocardial fibrotic response via inhibition of NADPH oxidase 4. Free Radic Biol Med. 2013;54:93–104.

40. Qin F, Simeone M, Patel R. Inhibition of NADPH oxidase reduces myocardial oxidative stress and apoptosis and improves cardiac function in heart failure after myocardial infarction. Free Radic Biol Med. 2007;43(2):271–81.
41. Cave A, Grieve D, Johar S, Zhang M, Shah AM. NADPH oxidase-derived reactive oxygen species in cardiac pathophysiology. Philos Trans R Soc Lond Ser B Biol Sci. 2005;360(1464):2327–34.
42. Irani K, Xia Y, Zweier JL, Sollott SJ, Der CJ, Fearon ER, et al. Mitogenic signaling mediated by oxidants in Ras-transformed fibroblasts. Science. 1997;275(5306):1649–52.
43. Hagler MA, Hadley TM, Zhang H, Mehra K, Roos CM, Schaff HV, et al. TGF-beta signalling and reactive oxygen species drive fibrosis and matrix remodelling in myxomatous mitral valves. Cardiovasc Res. 2013;99(1):175–84.
44. Bendall JK, Cave AC, Heymes C, Gall N, Shah AM. Pivotal role of a gp91(phox)-containing NADPH oxidase in angiotensin II-induced cardiac hypertrophy in mice. Circulation. 2002;105(3):293–6.
45. Johar D, Roth JC, Bay GH, Walker JN, Kroczak TJ, Los M. Inflammatory response, reactive oxygen species, programmed (necrotic-like and apoptotic) cell death and cancer. Rocz Akad Med Bialymst. 2004;49:31–9.
46. Aceves SS, Ackerman SJ. Relationships between eosinophilic inflammation, tissue remodeling, and fibrosis in eosinophilic esophagitis. Immunol Allergy Clin N Am. 2009;29(1):197–211. xiii–xiv.
47. Seguela PE, Iriart X, Acar P, Montaudon M, Roudaut R, Thambo JB. Eosinophilic cardiac disease: molecular, clinical and imaging aspects. Arch Cardiovasc Dis. 2015;108(4):258–68.
48. Wehling-Henricks M, Sokolow S, Lee JJ, Myung KH, Villalta SA, Tidball JG. Major basic protein-1 promotes fibrosis of dystrophic muscle and attenuates the cellular immune response in muscular dystrophy. Hum Mol Genet. 2008;17(15):2280–92.
49. Jongstra-Bilen J, Haidari M, Zhu SN, Chen M, Guha D, Cybulsky MI. Low-grade chronic inflammation in regions of the normal mouse arterial intima predisposed to atherosclerosis. J Exp Med. 2006;203(9):2073–83.
50. Millonig G, Niederegger H, Rabl W, Hochleitner BW, Hoefer D, Romani N, et al. Network of vascular-associated dendritic cells in intima of healthy young individuals. Arterioscler Thromb Vasc Biol. 2001;21(4):503–8.
51. Dopheide JF, Sester U, Schlitt A, Horstick G, Rupprecht HJ, Munzel T, et al. Monocyte-derived dendritic cells of patients with coronary artery disease show an increased expression of costimulatory molecules CD40, CD80 and CD86 in vitro. Coron Artery Dis. 2007;18(7):523–31.
52. Hart DN, Fabre JW. Demonstration and characterization of Ia-positive dendritic cells in the interstitial connective tissues of rat heart and other tissues, but not brain. J Exp Med. 1981;154(2):347–61.
53. Choi JH, Do Y, Cheong C, Koh H, Boscardin SB, Oh YS, et al. Identification of antigen-presenting dendritic cells in mouse aorta and cardiac valves. J Exp Med. 2009;206(3):497–505.
54. Asadi M, Farokhi F, Delirezh N, Ganji Bakhsh M, Nejati V, Golami K. Fibroblast and T cells conditioned media induce maturation dendritic cell and promote T helper immune response. Vet Res Forum. 2012;3(2):111–8.
55. Kitamura H, Cambier S, Somanath S, Barker T, Minagawa S, Markovics J, et al. Mouse and human lung fibroblasts regulate dendritic cell trafficking, airway inflammation, and fibrosis through integrin alphavbeta8-mediated activation of TGF-beta. J Clin Invest. 2011;121(7):2863–75.
56. Dixon KO, Rossmann L, Kamerling SW, van Kooten C. Human renal fibroblasts generate dendritic cells with a unique regulatory profile. Immunol Cell Biol. 2014;92(8):688–98.
57. Saalbach A, Klein C, Sleeman J, Sack U, Kauer F, Gebhardt C, et al. Dermal fibroblasts induce maturation of dendritic cells. J Immunol. 2007;178(8):4966–74.
58. Newby AC. Metalloproteinase production from macrophages - a perfect storm leading to atherosclerotic plaque rupture and myocardial infarction. Exp Physiol. 2016;101(11):1327–37.

59. Lim DH, Cho JY, Miller M, McElwain K, McElwain S, Broide DH. Reduced peribronchial fibrosis in allergen-challenged MMP-9-deficient mice. Am J Physiol Lung Cell Mol Physiol. 2006;291(2):L265–71.
60. Matsumoto Y, Park IK, Kohyama K. Matrix metalloproteinase (MMP)-9, but not MMP-2, is involved in the development and progression of C protein-induced myocarditis and subsequent dilated cardiomyopathy. J Immunol. 2009;183(7):4773–81.
61. Ducharme A, Frantz S, Aikawa M, Rabkin E, Lindsey M, Rohde LE, et al. Targeted deletion of matrix metalloproteinase-9 attenuates left ventricular enlargement and collagen accumulation after experimental myocardial infarction. J Clin Invest. 2000;106(1):55–62.
62. Munch J, Avanesov M, Bannas P, Saring D, Kramer E, Mearini G, et al. Serum matrix metalloproteinases as quantitative biomarkers for myocardial fibrosis and sudden cardiac death risk stratification in patients with hypertrophic cardiomyopathy. J Card Fail. 2016;22(10):845–50.
63. Westermann D, Savvatis K, Lindner D, Zietsch C, Becher PM, Hammer E, et al. Reduced degradation of the chemokine MCP-3 by matrix metalloproteinase-2 exacerbates myocardial inflammation in experimental viral cardiomyopathy. Circulation. 2011;124(19):2082–93.
64. Murray LA, Chen Q, Kramer MS, Hesson DP, Argentieri RL, Peng X, et al. TGF-beta driven lung fibrosis is macrophage dependent and blocked by serum amyloid P. Int J Biochem Cell Biol. 2011;43(1):154–62.
65. Rockey DC, Bell PD, Hill JA. Fibrosis--a common pathway to organ injury and failure. N Engl J Med. 2015;373(1):96.
66. Mewhort HE, Lipon BD, Svystonyuk DA, Teng G, Guzzardi DG, Silva C, et al. Monocytes increase human cardiac myofibroblast-mediated extracellular matrix remodeling through TGF-beta1. Am J Physiol Heart Circ Physiol. 2016;310(6):H716–24.
67. Bronnum H, Eskildsen T, Andersen DC, Schneider M, Sheikh SP. IL-1beta suppresses TGF-beta-mediated myofibroblast differentiation in cardiac fibroblasts. Growth Factors. 2013;31(3):81–9.
68. Chen SJ, Yuan W, Mori Y, Levenson A, Trojanowska M, Varga J. Stimulation of type I collagen transcription in human skin fibroblasts by TGF-beta: involvement of Smad 3. J Invest Dermatol. 1999;112(1):49–57.
69. Leask A, Abraham DJ. TGF-beta signaling and the fibrotic response. FASEB J. 2004;18(7):816–27.
70. Meyer-Ter-Vehn T, Gebhardt S, Sebald W, Buttmann M, Grehn F, Schlunck G, et al. p38 inhibitors prevent TGF-beta-induced myofibroblast transdifferentiation in human tenon fibroblasts. Invest Ophthalmol Vis Sci. 2006;47(4):1500–9.
71. Overall CM, Wrana JL, Sodek J. Independent regulation of collagenase, 72-kDa progelatinase, and metalloendoproteinase inhibitor expression in human fibroblasts by transforming growth factor-beta. J Biol Chem. 1989;264(3):1860–9.
72. Varga J, Jimenez SA. Stimulation of normal human fibroblast collagen production and processing by transforming growth factor-beta. Biochem Biophys Res Commun. 1986;138(2):974–80.
73. Verrecchia F, Mauviel A. Transforming growth factor-beta and fibrosis. World J Gastroenterol. 2007;13(22):3056–62.
74. Kuwahara F, Kai H, Tokuda K, Kai M, Takeshita A, Egashira K, et al. Transforming growth factor-beta function blocking prevents myocardial fibrosis and diastolic dysfunction in pressure-overloaded rats. Circulation. 2002;106(1):130–5.
75. Okada H, Takemura G, Kosai K, Li Y, Takahashi T, Esaki M, et al. Postinfarction gene therapy against transforming growth factor-beta signal modulates infarct tissue dynamics and attenuates left ventricular remodeling and heart failure. Circulation. 2005;111(19):2430–7.
76. Kulkarni AB, Karlsson S. Transforming growth factor-beta 1 knockout mice. A mutation in one cytokine gene causes a dramatic inflammatory disease. Am J Pathol. 1993;143(1):3–9.
77. Ikeuchi M, Tsutsui H, Shiomi T, Matsusaka H, Matsushima S, Wen J, et al. Inhibition of TGF-beta signaling exacerbates early cardiac dysfunction but prevents late remodeling after infarction. Cardiovasc Res. 2004;64(3):526–35.

78. Hatamochi A, Mori K, Ueki H. Role of cytokines in controlling connective tissue gene expression. Arch Dermatol Res. 1994;287(1):115–21.
79. Sullivan DE, Ferris M, Nguyen H, Abboud E, Brody AR. TNF-alpha induces TGF-beta1 expression in lung fibroblasts at the transcriptional level via AP-1 activation. J Cell Mol Med. 2009;13(8B):1866–76.
80. Hamid T, Gu Y, Ortines RV, Bhattacharya C, Wang G, Xuan YT, et al. Divergent tumor necrosis factor receptor-related remodeling responses in heart failure: role of nuclear factor-kappaB and inflammatory activation. Circulation. 2009;119(10):1386–97.
81. Duerrschmid C, Crawford JR, Reineke E, Taffet GE, Trial J, Entman ML, et al. TNF receptor 1 signaling is critically involved in mediating angiotensin-II-induced cardiac fibrosis. J Mol Cell Cardiol. 2013;57:59–67.
82. Levick SP, Melendez GC, Plante E, McLarty JL, Brower GL, Janicki JS. Cardiac mast cells: the centrepiece in adverse myocardial remodelling. Cardiovasc Res. 2011;89(1):12–9.
83. Kinet JP. The essential role of mast cells in orchestrating inflammation. Immunol Rev. 2007;217:5–7.
84. Kim J, Ogai A, Nakatani S, Hashimura K, Kanzaki H, Komamura K, et al. Impact of blockade of histamine H2 receptors on chronic heart failure revealed by retrospective and prospective randomized studies. J Am Coll Cardiol. 2006;48(7):1378–84.
85. Asanuma H, Minamino T, Ogai A, Kim J, Asakura M, Komamura K, et al. Blockade of histamine H2 receptors protects the heart against ischemia and reperfusion injury in dogs. J Mol Cell Cardiol. 2006;40(5):666–74.
86. Brower GL, Chancey AL, Thanigaraj S, Matsubara BB, Janicki JS. Cause and effect relationship between myocardial mast cell number and matrix metalloproteinase activity. Am J Physiol Heart Circ Physiol. 2002;283(2):H518–25.
87. Brower GL, Janicki JS. Pharmacologic inhibition of mast cell degranulation prevents left ventricular remodeling induced by chronic volume overload in rats. J Card Fail. 2005;11(7):548–56.
88. Levick SP, Gardner JD, Holland M, Hauer-Jensen M, Janicki JS, Brower GL. Protection from adverse myocardial remodeling secondary to chronic volume overload in mast cell deficient rats. J Mol Cell Cardiol. 2008;45(1):56–61.
89. Frangogiannis NG, Lindsey ML, Michael LH, Youker KA, Bressler RB, Mendoza LH, et al. Resident cardiac mast cells degranulate and release preformed TNF-alpha, initiating the cytokine cascade in experimental canine myocardial ischemia/reperfusion. Circulation. 1998;98(7):699–710.
90. Seguin CA, Pilliar RM, Madri JA, Kandel RA. TNF-alpha induces MMP2 gelatinase activity and MT1-MMP expression in an in vitro model of nucleus pulposus tissue degeneration. Spine (Phila Pa 1976). 2008;33(4):356–65.
91. Gilles S, Zahler S, Welsch U, Sommerhoff CP, Becker BF. Release of TNF-alpha during myocardial reperfusion depends on oxidative stress and is prevented by mast cell stabilizers. Cardiovasc Res. 2003;60(3):608–16.
92. Bhattacharya K, Farwell K, Huang M, Kempuraj D, Donelan J, Papaliodis D, et al. Mast cell deficient W/Wv mice have lower serum IL-6 and less cardiac tissue necrosis than their normal littermates following myocardial ischemia-reperfusion. Int J Immunopathol Pharmacol. 2007;20(1):69–74.
93. Cimini M, Fazel S, Zhuo S, Xaymardan M, Fujii H, Weisel RD, et al. c-kit dysfunction impairs myocardial healing after infarction. Circulation. 2007;116(11 Suppl):I77–82.
94. Hara M, Ono K, Hwang MW, Iwasaki A, Okada M, Nakatani K, et al. Evidence for a role of mast cells in the evolution to congestive heart failure. J Exp Med. 2002;195(3):375–81.
95. Levick SP, McLarty JL, Murray DB, Freeman RM, Carver WE, Brower GL. Cardiac mast cells mediate left ventricular fibrosis in the hypertensive rat heart. Hypertension. 2009;53(6):1041–7.
96. Gailit J, Marchese MJ, Kew RR, Gruber BL. The differentiation and function of myofibroblasts is regulated by mast cell mediators. J Invest Dermatol. 2001;117(5):1113–9.

97. Skrabal CA, Thompson LO, Southard RE, Joyce DL, Noon GP, Loebe M, et al. Interaction between isolated human myocardial mast cells and cultured fibroblasts. J Surg Res. 2004;118(1):66–70.

98. Boerma M, Fiser WP, Hoyt G, Berry GJ, Joseph L, Joseph J, et al. Influence of mast cells on outcome after heterotopic cardiac transplantation in rats. Transpl Int. 2007;20(3):256–65.

99. Genovese A, Rossi FW, Spadaro G, Galdiero MR, Marone G. Human cardiac mast cells in anaphylaxis. Chem Immunol Allergy. 2010;95:98–109.

100. Li QY, Raza-Ahmad A, MacAulay MA, Lalonde LD, Rowden G, Trethewey E, et al. The relationship of mast cells and their secreted products to the volume of fibrosis in posttransplant hearts. Transplantation. 1992;53(5):1047–51.

101. Zweifel M, Hirsiger H, Matozan K, Welle M, Schaffner T, Mohacsi P. Mast cells in ongoing acute rejection: increase in number and expression of a different phenotype in rat heart transplants. Transplantation. 2002;73(11):1707–16.

102. Koskinen PK, Kovanen PT, Lindstedt KA, Lemstrom KB. Mast cells in acute and chronic rejection of rat cardiac allografts--a major source of basic fibroblast growth factor. Transplantation. 2001;71(12):1741–7.

103. McLarren KW, Cole AE, Weisser SB, Voglmaier NS, Conlin VS, Jacobson K, et al. SHIP-deficient mice develop spontaneous intestinal inflammation and arginase-dependent fibrosis. Am J Pathol. 2011;179(1):180–8.

104. Monroe JG, Rothenberg EV, editors. Molecular biology of B-cell and T-cell development. New York: Springer Science and Business Media, LLC; 1998.

105. Yoshizaki A, Yanaba K, Iwata Y, Komura K, Ogawa A, Akiyama Y, et al. Cell adhesion molecules regulate fibrotic process via Th1/Th2/Th17 cell balance in a bleomycin-induced scleroderma model. J Immunol. 2010;185(4):2502–15.

106. Gurujeyalakshmi G, Giri SN. Molecular mechanisms of antifibrotic effect of interferon gamma in bleomycin-mouse model of lung fibrosis: downregulation of TGF-beta and procollagen I and III gene expression. Exp Lung Res. 1995;21(5):791–808.

107. Oldroyd SD, Thomas GL, Gabbiani G, El Nahas AM. Interferon-gamma inhibits experimental renal fibrosis. Kidney Int. 1999;56(6):2116–27.

108. Borthwick LA, Barron L, Hart KM, Vannella KM, Thompson RW, Oland S, et al. Macrophages are critical to the maintenance of IL-13-dependent lung inflammation and fibrosis. Mucosal Immunol. 2016;9(1):38–55.

109. Borthwick LA, Wynn TA, Fisher AJ. Cytokine mediated tissue fibrosis. Biochim Biophys Acta. 2013;1832(7):1049–60.

110. Chiaramonte MG, Donaldson DD, Cheever AW, Wynn TA. An IL-13 inhibitor blocks the development of hepatic fibrosis during a T-helper type 2-dominated inflammatory response. J Clin Invest. 1999;104(6):777–85.

111. Wilson MS, Wynn TA. Pulmonary fibrosis: pathogenesis, etiology and regulation. Mucosal Immunol. 2009;2(2):103–21.

112. Jimenez SA, Freundlich B, Rosenbloom J. Selective inhibition of human diploid fibroblast collagen synthesis by interferons. J Clin Invest. 1984;74(3):1112–6.

113. Fairweather D, Frisancho-Kiss S, Yusung SA, Barrett MA, Davis SE, Gatewood SJ, et al. Interferon-gamma protects against chronic viral myocarditis by reducing mast cell degranulation, fibrosis, and the profibrotic cytokines transforming growth factor-beta 1, interleukin-1 beta, and interleukin-4 in the heart. Am J Pathol. 2004;165(6):1883–94.

114. Nathan CF, Prendergast TJ, Wiebe ME, Stanley ER, Platzer E, Remold HG, et al. Activation of human macrophages. Comparison of other cytokines with interferon-gamma. J Exp Med. 1984;160(2):600–5.

115. Piguet PF, Collart MA, Grau GE, Kapanci Y, Vassalli P. Tumor necrosis factor/cachectin plays a key role in bleomycin-induced pneumopathy and fibrosis. J Exp Med. 1989;170(3):655–63.

116. Han YL, Li YL, Jia LX, Cheng JZ, Qi YF, Zhang HJ, et al. Reciprocal interaction between macrophages and T cells stimulates IFN-gamma and MCP-1 production in Ang II-induced cardiac inflammation and fibrosis. PLoS One. 2012;7(5):e35506.

117. Wynn TA. Fibrotic disease and the T(H)1/T(H)2 paradigm. Nat Rev Immunol. 2004;4(8):583–94.
118. Chen ES, Greenlee BM, Wills-Karp M, Moller DR. Attenuation of lung inflammation and fibrosis in interferon-gamma-deficient mice after intratracheal bleomycin. Am J Respir Cell Mol Biol. 2001;24(5):545–55.
119. Marko L, Kvakan H, Park JK, Qadri F, Spallek B, Binger KJ, et al. Interferon-gamma signaling inhibition ameliorates angiotensin II-induced cardiac damage. Hypertension. 2012;60(6):1430–6.
120. Sandler NG, Mentink-Kane MM, Cheever AW, Wynn TA. Global gene expression profiles during acute pathogen-induced pulmonary inflammation reveal divergent roles for Th1 and Th2 responses in tissue repair. J Immunol. 2003;171(7):3655–67.
121. Yu Q, Horak K, Larson DF. Role of T lymphocytes in hypertension-induced cardiac extracellular matrix remodeling. Hypertension. 2006;48(1):98–104.
122. Fichtner-Feigl S, Strober W, Kawakami K, Puri RK, Kitani A. IL-13 signaling through the IL-13alpha2 receptor is involved in induction of TGF-beta1 production and fibrosis. Nat Med. 2006;12(1):99–106.
123. Mosser DM, Edwards JP. Exploring the full spectrum of macrophage activation. Nat Rev Immunol. 2008;8(12):958–69.
124. Fallon PG, Richardson EJ, McKenzie GJ, McKenzie AN. Schistosome infection of transgenic mice defines distinct and contrasting pathogenic roles for IL-4 and IL-13: IL-13 is a profibrotic agent. J Immunol. 2000;164(5):2585–91.
125. Yang G, Volk A, Petley T, Emmell E, Giles-Komar J, Shang X, et al. Anti-IL-13 monoclonal antibody inhibits airway hyperresponsiveness, inflammation and airway remodeling. Cytokine. 2004;28(6):224–32.
126. Hashimoto S, Gon Y, Takeshita I, Maruoka S, Horie T. IL-4 and IL-13 induce myofibroblastic phenotype of human lung fibroblasts through c-Jun NH2-terminal kinase-dependent pathway. J Allergy Clin Immunol. 2001;107(6):1001–8.
127. Bailey JR, Bland PW, Tarlton JF, Peters I, Moorghen M, Sylvester PA, et al. IL-13 promotes collagen accumulation in Crohn's disease fibrosis by down-regulation of fibroblast MMP synthesis: a role for innate lymphoid cells? PLoS One. 2012;7(12):e52332.
128. Mentink-Kane MM, Wynn TA. Opposing roles for IL-13 and IL-13 receptor alpha 2 in health and disease. Immunol Rev. 2004;202:191–202.
129. Brunner SM, Schiechl G, Kesselring R, Martin M, Balam S, Schlitt HJ, et al. IL-13 signaling via IL-13Ralpha2 triggers TGF-beta1-dependent allograft fibrosis. Transplant Res. 2013;2(1):16.
130. Karo-Atar D, Bordowitz A, Wand O, Pasmanik-Chor M, Fernandez IE, Itan M, et al. A protective role for IL-13 receptor alpha 1 in bleomycin-induced pulmonary injury and repair. Mucosal Immunol. 2016;9(1):240–53.
131. Feng W, Li W, Liu W, Wang F, Li Y, Yan W. IL-17 induces myocardial fibrosis and enhances RANKL/OPG and MMP/TIMP signaling in isoproterenol-induced heart failure. Exp Mol Pathol. 2009;87(3):212–8.
132. Wang L, Chen S, Xu K. IL-17 expression is correlated with hepatitis B-related liver diseases and fibrosis. Int J Mol Med. 2011;27(3):385–92.
133. Wilson MS, Madala SK, Ramalingam TR, Gochuico BR, Rosas IO, Cheever AW, et al. Bleomycin and IL-1beta-mediated pulmonary fibrosis is IL-17A dependent. J Exp Med. 2010;207(3):535–52.
134. Ouyang W, Kolls JK, Zheng Y. The biological functions of T helper 17 cell effector cytokines in inflammation. Immunity. 2008;28(4):454–67.
135. Liu Y, Zhu H, Su Z, Sun C, Yin J, Yuan H, et al. IL-17 contributes to cardiac fibrosis following experimental autoimmune myocarditis by a PKCbeta/Erk1/2/NF-kappaB-dependent signaling pathway. Int Immunol. 2012;24(10):605–12.
136. Yamashita T, Iwakura T, Matsui K, Kawaguchi H, Obana M, Hayama A, et al. IL-6-mediated Th17 differentiation through RORgammat is essential for the initiation of experimental autoimmune myocarditis. Cardiovasc Res. 2011;91(4):640–8.

137. Hofmann U, Beyersdorf N, Weirather J, Podolskaya A, Bauersachs J, Ertl G, et al. Activation of CD4+ T lymphocytes improves wound healing and survival after experimental myocardial infarction in mice. Circulation. 2012;125(13):1652–63.
138. Yamashita T, Obana M, Hayama A, Iwakura T, Komuro I, Nakayama H, et al. Th17 cells exhibit protective effects against cardiac fibrosis after myocardial infarction. Circulation. 2011;124(Suppl 21):A14566. Core 5.
139. Liu F, Liu J, Weng D, Chen Y, Song L, He Q, et al. CD4+CD25+Foxp3+ regulatory T cells depletion may attenuate the development of silica-induced lung fibrosis in mice. PLoS One. 2010;5(11):e15404.
140. Kanellakis P, Dinh TN, Agrotis A, Bobik A. CD4(+)CD25(+)Foxp3(+) regulatory T cells suppress cardiac fibrosis in the hypertensive heart. J Hypertens. 2011;29(9):1820–8.
141. Cao Y, Xu W, Xiong S. Adoptive transfer of regulatory T cells protects against Coxsackievirus B3-induced cardiac fibrosis. PLoS One. 2013;8(9):e74955.
142. Zimmermann O, Homann JM, Bangert A, Muller AM, Hristov G, Goeser S, et al. Successful use of mRNA-nucleofection for overexpression of interleukin-10 in murine monocytes/macrophages for anti-inflammatory therapy in a murine model of autoimmune myocarditis. J Am Heart Assoc. 2012;1(6):e003293.
143. Saxena A, Dobaczewski M, Rai V, Haque Z, Chen W, Li N, et al. Regulatory T cells are recruited in the infarcted mouse myocardium and may modulate fibroblast phenotype and function. Am J Physiol Heart Circ Physiol. 2014;307(8):H1233–42.
144. Weirather J, Hofmann UD, Beyersdorf N, Ramos GC, Vogel B, Frey A, et al. Foxp3+ CD4+ T cells improve healing after myocardial infarction by modulating monocyte/macrophage differentiation. Circ Res. 2014;115(1):55–67.
145. Matsumoto K, Ogawa M, Suzuki J, Hirata Y, Nagai R, Isobe M. Regulatory T lymphocytes attenuate myocardial infarction-induced ventricular remodeling in mice. Int Heart J. 2011;52(6):382–7.
146. Sharir R, Semo J, Shimoni S, Ben-Mordechai T, Landa-Rouben N, Maysel-Auslender S, et al. Experimental myocardial infarction induces altered regulatory T cell hemostasis, and adoptive transfer attenuates subsequent remodeling. PLoS One. 2014;9(12):e113653.
147. Skorska A, von Haehling S, Ludwig M, Lux CA, Gaebel R, Kleiner G, et al. The CD4(+) AT2R(+) T cell subpopulation improves post-infarction remodelling and restores cardiac function. J Cell Mol Med. 2015;19(8):1975–85.
148. Tang TT, Yuan J, Zhu ZF, Zhang WC, Xiao H, Xia N, et al. Regulatory T cells ameliorate cardiac remodeling after myocardial infarction. Basic Res Cardiol. 2012;107(1):232.
149. Wang YP, Xie Y, Ma H, Su SA, Wang YD, Wang JA, et al. Regulatory T lymphocytes in myocardial infarction: a promising new therapeutic target. Int J Cardiol. 2016;203:923–8.
150. Chen WC, Lee BG, Park DW, Kim K, Chu H, Kim K, et al. Controlled dual delivery of fibroblast growth factor-2 and interleukin-10 by heparin-based coacervate synergistically enhances ischemic heart repair. Biomaterials. 2015;72:138–51.
151. Verma SK, Krishnamurthy P, Barefield D, Singh N, Gupta R, Lambers E, et al. Interleukin-10 treatment attenuates pressure overload-induced hypertrophic remodeling and improves heart function via signal transducers and activators of transcription 3-dependent inhibition of nuclear factor-kappaB. Circulation. 2012;126(4):418–29.
152. Kesherwani V, Chavali V, Hackfort BT, Tyagi SC, Mishra PK. Exercise ameliorates high fat diet induced cardiac dysfunction by increasing interleukin 10. Front Physiol. 2015;6:124.
153. Franz M, Doll F, Grun K, Richter P, Kose N, Ziffels B, et al. Targeted delivery of interleukin-10 to chronic cardiac allograft rejection using a human antibody specific to the extra domain a of fibronectin. Int J Cardiol. 2015;195:311–22.
154. Holt AP, Stamataki Z, Adams DH. Attenuated liver fibrosis in the absence of B cells. Hepatology. 2006;43(4):868–71.
155. Novobrantseva TI, Majeau GR, Amatucci A, Kogan S, Brenner I, Casola S, et al. Attenuated liver fibrosis in the absence of B cells. J Clin Invest. 2005;115(11):3072–82.

156. Zhou X, Tan FK, Milewicz DM, Guo X, Bona CA, Arnett FC. Autoantibodies to fibrillin-1 activate normal human fibroblasts in culture through the TGF-beta pathway to recapitulate the "scleroderma phenotype". J Immunol. 2005;175(7):4555–60.

157. Francois A, Chatelus E, Wachsmann D, Sibilia J, Bahram S, Alsaleh G, et al. B lymphocytes and B-cell activating factor promote collagen and profibrotic markers expression by dermal fibroblasts in systemic sclerosis. Arthritis Res Ther. 2013;15(5):R168.

158. Frank R, Dean SA, Molina MR, Kamoun M, Lal P. Correlations of lymphocyte subset infiltrates with donor-specific antibodies and acute antibody-mediated rejection in endomyocardial biopsies. Cardiovasc Pathol. 2015;24(3):168–72.

159. Russell PS, Chase CM, Colvin RB. Alloantibody- and T cell-mediated immunity in the pathogenesis of transplant arteriosclerosis: lack of progression to sclerotic lesions in B cell-deficient mice. Transplantation. 1997;64(11):1531–6.

160. Zeng Q, Ng YH, Singh T, Jiang K, Sheriff KA, Ippolito R, et al. B cells mediate chronic allograft rejection independently of antibody production. J Clin Invest. 2014;124(3):1052–6.

161. Serreze DV, Silveira PA. The role of B lymphocytes as key antigen-presenting cells in the development of T cell-mediated autoimmune type 1 diabetes. Curr Dir Autoimmun. 2003;6:212–27.

162. Krebs P, Kurrer MO, Kremer M, De Giuli R, Sonderegger I, Henke A, et al. Molecular mapping of autoimmune B cell responses in experimental myocarditis. J Autoimmun. 2007;28(4):224–33.

163. Liu PP, Mason JW. Advances in the understanding of myocarditis. Circulation. 2001;104(9):1076–82.

164. Matsumoto Y, Park IK, Kohyama K. B-cell epitope spreading is a critical step for the switch from C-protein-induced myocarditis to dilated cardiomyopathy. Am J Pathol. 2007;170(1):43–51.

165. Yu M, Wen S, Wang M, Liang W, Li HH, Long Q, et al. TNF-alpha-secreting B cells contribute to myocardial fibrosis in dilated cardiomyopathy. J Clin Immunol. 2013;33(5):1002–8.

166. Zouggari Y, Ait-Oufella H, Bonnin P, Simon T, Sage AP, Guerin C, et al. B lymphocytes trigger monocyte mobilization and impair heart function after acute myocardial infarction. Nat Med. 2013;19(10):1273–80.

167. Pinto AR, Paolicelli R, Salimova E, Gospocic J, Slonimsky E, Bilbao-Cortes D, et al. An abundant tissue macrophage population in the adult murine heart with a distinct alternatively-activated macrophage profile. PLoS One. 2012;7(5):e36814.

168. Nash GB, Buckley CD, Ed Rainger G. The local physicochemical environment conditions the proinflammatory response of endothelial cells and thus modulates leukocyte recruitment. FEBS Lett. 2004;569(1–3):13–7.

169. Tieu BC, Lee C, Sun H, Lejeune W, Recinos A 3rd, Ju X, et al. An adventitial IL-6/MCP1 amplification loop accelerates macrophage-mediated vascular inflammation leading to aortic dissection in mice. J Clin Invest. 2009;119(12):3637–51.

170. Turner NA. Inflammatory and fibrotic responses of cardiac fibroblasts to myocardial damage associated molecular patterns (DAMPs). J Mol Cell Cardiol. 2016;94:189–200.

171. Lugrin J, Parapanov R, Rosenblatt-Velin N, Rignault-Clerc S, Feihl F, Waeber B, et al. Cutting edge: IL-1alpha is a crucial danger signal triggering acute myocardial inflammation during myocardial infarction. J Immunol. 2015;194(2):499–503.

172. Rohde D, Schon C, Boerries M, Didrihsone I, Ritterhoff J, Kubatzky KF, et al. S100A1 is released from ischemic cardiomyocytes and signals myocardial damage via toll-like receptor 4. EMBO Mol Med. 2014;6(6):778–94.

173. Zhang W, Lavine K, Epelman S, Evans S, Weinheimer C, Barger P, et al. Necrotic myocardial cells release damage-associated molecular patterns that provoke fibroblast activation in vitro and trigger myocardial inflammation and fibrosis in vivo. J Am Heart Assoc. 2015;4(6):e001993.

174. Arslan F, de Kleijn DP, Pasterkamp G. Innate immune signaling in cardiac ischemia. Nat Rev Cardiol. 2011;8(5):292–300.
175. Frangogiannis NG. The immune system and cardiac repair. Pharmacol Res. 2008;58(2):88–111.
176. Middleton J, Patterson AM, Gardner L, Schmutz C, Ashton BA. Leukocyte extravasation: chemokine transport and presentation by the endothelium. Blood. 2002;100(12):3853–60.
177. McGettrick HM, Smith E, Filer A, Kissane S, Salmon M, Buckley CD, et al. Fibroblasts from different sites may promote or inhibit recruitment of flowing lymphocytes by endothelial cells. Eur J Immunol. 2009;39(1):113–25.
178. Weih F, Carrasco D, Durham SK, Barton DS, Rizzo CA, Ryseck RP, et al. Multiorgan inflammation and hematopoietic abnormalities in mice with a targeted disruption of RelB, a member of the NF-kappa B/Rel family. Cell. 1995;80(2):331–40.
179. Zickus C, Kunkel SL, Simpson K, Evanoff H, Glass M, Strieter RM, et al. Differential regulation of C-C chemokines during fibroblast-monocyte interactions: adhesion vs. inflammatory cytokine pathways. Mediat Inflamm. 1998;7(4):269–74.
180. Steinhauser ML, Kunkel SL, Hogaboam CM, Evanoff H, Strieter RM, Lukacs NW. Macrophage/fibroblast coculture induces macrophage inflammatory protein-1alpha production mediated by intercellular adhesion molecule-1 and oxygen radicals. J Leukoc Biol. 1998;64(5):636–41.
181. Hogaboam CM, Steinhauser ML, Chensue SW, Kunkel SL. Novel roles for chemokines and fibroblasts in interstitial fibrosis. Kidney Int. 1998;54(6):2152–9.
182. Gharaee-Kermani M, Denholm EM, Phan SH. Costimulation of fibroblast collagen and transforming growth factor beta1 gene expression by monocyte chemoattractant protein-1 via specific receptors. J Biol Chem. 1996;271(30):17779–84.
183. Yamamoto T, Eckes B, Mauch C, Hartmann K, Krieg T. Monocyte chemoattractant protein-1 enhances gene expression and synthesis of matrix metalloproteinase-1 in human fibroblasts by an autocrine IL-1 alpha loop. J Immunol. 2000;164(12):6174–9.
184. Morimoto H, Takahashi M, Izawa A, Ise H, Hongo M, Kolattukudy PE, et al. Cardiac overexpression of monocyte chemoattractant protein-1 in transgenic mice prevents cardiac dysfunction and remodeling after myocardial infarction. Circ Res. 2006;99(8):891–9.
185. Dewald O, Zymek P, Winkelmann K, Koerting A, Ren G, Abou-Khamis T, et al. CCL2/monocyte chemoattractant protein-1 regulates inflammatory responses critical to healing myocardial infarcts. Circ Res. 2005;96(8):881–9.
186. Lee SK, Seo SH, Kim BS, Kim CD, Lee JH, Kang JS, et al. IFN-gamma regulates the expression of B7-H1 in dermal fibroblast cells. J Dermatol Sci. 2005;40(2):95–103.
187. Smith RS, Smith TJ, Blieden TM, Phipps RP. Fibroblasts as sentinel cells. Synthesis of chemokines and regulation of inflammation. Am J Pathol. 1997;151(2):317–22.
188. Yellin MJ, Winikoff S, Fortune SM, Baum D, Crow MK, Lederman S, et al. Ligation of CD40 on fibroblasts induces CD54 (ICAM-1) and CD106 (VCAM-1) up-regulation and IL-6 production and proliferation. J Leukoc Biol. 1995;58(2):209–16.
189. Buckley CD, Amft N, Bradfield PF, Pilling D, Ross E, Arenzana-Seisdedos F, et al. Persistent induction of the chemokine receptor CXCR4 by TGF-beta 1 on synovial T cells contributes to their accumulation within the rheumatoid synovium. J Immunol. 2000;165(6):3423–9.
190. Li M, Riddle SR, Frid MG, El Kasmi KC, McKinsey TA, Sokol RJ, et al. Emergence of fibroblasts with a proinflammatory epigenetically altered phenotype in severe hypoxic pulmonary hypertension. J Immunol. 2011;187(5):2711–22.
191. Abendroth A, Slobedman B, Lee E, Mellins E, Wallace M, Arvin AM. Modulation of major histocompatibility class II protein expression by varicella-zoster virus. J Virol. 2000;74(4):1900–7.
192. Scott S, Pandolfi F, Kurnick JT. Fibroblasts mediate T cell survival: a proposed mechanism for retention of primed T cells. J Exp Med. 1990;172(6):1873–6.
193. Zuliani T, Saiagh S, Knol AC, Esbelin J, Dreno B. Fetal fibroblasts and keratinocytes with immunosuppressive properties for allogeneic cell-based wound therapy. PLoS One. 2013;8(7):e70408.

194. Boots AM, Wimmers-Bertens AJ, Rijnders AW. Antigen-presenting capacity of rheumatoid synovial fibroblasts. Immunology. 1994;82(2):268–74.
195. Pilling D, Akbar AN, Girdlestone J, Orteu CH, Borthwick NJ, Amft N, et al. Interferon-beta mediates stromal cell rescue of T cells from apoptosis. Eur J Immunol. 1999;29(3):1041–50.
196. Cowie MR, Anker SD, Felker GM, Filippatos G, Jaarsma T, Jourdain P, et al. Improving care for patients with acute heart failure: before, during and after hospitalization. ESC Heart Fail. 2014;1:110–45.

Chapter 4
Endothelial Cells

Caterina Sturtzel

4.1 Introduction

The commonly accepted roles of endothelial cells (EC) in homeostasis of body physiology are to safeguard transport logistics, control vascular permeability, and regulate vascular tone. In the immunology of cardiovascular homeostasis and pathology, EC can be regarded from two perspectives: on the one hand, they are a constitutive and integral part of the cardiovascular system and therefore intrinsically causing disease if dysfunctional, and on the other hand, they actively mediate immune responses at places of injury or infection [1].

Cobblestone shape is a main histological characteristic of EC, but they constitute more than static mechano-protective plates. EC that line the inner vessel wall are not at all inert bystander cells but central and active parts of two major systems in the body—the immune and the vascular system. As a consequence, damage, (hyper) activation, and dysfunction of EC are frequently part of the etiology of cardiovascular diseases. These two systems often act in concert, for example, during wound healing, but there are also conditions where EC engage in distinctive roles in each of them, such as during development and tissue regeneration.

The vascular system is composed of EC lining the inside of vessels and of smooth muscle cells or pericytes supporting the vessel structure. Strongly adapted to the various tissues, the lymphatic and the blood vessel system pervade the entire body. Lymphatic vessels are blind-ended tubes equipped with valves to fulfill efficiently their major task of collecting and draining interstitial fluid leaking out of blood vessels. Thereby, they are also a transport route for nutrients or mobile cells, such as white blood cells, again interlinking function with the immune system [2]. Blood vessels

C. Sturtzel, PhD
Innovative Cancer Models, Children's Cancer Research Institute,
St. Anna Kinderkrebsforschung e.V, Vienna, Austria
e-mail: caterina.sturtzel@ccri.at

© Springer International Publishing AG 2017   71
S. Sattler, T. Kennedy-Lydon (eds.), *The Immunology of Cardiovascular*
Homeostasis and Pathology, Advances in Experimental Medicine and Biology 1003,
DOI 10.1007/978-3-319-57613-8_4

exist as capillaries, veins, or arteries, covered by supporting cells, and their major tasks are the transport of oxygen as well as nutrients and immune cells to the various tissues of the body [3]. Therefore, genesis of the lymphatic system in the developing embryo is triggered by rising fluid pressure, whereas blood vessel vasculogenesis and angiogenesis are driven by hypoxia [4, 5]. During embryonic development, the first vascular plexus is established by coalescing hemangioblasts from which eventually vessels are built by sprouting of EC, the process defined as angiogenesis [3, 6].

EC isolated from different tissues will exhibit organ-specific adaptations and adjustments in shape and function. For example, EC of the central nervous system form the blood-brain barrier, uterine EC express estrogen receptors, EC of the high endothelial venules allow for transcellular routes for leukocyte extravasation during homing, EC of the endocardium fold up and adapt to the constant heartbeat, and EC committed for either arterial or venous vessels show different sprouting capacities [7–10].

As active part of the immune system, EC not only function as a transport device for mobile immune cells and form a mechanical barrier against intruders, but they also (1) have essential paracrine function by secreting chemokines, interleukins, interferons, and growth factors; (2) organize recruitment of immune cells and regulate leukocyte extravasation at places of inflammation by inducible expression of adhesion molecules like E-selectin, P-selectin, ICAM, or VCAM [11]; as well as (3) maintain appropriate hemostasis or coagulation.

The classical four signs of inflammation described by Celsus (30 BC–38 AD), dolor (pain), calor (heat), rubor (reddishness), and tumor (swelling), already illustrated the significant role of EC during inflammation, since these reactions are all mediated by EC through local changes of vessel barrier function. Although EC are not immune cells in the classical sense, as they cannot kill, phagocytose, and produce antibodies or similar, they essentially coordinate the immune response.

4.2 Classical Functions of Endothelial Cells and Their Immunological Relevance

4.2.1 Hemostasis

To maintain barrier function and to prevent intrusion of pathogens and their quick systemic spread, junctions need to be kept tight and repaired quickly after vessels rupture. During tissue trauma vessels are often damaged, and, in cooperation with platelets, the endothelium initiates processes aiming to stop bleeding and close holes. Coagulation results in the formation of solid blood clots to plug the opening in the vessel. Thereby, hemostasis, the cessation of bleeding, is reached (Fig. 4.1). However, as crucial as this activity of the endothelium and the platelets is in the correct situation, as dangerous can it be when activated aberrantly, for example, during disseminated coagulation, which carries a high risk for fatal outcomes [12]. When clots are formed uncontrollably, they can occlude vessels, especially narrowing capillaries, and reach the state of thrombosis. Therefore, the endothelium in its basal state is anticoagulant.

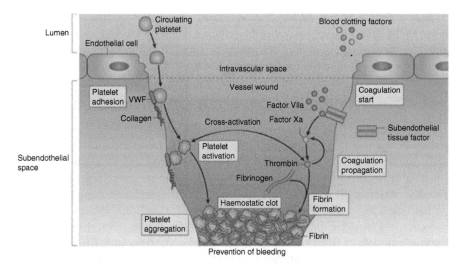

Fig. 4.1 Hemostasis involves two principle components: platelets and the coagulation system with its major product, fibrin. Both systems act in concert to generate a hemostatic clot that seals the wound. The efficient recruitment of platelets involves specific surface receptors, such as the platelet glycoprotein Ib (GPIb)-GPV-GPIX complex, GPVI, and several integrins (not shown). These platelet receptors recognize distinct ligands that are normally concealed by the endothelial barrier and become exposed only after vessel damage. These ligands include von Willebrand factor (VWF) and collagens, as well as fibrinogen, vitronectin, and fibronectin (not shown). Platelet recruitment does not induce hemostasis unless fibrin is also formed by the coagulation system. Coagulation requires the sequential activation of blood-based serine proteases and their cofactors (collectively known as blood clotting factors). The process is initiated by tissue factor, which is expressed by subendothelial cells and is therefore hidden in the intact vessel wall. In response to injury, however, tissue factor is exposed to blood and can interact with blood-based factor VIIa to trigger the coagulation cascade, which culminates in the formation of fibrin (Modified from [12])

To control and balance the homeostasis of hemostasis, the activation of coagulation is tightly regulated and depends on a full cascade of progressive protease activities on proenzymes [13]. Activation of the coagulation cascade culminates in the formation of fibrin from fibrinogen. Polymerized and cross-linked fibrinogen becomes a sticky substance providing a mesh on activated platelets, which supports formation of a clot. These thrombi can be degraded again by proteases, especially plasmin, when healing progresses [12–14].

During hemostasis, the endothelium provides a crucial base whereupon activities are organized and regulated. Procoagulant molecules, including von Willebrand factor (vWF) and tissue factor (TF), are expressed in subendothelial areas on collagen and fibroblasts and become exposed to blood upon injury of the vessel wall. There, platelet aggregation is induced by receptor binding of vWF, and TF binds circulating coagulation factor VII, which initiates the proteolytic coagulation cascade. The proteolysis of coagulation factor VII (fVII) generates fVIIa, which further supports cleavage of fX into fXa and forces thrombin generation from prothrombin. Other circulating factors including factor V, VIII, and IX contribute as cofactors to enhanced thrombin formation. Ultimately, thrombin releases fibrin from fibrinogen, which further strengthens clot formation of the platelets.

Weibel-Palade bodies (WPB) are preformed endothelial-specific first-aid kits, perfectly equipped to rapidly and highly efficiently respond to an insult to the vasculature, without losing time of activating the translational machinery. These rod-shaped subcellular organelles are filled with a whole battery of bioactive compounds such as their major component vWF to recruit platelets to close the wound, by concentrating them to the vessel wall by binding through their glycoprotein 1balpha [15].

They further contain P-selectin to recruit leukocytes to guard the wound, IL-8 to boost inflammation, endothelin-1 for vasoconstriction to close off the affected area, angiopoietin-2 to destabilize endothelial junctions and its barrier function for flexibility during tissue repair, and tPA to prevent excessive fibrin formation [16–18]. Relative allocation of the content of WPB is situation dependent, with an increased amount of IL-8 during inflammatory situations, mutual exclusive presence of P-selectin and angiopoietin-2 due to different transport sources, and varying amounts of tPA [17, 19]. Activation and exocytosis of WPB can be triggered by several stimuli including thrombin, vascular endothelial growth factor (VEGF), or epinephrine either through Ca^{2+}/calmodulin-dependent pathways or in response to cAMP-raising agonists distinctly influencing cytoskeletal function [20].

Tissue factor expression on EC increases upon pro-inflammatory stimulation with, e.g., TNF-alpha, oxidized phospholipids, pro-angiogenic factors, or shear stress [21–23]. During inflammation, clot formation can contribute to pathogen containment and regeneration of the vessel barrier function. However, this scenario also substantially contributes to atherosclerotic plaque formation [12].

Several pathways control aberrant initiation of the sequentially amplifying coagulation cascade. To prevent coagulation, it is necessary to interfere at the very top of the cascade. Tissue factor pathway inhibitor (TFPI) is a serine protease inhibitor that precludes complexing of TF to fVIIa and thus dampens coagulation. To form a clot now, fVIII and fX need to override this blockage. There are two main splice isoforms in humans; TFPIalpha is secreted by EC and present in the plasma but also stored in platelets. TFPIbeta is EC specific and anchored by GPI into the plasma membrane [14, 24]. Regulation of the coagulation cascade can thereby be spaciously differently controlled in the fluid phase and at the vessel wall.

Disruption of this intricate balance can cause severe disorders, such as the congenital bleeding disease hemophilia A or B, when the function of fVIII or fX is impaired, respectively. Still, acute conditions such as thrombosis or disseminated intravascular coagulation (DIC) are the result of uncontrolled activation. There is a high risk for developing this pathologic state during systemic inflammation when fibrin is over-consumed and clot formation is not effective [25].

To reconstitute unperturbed flow, removal of the thrombus is necessary once healing has progressed sufficiently. Fibrinolysis of clots is crucial to prevent thrombosis and is accomplished by plasmin. Plasmin is cleaved off its liver-secreted zymogen plasminogen by the serine proteases (serpins) tissue plasminogen activator (tPA), mainly produced by EC, or urokinase (uPA), secreted by many different cell types. The process of fibrin degradation needs to be as tightly controlled as its generation and includes several safety check points [26]. tPA requires fibrin as cofactor, and thus only cleaves clot associated plasminogen, and is irreversibly and rapidly inhibited by its specific plasminogen activator inhibitor (PAI-1) when circulating. Whereas tPA acts mostly in the bloodstream, uPA works mostly extravascularly. Furthermore, nonfibrin-bound plasmin is bound by alpha2-antiplasmin rendering it inactive through blocking its fibrin-binding site. Taking advantage of these specificities may allow for targeted therapy during clinical thrombotic events [27].

Acute occlusion of main vessels by thrombi is detrimental for the affected ischemic tissue, for example, during a myocardial infarct; however, rapid sealing of injured vessels is necessary to keep up vital nutrient support and protection from intruding pathogens. Therefore, depending on the specific situation, maintaining the appropriate balance between pro- and anticoagulative action of the endothelium is crucial for effective immunity of the human body.

4.2.2   Vascular Tone

Under homeostasis, the vascular tone is regulated in balance of vasodilative and vasoconstrictive signals to adapt blood pressure and flow to current activity requirements. EC control vascular tone by sending paracrine signals to smooth muscle cells surrounding the vessels, which can constrict vessels by contraction or dilate them by relaxation.

The most potent vasoconstrictor is endothelin (ET), a 21aa peptide existing in three isoforms mainly synthesized by EC [28]. Serum levels of ET-1, the predominant form of endothelin, are elevated by pro-inflammatory, EC-activating signaling, with transcription factor binding sites for AP1, NF-kB, GATA2, SMAD, or HIF1alpha detected in the endothelin gene [29]. However, ET-1 itself induces expression of pro-inflammatory signals. Constriction of a vessel in an inflamed area achieves a containment effect for pathogens and decelerates passing leukocytes for transmigration. ET-1 signaling increases expression of adhesion molecules such as VCAM (vascular cell adhesion molecule) on endothelial cells and supports the clustering of neutrophils, which contributes to the massive neutrophil infiltration observed in ischemic myocardium [28].

The main counter-player against vasodilation is nitric oxide (NO), a gasotransmitter, produced by NO synthases (NOS) in a stepwise redox reaction from L-arginine. There are three isoforms of NO synthase, nNOS (neuronal), eNOS (endothelial), and iNOS (cytokine-inducible). Under healthy conditions, eNOS in the endothelium provides NO to keep the vascular tone to adjusted levels under altering blood pressure and blood flow conditions [30, 31]. Endothelial dysfunction is a state of impaired NO bioavailability and linked to development of atherosclerosis and cardiovascular disease [32]. Flow-mediated dilation (FMD) is typically measured to determine endothelial dysfunction in patients, where a reduction can be used as prognostic marker for heart failure and presents concomitantly with vascular remodeling of arterial vessels [33]. Capacity overload of the system or depletion of L-arginine or the essential cofactor tetrahydrobiopterin leads to eNOS uncoupling, a switch in the NO generation process that also produces reactive oxygen species (ROS). This oxidative stress in the long term causes subtle remodeling of the vasculature to a chronic pro-inflammatory state and contributes to atherosclerotic plaque formation [34].

In contrast, iNOS, as reflected by the name, is steeply induced by cytokines under inflammatory conditions, especially to generate ROS to combat pathogens. NO itself has radical potential and exerts microbicidal function. iNOS is also expressed in EC, but the main source are leukocytes, especially macrophages [35]. Under sterile inflammatory conditions, iNOS activation constitutes a significant threat to the cardiovascular system and may lead to the detrimental development of septic shock.

4.3   Endothelial Cells as Part of the Immune Response

4.3.1   Expression of Innate Immune Receptors

Toll-Like Receptors EC express several innate immune receptors including the toll-like receptor (TLR) family recognizing pathogen-associated molecular patterns (PAMPs) [36, 37]. Expression of all TLRs is detectable in EC. TLR1, TLR2, TLR3, TLR4, TLR5, TLR6, and TLR9 are found in all different kinds of tissue-specific EC. In resting EC, TLR7, TLR8, and TLR10 are absent, but they are inducible under inflammatory activation [38]. Upon agonist binding, dimerization, and activation of TLRs, NF-kappaB and MAPK signaling are initiated via MyD88 and/or TRIF. This leads to a pro-inflammatory cell response, which in EC means structural changes of adhesion molecules in order to increase vascular permeability, production of inflammatory cytokines, presentation of adhesion molecules to recruit leukocytes, and the switch to a procoagulant state [36]. Specifically, direct activation of TLR1/2, TLR3, and TLR4, by their respective agonists Pam3CSK4, Poly(I:C), or LPS, elicits a strong pro-inflammatory response by stimulating the production of cytokines such as IL-6, IL-8, TNF-alpha, and IL-1 beta, altering adhesion molecule expression, including E-selectin, P-selectin, ICAM, and VCAM, elevating vascular permeability through reduced junction protein claudin-5 as well as secretion of procoagulant factors like tissue factor, PAI-1, uPa, and vWF [38–40].

Notably, there are crucial functional differences between TLR responses in monocytes and EC. Some are mediated via different routes of NF-kB and MAPK signaling, as ERK5 seems to regulate endothelial TLR2-dependent transcriptional response including its own upregulation, whereas MEK1 controls monocytic activation [41]. TLR2 in endothelial cells is expressed only at low level at baseline but is strongly upregulated by initial contact with its ligand. In contrast, leukocytes show a constitutively high TLR2 expression. This seems to be a functional adaptation to prevent overshooting endothelial activation and in consequence harmful vascular hyperpermeability, thrombosis, or septic shock [39].

Vascular TLR2 and TLR4 do not only sense pathogens but also tissue damage, for example, by the presence of extracellular histones, and respond with elevated tissue factor production, which may challenge the balance between beneficial local microthrombus formation and the risk for sepsis [42]. In contrast to other reports, this study also describes the TLR2 and TLR4 to be displayed on the endothelial surface as on leukocytes. However, in EC TLR2 and TLR4 are often found intracellularly [43]. This discrepancy might be correlated with the activation state of the EC.

Hyperglycemia is another pro-inflammatory stimulus for the activation of EC. It is also mediated via TLR2 and TLR4/MyD88/NF-kB/AP1, leading to shedding of the repellent glycocalyx of the endothelium. This enables improved leukocyte adhesion and increased ROS production. In a chronic state, this contributes to the vascular complications of diabetes patients [44].

Circulating endothelial progenitor cells also present certain levels of TLRs. They are responsive to agonist stimulation, which, however, only induces cytokine production, but not differentiation, excluding TLR activation as a trigger for endothelial progenitor cell differentiation at sites of injury [45].

In addition to TLR, various other types of pattern recognition receptors exist in EC. NOD1 and NOD2, containing a nucleotide-binding oligomerization domain (NOD) and caspase recruitment domain (CARD), sense degraded bacterial components released from endosomes in the endothelial cytosol and activate NF-kB signaling [46]. The RNA helicase retinoic acid-inducible gene-I (RIG-I) recognizes particular viral ssRNA structures [47].

Lectin-like oxidized low-density lipoprotein receptor-1 (LOX-1) of EC mediates uptake of the glycation end-product oxidized LDL, which is generated under oxidative stress during inflammatory events. Its activation leads to exacerbation of the inflammatory response, chronic inflammation, endothelial dysfunction, and atherosclerosis [48]. LOX-1 is a member of a lectin-like receptor family, encoded in the natural killer (NK) gene complex together with dectin-1 and CLEC-1 [49]. C-type lectin-like receptor 1 (CLEC-1), which is also expressed in EC, is not known to be involved in leukopheresis, as other C-type lectins described later, but represents an intracellular pattern recognition receptor. It is upregulated by immune regulation TGF-beta and is involved in control of immune response to transplants [50, 51].

4.3.2 Endothelial Cells in Leukopheresis

One of the most crucial functions of EC during an inflammatory response is to organize and coordinate controlled transition of leukocytes through the vessel wall for recruitment into damaged/infected tissue. It is a major challenge for EC to keep up the balance between tightly sealing vessel walls to prevent leakage of transported fluids on the one hand and to facilitate extravasation of mobile immune cells on the other hand. However, during inflammation, increased vascular permeability and transendothelial migration (TEM), reflecting innate and adaptive immunity, are required at different time points.

Release of molecules such as antibodies or complement components to injured tissue should constrain infections. As a second line of defense, leukocytes join in. For this purpose, EC express adhesion molecules on their surface with various operative specializations to direct the leukocyte extravasation cascade. In general, TEM can be pictured as leukocytes migrating through the vessel wall in sequential steps of (1) tethering, (2) rolling, (3) firm adhesion, (4) crawling, and (5) eventually diapedesis (Fig. 4.2) [52]. L-, P-, and E-selectin constitute one main group of adhesion

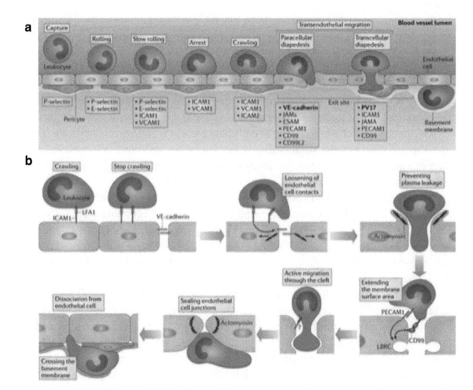

Fig. 4.2 (**a**) A range of cell adhesion receptors on endothelial cells (as shown at the *bottom* of the *panel*) mediates the capture, rolling, arrest, and crawling of leukocytes on the luminal endothelial cell surface. This is the prelude for the actual transmigration through the endothelial barrier—the diapedesis process. Leukocyte diapedesis is usually paracellular but can also occur in a minority of cases through a transcellular route. Whereas transmigration through the endothelial barrier takes about 2–3 min, leukocytes take up to 15–20 min to overcome the basement membrane, leading to the transient accumulation of leukocytes between endothelial cells and the basement membrane. Some of the adhesion receptors that participate in paracellular diapedesis are also relevant for transcellular diapedesis. Vascular endothelial cadherin (VE-cadherin) is exclusively involved in the paracellular route, functioning as a barrier to transmigration. The only candidate for a cell surface protein that might be exclusively involved in transcellular diapedesis is plasmalemma vesicle protein 1 (PV1), which is an essential component of fenestral and stomatal diaphragms. Owing to space limitations, the list of endothelial cell adhesion receptors shown here is not exhaustive but represents the most well studied. (**b**) The diapedesis process requires many functions mediated by leukocytes and endothelial cells: stopping intraluminal crawling at suitable exit sites, loosening of endothelial cell contacts, preventing plasma leakage, extending the membrane surface area at endothelial cell junctions through mobilization of the lateral border recycling compartment (LBRC), active leukocyte migration through the junctional cleft, and sealing of the junction after diapedesis. Finally, leukocytes dissociate from endothelial cells followed by transmigration through the basement membrane. *CD99L2* CD99 antigen-like protein 2, *ESAM* endothelial cell-selective adhesion molecule, *ICAM* intercellular adhesion molecule, *JAM* junctional adhesion molecule, *LFA-1* lymphocyte function-associated antigen 1, *PECAM1* platelet endothelial cell adhesion molecule 1, *VCAM1* vascular cell adhesion molecule 1 (Modified from [52])

molecules. They are C-type (Ca^{2+}-dependent) lectins binding to glycoconjugated ligands. These three closely related selectins recruit leukocytes out of blood flow toward an inflamed area by establishing first specific but dynamic contacts with EC [53]. This initial step of leukocyte tethering to EC is preceded by local EC glycocalyx shedding executed by heparinase, matrix metalloproteinases (MMPs), and ROS, as this charged cell surface coating prevents adhesion molecule and carbohydrate ligand presentation under normal conditions as a barrier for unintended extravasation [54].

E-selectin has to be synthesized de novo and is accordingly steeply induced by pro-inflammatory signals such as TNF-alpha or IL-1, whereas P-selectin is stored in Weibel-Palade bodies, which fuse upon stimulation with the cell membrane. L-selectin in contrast is constitutively expressed on leukocytes, and its main purpose is to guide them toward high endothelial venule structures during regular homing processes, where expression of the ligands glycosylated cell adhesion molecule-1 (GlyCAM1) and P-selectin glycoprotein ligand-1 (PSGL-1) captures them. However, similar structures are also present in atherosclerotic-prone vascular walls [55]. PSGL-1 is a low-affinity ligand for all selectins, thereby decelerating leukocytes close to extravasation sites, but firm adhesion has still to be established [56, 57].

PSGL-1 is resident in lipid rafts on the tips of microvilli, and simultaneous binding of several PSGL-1 molecules leads to formation of secondary structures to further supporting adhesion, whereby transition of tethering to rolling is smoothly proceeding [53].

CD44 is another versatile glycoprotein binding to L- or E-selectin when fitted with the appropriate posttranslational modification of certain carbohydrate residues. Furthermore, CD44 protein harbors docking sites for the interaction with components of the extracellular matrix, contributing to fixation of leukocytes in damaged areas. CD44 can regulate rolling velocity by cooperation with PSGL-1, thereby especially recruiting T cells [53].

E-selectin ligand-1 (ESL-1) can further support binding of PSGL-1 to P-selectin when ESL-1 is recognizing E-selectin in parallel [53].

All these molecules in their different combination and density can fine-tune the tethering/rolling process and indeed regulate which subsets of leukocytes are eventually recruited. Chemokines were found to decisively influence the type of captured immune cells due to distinct spatiotemporal regulation of expression of selectins and their ligands. The chemokine CCL2 elicits a rapid surface presence of L-selectin, PGSL-1, and CD44, crucial for neutrophil recruitment, and subsequently induces E-selectin expression to attach monocytes. This is in accordance with the observed phenomenon of a first wave of infiltrating neutrophils and a second wave of imigrating monocytes at sites of cardiovascular pathologies [58]. This study also depicts that E-selectin is coexpressed with CD31/PECAM at cell-cell endothelial junctions. Such junctions have to be opened in places where leukocytes should squeeze through, and E-selectin seems to pull them directly toward the lateral cell-cell borders.

The processes of arrest and crawling are mediated by stronger anchoring through interaction of adhesion molecules and their various integrin ligands, intercellular adhesion molecule (ICAM-1) and lymphocyte function-associated antigen-1 (LFA-1), vascular cell adhesion molecule-1 (VCAM-1) and VLA-4 (very late antigen-4), and platelet endothelial cell adhesion molecule (PECAM), respectively [59]. Binding of these ligands to integrins, transmembrane receptors for cell-cell and cell-ECM interactions, leads to conformational changes, inducing downstream intracellular signaling to alter cytoskeleton structures [60]. Thereby fixation and crawling of leukocytes even against of flow direction are supported. Inside-out signaling induces transition from ICAM-1 binding to LFA-1 for an anchoring arrest toward crawling mediating binding of macrophage antigen 1 (Mac-1).

ICAM-1/-2 and VCAM-1 are inducible by various inflammatory stimuli, such as TNF-alpha, IL-1beta, oxLDL, or C-reactive protein. This is regulated by signaling via the transcription factors NF-kB and AP1 for which several binding sites were discovered, for example, in the VCAM promoter [61, 62]. Detection of ICAM-1 or VCAM-1 on EC and on endothelial microparticles was shown to constitute a prognostic marker for cardiovascular diseases with a severe outcome [63]. Highly expressed ICAM-1 is an indication for activated EC as well as increased infiltration, and thereby attracted leukocytes destabilize atherosclerotic plaques [64]. Further, ICAM-1 is involved in the formation of unstable plaques through mineralocorticoid aldosterone, which normally regulates blood volume by shifting electrolyte concentrations. Mineralocorticoid receptor-responsive elements were found in the ICAM-1 promoter, and increased leukocyte infiltration destabilizes atherosclerotic plaques [65]. In addition, EC-derived ICAM-1 induced by IL-1b and IL-6 in circulation is responsible for attracting T-cell and monocyte infiltration into the left ventricle subsequent to heart failure [66].

PECAM-1 is an endothelial cell adhesion molecule that can be found at the lateral borders of an EC monolayer but is also expressed on leukocytes. In a complex with VEGFR2 and VE-cadherin, it functions as shear stress sensor and thereby activates signaling to further induce ICAM-1 expression [67].

The described adhesion molecules transiently attach leukocytes to endothelial cells, whereas connections between EC are tight and adherent junctions. The involved protein complexes regulate the barrier function of the endothelium under noninflamed conditions. To cross this sealed cell wall for leukocytes during inflammation, two routes are conceivable: either trans- or paracellular. Although data are yet controversial due to limitations of live microscopy of this complex cellular process, there is consent that transcellular passage of leukocytes through EC is happening, with an approximate proportion of 10% trans- and 90% paracellular TEM also depending on blood vessel type and thickness as well as potentially the type of initial TEM stimulus [52].

For the paracellular route, adherent junctions have to loosen and open up in a harmonized way as to not completely disband the vessel but just to decrease barrier function. In EC adherent junctions are constituted by the single membrane protein VE-cadherin (cadherin 5) which forms homodimers with molecules on neighboring cells [68]. To anchor these junctions, VE-cadherins associate with beta- and alpha-catenin, and these further interconnect to the cytoskeleton. Experiments using constitutively stabilized VE-cadherin-catenin proteins revealed that leukocyte transmigration is strongly prevented then [69]. It is suggested that phosphorylation of VE-cadherin by tyrosine kinases and dissociation of vascular endothelial protein tyrosine phosphatase (VE-PTP) are prerequisite for opening the junctions through conformational changes and by internalization. There are tyrosine residues specific for induction of vascular leakage, while others are responsible for destabilizing junctions as preparation of diapedesis [70–72]. Leukocytes are required to unwrap junctions before passing through. When ICAM-1 molecules ligate and cluster, phosphorylation of VE-cadherin is induced, which also involves proteins of the Rho family [73]. This system is also responsible for the actin stress fiber rearrangements that pull apart the adherent junctions. Dissociation of VE-PTP can be triggered by binding of leukocytes but also by VEGF. It is also necessary to loosen contacts during vessel growth [74].

A whole system of counteracting proteins is required for successful TEM: the molecules PECAM, CD155, and CD99 on the membrane system termed lateral border recycling compartment (LBRC). Homophilic interactions between PECAM and CD99 expressed on leukocytes and EC direct the leukocyte toward a junction and then through it, respectively [75, 76]. The LBRC is moved with the help of kinesins. Other junctional proteins such as junctional adhesion molecule (JAM-)A and C also function as counter-receptors for passaging leukocytes. These molecules seem to surround the leukocytes in circular structures, forming an orientation guide to prevent hesitant or even backward migration. During ischemic reperfusion conditions, JAM-C expression is reduced at EC junctions, and disrupted polarized TEM of neutrophils but not of monocytes has been observed [77].

All these different proteins involved in TEM reflect the critical point of opening up a normally tightly sealed tissue structure to enable transition of whole cells without perturbing the entire vessel system [11, 78]. Furthermore the endothelium preserves a crucial selective capacity by regulating the recruited leukocyte type by differential expression of chemokines and adhesion molecules [79]. Knowing the different molecules involved in recruitment of different leukocytes to atherosclerotic plaques or damaged tissue after an ischemic event might offer more targeted therapeutic strategies.

4.3.3 Angiogenesis

Angiogenesis, defined as the formation of new blood vessels from preexisting vessels, is not only required during development and growth but is necessarily linked to tissue repair and restoration of oxygen and metabolite supply as well as barrier function in wounded, ischemic, or inflamed areas. During angiogenesis, EC are activated, and single lines of cells start to migrate out of a preexisting vessel toward a gradient of vascular endothelial growth factor (VEGF), a growth factor produced under hypoxic conditions [80]. However, a lot of factors including chemokines are known to have pro-angiogenic capacity, reflecting the interlinked need for new vessels during an immune response. For example, IL-8 is highly angiogenic, and its expression is associated with poor prognosis in different cancers but induces EC proliferation in ischemic myocardium [81, 82].

It is commonly accepted that new vessels are formed as outgrowing sprouts of tip/stalk cells. The leading tip cell is highly migratory and protrudes many filopodia, which express VEGF receptors to sense the VEGF gradient. So-called stalk cells follow behind the tip cell. These are highly proliferative and will eventually form a new, lumenized vessel. Delta-like 4 (Dll4), a Notch receptor ligand, expressed on tip cells, induces Notch signaling in the neighboring cell, upon which surface expression of KDR/VEGF receptor 2 is downregulated implementing the stalk cell phenotype [83, 84]. Several factors might select for a cell to become a tip cell, including random local overexpression of KDR, metabolic advantages of some cells in terms of elevated glycolysis conferring higher motility, or cell arrangements orientating cells into certain directions to facilitate migration [85, 86]. When a sprout encounters another, they will anastomose and blood can flow through a newly formed vessel [87, 88]. This process is often bridged by macrophages via conferring additional sources of Notch receptors especially at branching points [89]. Monocytes can also be an additional resource of VEGF, which is necessary for the process of arteriogenesis, the rapid maturation of collateral capillaries into arteries after an occlusion event of the arterial circulation [90, 91]. This involves NF-kB signaling that can stabilize hypoxia-inducible factor 1alpha under non-hypoxic conditions.

Stimulation and support of angiogenesis by macrophages is also a potential indirect mechanism induced by the immune-suppressive cytokine IL-19. IL-19, a member of the IL-10 family, is expressed by EC of inflamed coronary tissue. It boosts bFGF-dependent angiogenesis in the absence of hypoxia by effects exerted on vascular smooth muscle cells [92, 93].

Originally, VEGF was described as vascular permeabilization factor referring to one of its obvious physiological effects [94]. To allow vessel growth, junctional adhesion has to be destabilized, similar to inflammation-induced permeability, to allow for restructuring of the EC layer. VEGF usually stands for VEGF-A, the classical pro-angiogenic factor, representing a whole structurally related family. VEGF crucially sustains EC survival and promotes blood vessel angiogenesis. VEGF proteins are the ligands for the receptor tyrosine kinase family of VEGF receptors. There are three receptors, VEGFR1, VEGFR2, and VEGFR3, also known as Flt1, Flk1, and Flt4, respectively. VEGFR1 binds VEGF-A with higher affinity than VEGFR2, but VEGFR1 is hardly mitogenic and the intrinsic signaling kinase activity is very low. VEGFR1 and its soluble splice form sFlt1 are therefore regarded as decoy receptors, titrating out abundant VEGF at times of massive angiogenesis or to maintain avascularity of corneas [95].

VEFGR2 possesses high intrinsic tyrosine kinase activity upon ligand binding. Proliferation of EC is stimulated by VEGF primarily via phospholipase gamma and protein kinase C leading to RAF/ERK/MAPK pathway signaling. The pro-survival effect of VEGF-A-VEGFR2 signaling is mediated through PI3K/PIP3/PKB/AKT-dependent phosphorylation and blocking of proapoptotic caspases [96].

Inflammatory signals induce a qualitatively, partly overlapping transcription profile in EC compared to angiogenic stimuli, but quantitative differences reflect the fine-tuning potential of the system. For example, VCAM-1 is steeply induced by IL-1 as well as by VEGF, however, with a factor 100 difference in magnitude. This reflects the significantly greater need for leukocyte recruitment into inflamed/damaged tissue, than during sterile angiogenesis, where only a small number is needed for surveillance. However, some endothelial genes are specifically activated only under pro-angiogenic conditions, specifically required for the sprouting process itself, while numerous others are activated under pro-inflammatory conditions only, since hypoxic conditions are not always present when inflammation has to be triggered [97, 98].

As mentioned above, many cytokines also exert pro-angiogenic, EC-activating effects. Another prominent example, IL-33, especially exemplifies how entangled the different functions of EC are. IL-33, member of the IL-1 superfamily, is released during inflammatory tissue damage or trauma by necrotic or affected cells. IL-33 activates endothelial migration in a potentially pro-angiogenic way and increases vascular permeability by elevated eNOS-dependent NO levels [99]. At the same time, IL-33 upregulates TF expression in EC and downregulates TFPI, pushing them to a procoagulant state [100]. IL-33 and TF can be co-detected in atherosclerotic plaques, and levels of IL-33 correlate to disease activity in CAD [101].

All processes of EC activation, inflammation, hemostasis, and angiogenesis have one principle in common: the end is already part of the program. Therefore, VEGF inducible transcription factors control targets, which will neutralize the pro-angiogenic activation of EC if no restimulation occurs, as part of a negative-feedback mechanism when normoxia is restored. VEGF-dependent MEF2C induced A2M, which functions as a global serine protease inhibitor [102]. This likely prevents excessive extracellular matrix (ECM) and tissue degradation or aberrant angiogenesis [103]. Also the inflammatory response has to be brought back to a resting level to prevent excessive inflammatory damage. Strong pro-inflammatory stimuli such as IL-1 or TNF-alpha induce, during a second wave, inhibitors of the NF-kB, NFAT, and MAPK pathway to resolve activation [104].

4.3.4 EC in Cardiovascular Disease

In contrast to smooth muscle cells, EC can tolerate hypoxia very well, in culture even for weeks through different expression of HIF-1 and HIF-2, but, for example, in a myocardial infarct after occlusion of a vessel after 20–40 min, the clinically long observed wavefront phenomenon of necrotic areas sets in [105, 106]. However, they are very sensitive to reperfusion injury when blood flow is restored. Necrotic cardiomyocytes and hypoxia activate EC, rendering them targets for infiltrating leukocytes. Notably, however, EC seem not to tolerate hypothermia very well. Cardiac arrest patients treated with hypothermia to improve neurological prognosis show aggravated endothelial dysfunction and elevated levels of sVCAM-1 [107].

ROS are commonly considered detrimental to cells, and EC are also very vulnerable for their destructive potential. However, there are conflicting reports regarding this aspect, as antioxidant treatment by diet or drugs was not effective in EC-dependent CVD risk factor prevention [108]. Elucidating this phenomenon on molecular level revealed that coronary EC become proapoptotic upon long-term ROS burden in the mitochondrial cell compartment but need short-term ROS stimuli for survival [109].

Further, EC are very sensitive to flow and adapt to different flow conditions. Flow-mediated dilation and low-flow-mediated vasoconstriction are regulated by healthy responsive EC to balance homeostasis, but loss of these functions is indicative for endothelial dysfunction and correlates with an adverse prognosis for CVD [110].

Pulsatile laminar flow is atheroprotective, especially at vessel branches, as it induces eNOS and consequently elevates the level of NO and suppresses endothelin-1 [111]. Shear stress is decisive for the balanced expression of these two counterplayers in the vascular system, but the potential of high wall shear stress to remodel the endothelium is also considered as a driver of formation of non-stable atherosclerotic plaques. However, imaging possibilities are not yet meaningful enough for correlating shear stress, morphologic changes of plaque, and adverse events [112, 113].

As extensively reviewed by Heusch et al., after myocardial infarction, the area of risk is the critical region that determines the outcome of adverse events [114]. Reperfusion injury manifests as increased vascular permeability along with edema formation, which is not only caused by lost barrier function and glycocalyx loss upon inflammation but also by electrolyte concentration shifts due to loss of energy-dependent ion pumps. Edema impairs further microvascular perfusion by compression. Nitric oxide can attenuate deprivation of the barrier function; however, vasomotion in infarcted areas is often shifted to hyperconstriction through endothelin, leading to vascular remodeling. Microembolisms resulting from atherothrombotic debris or after percutaneous coronary intervention, or cell aggregates assembled through the increased expression of adhesion molecules, can further reduce circulation. If the swelling of the vessels is too severe, these might rupture, and the resulting hemorrhage leads to severe myocardial necrosis. The area of risk can be reduced by cardioprotective interventions like pre- or postischemic conditioning but only if some collateral flow is preserved to transfer protective factors [114]. Remote ischemic preconditioning can be cardioprotective in animal models where several cycles of few minutes ischemia seem to be an effective schedule [115]. Detailed definition of the involved molecular mediators sent and received by EC poses a new therapeutic target to treat ischemic maladies.

4.4 Conclusion

EC are culprits and victims during myocardial infarction at the same time. Although EC tolerate hypoxia better than other cardiac resident cell types, their pro-angiogenic activation causes loss of barrier function and edema formation. Furthermore their pro-inflammatory activation increases expression of adhesion molecules and causes leukocyte influx. Excessive immune cell infiltration can be detrimental to the already damaged tissue. Loss of vasodilative NO synthesis by EC further aggravates vessel occlusion in the heart. In addition, endothelial activation shifts them toward a hazardous prothrombotic state.

In summary, disruption of the classical endothelial functions of vessel formation, hemostasis, and regulation of vascular tone underlies most cardiovascular pathologies, and their central role in immune response organization exacerbates damage. Therefore it is necessary to also therapeutically target EC during cardiovascular diseases.

References

1. Pober JS, Sessa WC. Evolving functions of endothelial cells in inflammation. Nat Rev Immunol. 2007;7:803–15.
2. Alitalo K. The lymphatic vasculature in disease. Nat Med. 2011;17:1371–80.
3. Potente M, Gerhardt H, Carmeliet P. Basic and therapeutic aspects of angiogenesis. Cell. 2011;146:873–87.
4. Planas-Paz L, Strilic B, Goedecke A, Breier G, Fassler R, Lammert E. Mechanoinduction of lymph vessel expansion. EMBO J. 2012;31:788–804.
5. Semenza GL. Targeting HIF-1 for cancer therapy. Nat Rev Cancer. 2003;3:721–32.
6. Risau W. Differentiation of endothelium. FASEB J. 1995;9:926–33.
7. Domigan CK, Iruela-Arispe ML. Recent advances in vascular development. Curr Opin Hematol. 2012;19:176–83.
8. Adams RH, Alitalo K. Molecular regulation of angiogenesis and lymphangiogenesis. Nat Rev Mol Cell Biol. 2007;8:464–78.
9. Mickoleit M, Schmid B, Weber M, Fahrbach FO, Hombach S, Reischauer S, Huisken J. High-resolution reconstruction of the beating zebrafish heart. Nat Methods. 2014;11:919–22.
10. Haack T, Abdelilah-Seyfried S. The force within: endocardial development, mechanotransduction and signalling during cardiac morphogenesis. Development. 2016;143:373–86.
11. Vestweber D. Relevance of endothelial junctions in leukocyte extravasation and vascular permeability. Ann N Y Acad Sci. 2012;1257:184–92.
12. Engelmann B, Massberg S. Thrombosis as an intravascular effector of innate immunity. Nat Rev Immunol. 2013;13:34–45.
13. Kazmi RS, Boyce S, Lwaleed BA. Homeostasis of hemostasis: the role of endothelium. Semin Thromb Hemost. 2015;41:549–55.
14. Yau JW, Teoh H, Verma S. Endothelial cell control of thrombosis. BMC Cardiovasc Disord. 2015;15:130.
15. Andre P, Denis CV, Ware J, Saffaripour S, Hynes RO, Ruggeri ZM, Wagner DD. Platelets adhere to and translocate on von Willebrand factor presented by endothelium in stimulated veins. Blood. 2000;96:3322–8.
16. Weibel ER. Fifty years of Weibel-Palade bodies: the discovery and early history of an enigmatic organelle of endothelial cells. J Thromb Haemost. 2012;10:979–84.
17. Rondaij MG, Bierings R, Kragt A, van Mourik JA, Voorberg J. Dynamics and plasticity of Weibel-Palade bodies in endothelial cells. Arterioscler Thromb Vasc Biol. 2006;26:1002–7.
18. Denis CV, Andre P, Saffaripour S, Wagner DD. Defect in regulated secretion of P-selectin affects leukocyte recruitment in von Willebrand factor-deficient mice. Proc. Natl. Acad. Sci. U.S.A. 2001;98:4072–7.
19. Utgaard JO, Jahnsen FL, Bakka A, Brandtzaeg P, Haraldsen G. Rapid secretion of prestored interleukin 8 from Weibel-Palade bodies of microvascular endothelial cells. J Exp Med. 1998;188:1751–6.

20. Vischer UM, Wollheim CB. Purine nucleotides induce regulated secretion of von Willebrand factor: involvement of cytosolic Ca^{2+} and cyclic adenosine monophosphate-dependent signaling in endothelial exocytosis. Blood. 1998;91:118–27.

21. Mechtcheriakova D, Schabbauer G, Lucerna M, Clauss M, De Martin R, Binder BR, Hofer E. Specificity, diversity, and convergence in VEGF and TNF-alpha signaling events leading to tissue factor up-regulation via EGR-1 in endothelial cells. FASEB J. 2001;15:230–42.

22. Bochkov VN, Mechtcheriakova D, Lucerna M, Huber J, Malli R, Graier WF, Hofer E, Binder BR, Leitinger N. Oxidized phospholipids stimulate tissue factor expression in human endothelial cells via activation of ERK/EGR-1 and Ca(++)/NFAT. Blood. 2002;99:199–206.

23. Houston P, Dickson MC, Ludbrook V, White B, Schwachtgen JL, McVey JH, Mackman N, Reese JM, Gorman DG, Campbell C, Braddock M. Fluid shear stress induction of the tissue factor promoter in vitro and in vivo is mediated by Egr-1. Arterioscler Thromb Vasc Biol. 1999;19:281–9.

24. Mast AE. Tissue factor pathway inhibitor: multiple anticoagulant activities for a single protein. Arterioscler Thromb Vasc Biol. 2016;36:9–14.

25. Levi M. Current understanding of disseminated intravascular coagulation. Br J Haematol. 2004;124:567–76.

26. Chapin JC, Hajjar KA. Fibrinolysis and the control of blood coagulation. Blood Rev. 2015;29:17–24.

27. Lippi G, Mattiuzzi C, Favaloro EJ. Novel and emerging therapies: thrombus-targeted fibrinolysis. Semin Thromb Hemost. 2013;39:48–58.

28. Davenport AP, Hyndman KA, Dhaun N, Southan C, Kohan DE, Pollock JS, Pollock DM, Webb DJ, Maguire JJ. Endothelin. Pharmacol Rev. 2016;68:357–418.

29. Stow LR, Jacobs ME, Wingo CS, Cain BD. Endothelin-1 gene regulation. FASEB J. 2011;25:16–28.

30. Siragusa M, Fleming I. The eNOS signalosome and its link to endothelial dysfunction. Arch Eur J Physiol. 2016;468:1125–37.

31. Shesely EG, Maeda N, Kim HS, Desai KM, Krege JH, Laubach VE, Sherman PA, Sessa WC, Smithies O. Elevated blood pressures in mice lacking endothelial nitric oxide synthase. Proc Natl Acad Sci USA. 1996;93:13176–81.

32. Kuhlencordt PJ, Gyurko R, Han F, Scherrer-Crosbie M, Aretz TH, Hajjar R, Picard MH, Huang PL. Accelerated atherosclerosis, aortic aneurysm formation, and ischemic heart disease in apolipoprotein E/endothelial nitric oxide synthase double-knockout mice. Circulation. 2001;104:448–54.

33. Kishimoto S, Kajikawa M, Maruhashi T, Iwamoto Y, Matsumoto T, Iwamoto A, Oda N, Matsui S, Hidaka T, Kihara Y, Chayama K, Goto C, Aibara Y, Nakashima A, Noma K, Higashi Y. Endothelial dysfunction and abnormal vascular structure are simultaneously present in patients with heart failure with preserved ejection fraction. Int J Cardiol. 2017;231:181–7.

34. McNeill E, Channon KM. The role of tetrahydrobiopterin in inflammation and cardiovascular disease. Thromb Haemost. 2012;108:832–9.

35. Uehara EU, Shida Bde S, de Brito CA. Role of nitric oxide in immune responses against viruses: beyond microbicidal activity. Inflamm Res. 2015;64:845–52.

36. Khakpour S, Wilhelmsen K, Hellman J. Vascular endothelial cell toll-like receptor pathways in sepsis. Innate Immun. 2015;21:827–46.

37. Opitz B, Eitel J, Meixenberger K, Suttorp N. Role of toll-like receptors, NOD-like receptors and RIG-I-like receptors in endothelial cells and systemic infections. Thromb Haemost. 2009;102:1103–9.

38. Fitzner N, Clauberg S, Essmann F, Liebmann J, Kolb-Bachofen V. Human skin endothelial cells can express all 10 TLR genes and respond to respective ligands. Clin Vaccine Immunol. 2008;15:138–46.

39. Shin HS, Xu F, Bagchi A, Herrup E, Prakash A, Valentine C, Kulkarni H, Wilhelmsen K, Warren S, Hellman J. Bacterial lipoprotein TLR2 agonists broadly modulate endothelial function and coagulation pathways in vitro and in vivo. J Immunol. 2011;186:1119–30.

40. Pegu A, Qin S, Fallert Junecko BA, Nisato RE, Pepper MS, Reinhart TA. Human lymphatic endothelial cells express multiple functional TLRs. J Immunol. 2008;180:3399–405.
41. Wilhelmsen K, Mesa KR, Lucero J, Xu F, Hellman J. ERK5 protein promotes, whereas MEK1 protein differentially regulates, the toll-like receptor 2 protein-dependent activation of human endothelial cells and monocytes. J Biol Chem. 2012;287:26478–94.
42. Yang X, Li L, Liu J, Lv B, Chen F. Extracellular histones induce tissue factor expression in vascular endothelial cells via TLR and activation of NF-kappaB and AP-1. Thromb Res. 2016;137:211–8.
43. Dunzendorfer S, Lee HK, Soldau K, Tobias PS. Toll-like receptor 4 functions intracellularly in human coronary artery endothelial cells: roles of LBP and sCD14 in mediating LPS responses. FASEB J. 2004;18:1117–9.
44. Pahwa R, Nallasamy P, Jialal I. Toll-like receptors 2 and 4 mediate hyperglycemia induced macrovascular aortic endothelial cell inflammation and perturbation of the endothelial glycocalyx. J Diabetes Complicat. 2016;30:563–72.
45. Mazzucchelli I, Lisini D, Garofoli F, Dragoni S, Angelini M, Pozzi M, Bonetti E, Tzialla C, Kramer BW, Spinillo A, Maccario R, Rosti V, Moccia F, Borghesi A, Stronati M. Expression and function of toll-like receptors in human circulating endothelial colony forming cells. Immunol Lett. 2015;168:98–104.
46. Opitz B, Puschel A, Beermann W, Hocke AC, Forster S, Schmeck B, van Laak V, Chakraborty T, Suttorp N, Hippenstiel S. *Listeria monocytogenes* activated p38 MAPK and induced IL-8 secretion in a nucleotide-binding oligomerization domain 1-dependent manner in endothelial cells. J Immunol. 2006;176:484–90.
47. Yoneyama M, Kikuchi M, Natsukawa T, Shinobu N, Imaizumi T, Miyagishi M, Taira K, Akira S, Fujita T. The RNA helicase RIG-I has an essential function in double-stranded RNA-induced innate antiviral responses. Nat Immunol. 2004;5:730–7.
48. Lubrano V, Balzan S. Roles of LOX-1 in microvascular dysfunction. Microvasc Res. 2016;105:132–40.
49. Sattler S, Ghadially H, Reiche D, Karas I, Hofer E. Evolutionary development and expression pattern of the myeloid lectin-like receptor gene family encoded within the NK gene complex. Scand J Immunol. 2010;72:309–18.
50. Sattler S, Reiche D, Sturtzel C, Karas I, Richter S, Kalb ML, Gregor W, Hofer E. The human C-type lectin-like receptor CLEC-1 is upregulated by TGF-beta and primarily localized in the endoplasmic membrane compartment. Scand J Immunol. 2012;75:282–92.
51. Thebault P, Lhermite N, Tilly G, Le Texier L, Quillard T, Heslan M, Anegon I, Soulillou JP, Brouard S, Charreau B, Cuturi MC, Chiffoleau E. The C-type lectin-like receptor CLEC-1, expressed by myeloid cells and endothelial cells, is up-regulated by immunoregulatory mediators and moderates T cell activation. J Immunol. 2009;183:3099–108.
52. Vestweber D. How leukocytes cross the vascular endothelium. Nat Rev Immunol. 2015;15:692–704.
53. Zarbock A, Ley K, McEver RP, Hidalgo A. Leukocyte ligands for endothelial selectins: specialized glycoconjugates that mediate rolling and signaling under flow. Blood. 2011;118:6743–51.
54. Becker BF, Jacob M, Leipert S, Salmon AH, Chappell D. Degradation of the endothelial glycocalyx in clinical settings: searching for the sheddases. Br J Clin Pharmacol. 2015;80:389–402.
55. Galkina E, Kadl A, Sanders J, Varughese D, Sarembock IJ, Ley K. Lymphocyte recruitment into the aortic wall before and during development of atherosclerosis is partially L-selectin dependent. J Exp Med. 2006;203:1273–82.
56. Vandendries ER, Furie BC, Furie B. Role of P-selectin and PSGL-1 in coagulation and thrombosis. Thromb Haemost. 2004;92:459–66.
57. Ramachandran V, Yago T, Epperson TK, Kobzdej MM, Nollert MU, Cummings RD, Zhu C, McEver RP. Dimerization of a selectin and its ligand stabilizes cell rolling and enhances tether strength in shear flow. Proc Natl Acad Sci U.S.A. 2001;98:10166–71.

58. Zuchtriegel G, Uhl B, Hessenauer ME, Kurz AR, Rehberg M, Lauber K, Krombach F, Reichel CA. Spatiotemporal expression dynamics of selectins govern the sequential extravasation of neutrophils and monocytes in the acute inflammatory response. Arterioscler Thromb Vasc Biol. 2015;35:899–910.

59. Galkina E, Ley K. Vascular adhesion molecules in atherosclerosis. Arterioscler Thromb Vasc Biol. 2007;27:2292–301.

60. van Wetering S, van den Berk N, van Buul JD, Mul FP, Lommerse I, Mous R, ten Klooster JP, Zwaginga JJ, Hordijk PL. VCAM-1-mediated Rac signaling controls endothelial cell-cell contacts and leukocyte transmigration. Am J Physiol Cell Physiol. 2003;285:C343–52.

61. Cybulsky MI, Fries JW, Williams AJ, Sultan P, Eddy R, Byers M, Shows T, Gimbrone MA Jr, Collins T. Gene structure, chromosomal location, and basis for alternative mRNA splicing of the human VCAM1 gene. Proc Natl Acad Sci U.S.A. 1991;88:7859–63.

62. Kawanami D, Maemura K, Takeda N, Harada T, Nojiri T, Saito T, Manabe I, Imai Y, Nagai R. C-reactive protein induces VCAM-1 gene expression through NF-kappaB activation in vascular endothelial cells. Atherosclerosis. 2006;185:39–46.

63. Radecke CE, Warrick AE, Singh GD, Rogers JH, Simon SI, Armstrong EJ. Coronary artery endothelial cells and microparticles increase expression of VCAM-1 in myocardial infarction. Thromb Haemost. 2015;113:605–16.

64. Hoke M, Winter MP, Wagner O, Exner M, Schillinger M, Arnold Z, Mlekusch W, Maurer G, Koppensteiner R, Minar E, Goliasch G. The impact of selectins on mortality in stable carotid atherosclerosis. Thromb Haemost. 2015;114:632–8.

65. Marzolla V, Armani A, Mammi C, Moss ME, Pagliarini V, Pontecorvo L, Antelmi A, Fabbri A, Rosano G, Jaffe IZ, Caprio M. Essential role of ICAM-1 in aldosterone-induced atherosclerosis. Int J Cardiol. 2017;232:233–42.

66. Salvador AM, Nevers T, Velazquez F, Aronovitz M, Wang B, Abadia Molina A, Jaffe IZ, Karas RH, Blanton RM, Alcaide P. Intercellular adhesion molecule 1 regulates left ventricular leukocyte infiltration, cardiac remodeling, and function in pressure overload-induced heart failure. J Am Heart Assoc. 2016;5:e003126.

67. Tzima E, Irani-Tehrani M, Kiosses WB, Dejana E, Schultz DA, Engelhardt B, Cao G, DeLisser H, Schwartz MA. A mechanosensory complex that mediates the endothelial cell response to fluid shear stress. Nature. 2005;437:426–31.

68. Corada M, Mariotti M, Thurston G, Smith K, Kunkel R, Brockhaus M, Lampugnani MG, Martin-Padura I, Stoppacciaro A, Ruco L, McDonald DM, Ward PA, Dejana E. Vascular endothelial-cadherin is an important determinant of microvascular integrity in vivo. Proc Natl Acad Sci U.S.A. 1999;96:9815–20.

69. Schulte D, Kuppers V, Dartsch N, Broermann A, Li H, Zarbock A, Kamenyeva O, Kiefer F, Khandoga A, Massberg S, Vestweber D. Stabilizing the VE-cadherin-catenin complex blocks leukocyte extravasation and vascular permeability. EMBO J. 2011;30:4157–70.

70. Wessel F, Winderlich M, Holm M, Frye M, Rivera-Galdos R, Vockel M, Linnepe R, Ipe U, Stadtmann A, Zarbock A, Nottebaum AF, Vestweber D. Leukocyte extravasation and vascular permeability are each controlled in vivo by different tyrosine residues of VE-cadherin. Nat Immunol. 2014;15:223–30.

71. Orsenigo F, Giampietro C, Ferrari A, Corada M, Galaup A, Sigismund S, Ristagno G, Maddaluno L, Koh GY, Franco D, Kurtcuoglu V, Poulikakos D, Baluk P, McDonald D, Grazia Lampugnani M, Dejana E. Phosphorylation of VE-cadherin is modulated by haemodynamic forces and contributes to the regulation of vascular permeability in vivo. Nat Commun. 2012;3:1208.

72. Adam AP, Sharenko AL, Pumiglia K, Vincent PA. Src-induced tyrosine phosphorylation of VE-cadherin is not sufficient to decrease barrier function of endothelial monolayers. J Biol Chem. 2010;285:7045–55.

73. Saito H, Minamiya Y, Saito S, Ogawa J. Endothelial rho and rho kinase regulate neutrophil migration via endothelial myosin light chain phosphorylation. J Leukoc Biol. 2002;72:829–36.

74. Broermann A, Winderlich M, Block H, Frye M, Rossaint J, Zarbock A, Cagna G, Linnepe R, Schulte D, Nottebaum AF, Vestweber D. Dissociation of VE-PTP from VE-cadherin is required for leukocyte extravasation and for VEGF-induced vascular permeability in vivo. J Exp Med. 2011;208:2393–401.

75. Schenkel AR, Mamdouh Z, Chen X, Liebman RM, Muller WA. CD99 plays a major role in the migration of monocytes through endothelial junctions. Nat Immunol. 2002;3:143–50.

76. Schenkel AR, Chew TW, Muller WA. Platelet endothelial cell adhesion molecule deficiency or blockade significantly reduces leukocyte emigration in a majority of mouse strains. J Immunol. 2004;173:6403–8.

77. Woodfin A, Voisin MB, Beyrau M, Colom B, Caille D, Diapouli FM, Nash GB, Chavakis T, Albelda SM, Rainger GE, Meda P, Imhof BA, Nourshargh S. The junctional adhesion molecule JAM-C regulates polarized transendothelial migration of neutrophils in vivo. Nat Immunol. 2011;12:761–9.

78. Chistiakov DA, Orekhov AN, Bobryshev YV. Endothelial barrier and its abnormalities in cardiovascular disease. Front Physiol. 2015;6:365.

79. Schnoor M, Alcaide P, Voisin MB, van Buul JD. Crossing the vascular wall: common and unique mechanisms exploited by different leukocyte subsets during extravasation. Mediat Inflamm. 2015;2015:946509.

80. Gerhardt H. VEGF and endothelial guidance in angiogenic sprouting. Organogenesis. 2008;4:241–6.

81. Inoue K, Slaton JW, Eve BY, Kim SJ, Perrotte P, Balbay MD, Yano S, Bar-Eli M, Radinsky R, Pettaway CA, Dinney CP. Interleukin 8 expression regulates tumorigenicity and metastases in androgen-independent prostate cancer. Clin Cancer Res. 2000;6:2104–19.

82. Xie Q, Sun Z, Chen M, Zhong Q, Yang T, Yi J. IL-8 up-regulates proliferative angiogenesis in ischemic myocardium in rabbits through phosphorylation of Akt/GSK-3beta(ser9) dependent pathways. Int J Clin Exp Med. 2015;8:12498–508.

83. Phng LK, Gerhardt H. Angiogenesis: a team effort coordinated by notch. Dev Cell. 2009;16:196–208.

84. Hellstrom M, Phng LK, Hofmann JJ, Wallgard E, Coultas L, Lindblom P, Alva J, Nilsson AK, Karlsson L, Gaiano N, Yoon K, Rossant J, Iruela-Arispe ML, Kalen M, Gerhardt H, Betsholtz C. Dll4 signalling through Notch1 regulates formation of tip cells during angiogenesis. Nature. 2007;445:776–80.

85. Fraisl P, Mazzone M, Schmidt T, Carmeliet P. Regulation of angiogenesis by oxygen and metabolism. Dev Cell. 2009;16:167–79.

86. Jakobsson L, Franco CA, Bentley K, Collins RT, Ponsioen B, Aspalter IM, Rosewell I, Busse M, Thurston G, Medvinsky A, Schulte-Merker S, Gerhardt H. Endothelial cells dynamically compete for the tip cell position during angiogenic sprouting. Nat Cell Biol. 2010;12:943–53.

87. Wacker A, Gerhardt H. Endothelial development taking shape. Curr Opin Cell Biol. 2011;23:676–85.

88. Blanco R, Gerhardt H. VEGF and notch in tip and stalk cell selection. Cold Spring Harb Perspect Med. 2013;3:a006569.

89. Outtz HH, Tattersall IW, Kofler NM, Steinbach N, Kitajewski J. Notch1 controls macrophage recruitment and notch signaling is activated at sites of endothelial cell anastomosis during retinal angiogenesis in mice. Blood. 2011;118:3436–9.

90. Grunewald M, Avraham I, Dor Y, Bachar-Lustig E, Itin A, Jung S, Chimenti S, Landsman L, Abramovitch R, Keshet E. VEGF-induced adult neovascularization: recruitment, retention, and role of accessory cells. Cell. 2006;124:175–89.

91. Tirziu D, Jaba IM, Yu P, Larrivee B, Coon BG, Cristofaro B, Zhuang ZW, Lanahan AA, Schwartz MA, Eichmann A, Simons M. Endothelial nuclear factor-kappaB-dependent regulation of arteriogenesis and branching. Circulation. 2012;126:2589–600.

92. Kako F, Gabunia K, Ray M, Kelemen SE, England RN, Kako B, Scalia RG, Autieri MV. Interleukin-19 induces angiogenesis in the absence of hypoxia by direct and indirect immune mechanisms. Am J Physiol Cell Physiol. 2016;310:C931–41.

93. Jain S, Gabunia K, Kelemen SE, Panetti TS, Autieri MV. The anti-inflammatory cytokine interleukin 19 is expressed by and angiogenic for human endothelial cells. Arterioscler Thromb Vasc Biol. 2011;31:167–75.

94. Dvorak HF, Brown LF, Detmar M, Dvorak AM. Vascular permeability factor/vascular endothelial growth factor, microvascular hyperpermeability, and angiogenesis. Am J Pathol. 1995;146:1029–39.

95. Rahimi N. VEGFR-1 and VEGFR-2: two non-identical twins with a unique physiognomy. Front Biosci. 2006;11:818–29.

96. Koch S, Tugues S, Li X, Gualandi L, Claesson-Welsh L. Signal transduction by vascular endothelial growth factor receptors. Biochem J. 2011;437:169–83.

97. Schweighofer B, Testori J, Sturtzel C, Sattler S, Mayer H, Wagner O, Bilban M, Hofer E. The VEGF-induced transcriptional response comprises gene clusters at the crossroad of angiogenesis and inflammation. Thromb Haemost. 2009;102:544–54.

98. Testori J, Schweighofer B, Helfrich I, Sturtzel C, Lipnik K, Gesierich S, Nasarre P, Hofer-Warbinek R, Bilban M, Augustin HG, Hofer E. The VEGF-regulated transcription factor HLX controls the expression of guidance cues and negatively regulates sprouting of endothelial cells. Blood. 2011;117:2735–44.

99. Choi YS, Choi HJ, Min JK, Pyun BJ, Maeng YS, Park H, Kim J, Kim YM, Kwon YG. Interleukin-33 induces angiogenesis and vascular permeability through ST2/TRAF6-mediated endothelial nitric oxide production. Blood. 2009;114:3117–26.

100. Stojkovic S, Kaun C, Basilio J, Rauscher S, Hell L, Krychtiuk KA, Bonstingl C, de Martin R, Groger M, Ay C, Holnthoner W, Eppel W, Neumayer C, Huk I, Huber K, Demyanets S, Wojta J. Tissue factor is induced by interleukin-33 in human endothelial cells: a new link between coagulation and inflammation. Sci Rep. 2016;6:25171.

101. Demyanets S, Konya V, Kastl SP, Kaun C, Rauscher S, Niessner A, Pentz R, Pfaffenberger S, Rychli K, Lemberger CE, de Martin R, Heinemann A, Huk I, Groger M, Maurer G, Huber K, Wojta J. Interleukin-33 induces expression of adhesion molecules and inflammatory activation in human endothelial cells and in human atherosclerotic plaques. Arterioscler Thromb Vasc Biol. 2011;31:2080–9.

102. Sturtzel C, Testori J, Schweighofer B, Bilban M, Hofer E. The transcription factor MEF2C negatively controls angiogenic sprouting of endothelial cells depending on oxygen. PLoS One. 2014;9:e101521.

103. Bhattacharjee G, Asplin IR, Wu SM, Gawdi G, Pizzo SV. The conformation-dependent interaction of alpha 2-macroglobulin with vascular endothelial growth factor. A novel mechanism of alpha 2-macroglobulin/growth factor binding. J Biol Chem. 2000;275:26806–11.

104. Winsauer G, de Martin R. Resolution of inflammation: intracellular feedback loops in the endothelium. Thromb Haemost. 2007;97:364–9.

105. Nauta TD, van den Broek M, Gibbs S, van der Pouw-Kraan TC, Oudejans CB, van Hinsbergh VW, Koolwijk P. Identification of HIF-2alpha-regulated genes that play a role in human microvascular endothelial sprouting during prolonged hypoxia in vitro. Angiogenesis. 2016;20(1):39–54.

106. Reimer KA, Lowe JE, Rasmussen MM, Jennings RB. The wavefront phenomenon of ischemic cell death. 1. Myocardial infarct size vs duration of coronary occlusion in dogs. Circulation. 1977;56:786–94.

107. Brugaletta S, Scalone G, Dantas AP, Ortega-Paz L, Garabito M, Roque M, Martin V, Masotti M, Freixa X, Sabate M. Endothelial function impairment in STEMI patients with out-of-hospital cardiac arrest under therapeutic hypothermia treatment. Int J Cardiol. 2017;232:70–5.

108. Willcox BJ, Curb JD, Rodriguez BL. Antioxidants in cardiovascular health and disease: key lessons from epidemiologic studies. Am J Cardiol. 2008;101:75D–86D.

109. Shafique E, Torina A, Reichert K, Colantuono B, Nur N, Zeeshan K, Ravichandran V, Liu Y, Feng J, Zeeshan K, Benjamin LE, Irani K, Harrington EO, Sellke FW, Abid MR. Mitochondrial redox plays a critical role in the paradoxical effects of NAPDH oxidase-derived ROS on coronary endothelium. Cardiovasc Res. 2017;113(2):234–46.

110. Gori T, von Henning U, Muxel S, Schaefer S, Fasola F, Vosseler M, Schnorbus B, Binder H, Parker JD, Munzel T. Both flow-mediated dilation and constriction are associated with changes in blood flow and shear stress: two complementary perspectives on endothelial function. Clin Hemorheol Microcirc. 2016;64(3):255–66.
111. Young A, Wu W, Sun W, Benjamin Larman H, Wang N, Li YS, Shyy JY, Chien S, Garcia-Cardena G. Flow activation of AMP-activated protein kinase in vascular endothelium leads to Kruppel-like factor 2 expression. Arterioscler Thromb Vasc Biol. 2009;29:1902–8.
112. Eshtehardi P, Brown AJ, Bhargava A, Costopoulos C, Hung OY, Corban MT, Hosseini H, Gogas BD, Giddens DP, Samady H. High wall shear stress and high-risk plaque: an emerging concept. Int J Cardiovasc Imaging. 2017; doi:10.1007/s10554-016-1055-1.
113. Dolan JM, Kolega J, Meng H. High wall shear stress and spatial gradients in vascular pathology: a review. Ann Biomed Eng. 2013;41:1411–27.
114. Heusch G. The coronary circulation as a target of cardioprotection. Circ Res. 2016;118:1643–58.
115. Johnsen J, Pryds K, Salman R, Lofgren B, Kristiansen SB, Botker HE. The remote ischemic preconditioning algorithm: effect of number of cycles, cycle duration and effector organ mass on efficacy of protection. Basic Res Cardiol. 2016;111:10.

Chapter 5
Immune Functions and Properties of Resident Cells in the Heart and Cardiovascular System: Pericytes

Teresa Kennedy-Lydon

5.1 Introduction

Pericytes were first described in the late nineteenth century, by two distinguished anatomists of the time, Carl Eberth and Charles Rouget, who independently noted distinct populations of adventitial cells adjacent to capillaries that were continuous with vascular smooth muscle cells (VSMCs) of arteries and veins. Subsequently, the Nobel laureate and physiologist August Krogh termed the cells Rouget cells and suggested they functioned as contractile cells of capillaries. Since then, Rouget cells have been renamed 'pericytes', and a myriad of research articles pertaining to pericyte cell anatomy, localisation and function(s) have followed.

Pericytes are singular smooth muscle-like cells residing on the abluminal side of the endothelium. As their name infers, pericytes are perivascular cells comprising of a cell body with several claw-like processes that extend from the cell body and 'wrap around' microvessels, including arterioles, capillaries and venules [1–4]. Pericytes originate from mesenchymal stem cells (MSCs), which migrate to the outer walls of capillaries. During development they have large, euchromatic nuclei which later become heterochromatic and round. Subsequently, their morphology has been described as a 'bump on a log' due to this distinctly round nucleus and restricted perinuclear cytoplasm [5, 6]. Pericytes share many properties with vascular smooth muscle cells (VSMCs), including the expression of smooth muscle α-actin and myosin [7–9]. They have cellular processes which extend from the cell body and wrap around and envelope the vessel, in primary, secondary and tertiary formations. Primary processes are aligned directly from cell bodies, secondary processes branch off from the primary processes and encircle the vessel vertically and tertiary processes branch off from secondary processes and grip the vessel (Fig. 5.1a)

T. Kennedy-Lydon
Heart Science, NHLI, Imperial College London, London, UK
e-mail: teresa.kennedy-lydon@imperial.ac.uk

© Springer International Publishing AG 2017   93
S. Sattler, T. Kennedy-Lydon (eds.), *The Immunology of Cardiovascular Homeostasis and Pathology*, Advances in Experimental Medicine and Biology 1003, DOI 10.1007/978-3-319-57613-8_5

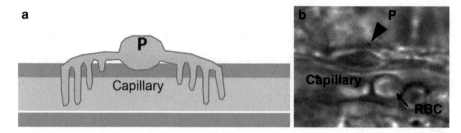

Fig. 5.1 Pericyte morphology: Schematic diagram depicting basic structure of a pericyte. (**a**) The 'bump-on-a-log' morphology is shown in a bright field image; (**b**) the pericytes are depicted by P, *arrowhead* adjacent to a vasa recta capillary filled with red blood cells (RBC, *arrow*) (Images adapted from [13])

[4]. These processes serve to increase the area of communication between pericytes and the vessel wall and indeed other juxtaposed vessels of the microcirculation.

Pericyte cell identification is complicated by their dynamic nature; as pericytes evolve continually throughout development, particularly during angiogenesis, they express markers at different intervals, and once a pericyte is committed to a particular tissue type, they cease to express immature or developmental markers [10]. Nonetheless, there are a number of accepted markers, namely, neuron-glial 2 (NG2), α-smooth muscle actin (α-SMA), desmin, regulator of G-protein signalling 5 (RGS-5) and platelet-derived growth factor receptor β (PDGFR β) [1, 10].

5.1.1 Function and Distribution

Pericytes have been identified in all organs and tissues in a wide range of species, and as such they have a variety of contrasting functional roles including vessel stabilisation, endothelial cell regulation, angiogenesis, phagocytosis and regulation of capillary blood flow [1–5].

Pericyte regulation of capillary blood flow was first described by Krogh as early as 1929 and was later confirmed by other studies investigating the ultrastructure of these ubiquitous cells. Furthermore, the concept of pericyte regulation of capillary blood flow has gained momentum with many studies [6, 11–14].

Pericytes contain the contractile proteins α-SMA, tropomyosin and myosin. These proteins are also found in smooth muscle cells, and it is suggested that they contribute to pericyte contractile function [1, 15]. Furthermore, receptor sites for cholinergic (nicotinic and muscarinic)[14, 16, 17] and adrenergic (α-2) receptors are present on pericytes, further enhancing their contractile ability. Studies have shown that cholinergic responses in pericytes cause contraction, whilst adrenergic responses result in relaxation [14].

Similarly to vascular smooth muscle cells (VSMCs), pericyte constriction is regulated by the intracellular calcium ($[Ca^{2+}]_i$) concentration [18]. This was further demonstrated by the removal of extracellular calcium from electrically stimulated pericytes in the central nervous system (CNS) which inhibited constriction [6]. It is suggested that a rise of $[Ca^{2+}]_i$ can depolarise the pericyte cell membrane from resting voltage (usually between -35 and -60) to a voltage that stimulates L-type voltage-operated calcium channels (VOCCs) [18]. A rise of $[Ca^{2+}]_i$ can activate downstream signalling pathways (such as myosin light chain kinases (MLCK) and mitogen-activated protein (MAP) kinases) via activation of intracellular calcium stores that culminate in alignment of the actin filaments along pericyte foot processes, resulting in constriction. Conversely, pericyte dilation is mediated by hyperpolarisation brought about by a decrease in $[Ca^{2+}]_i$. Hyperpolarisation in VSMCs is brought about by activation of potassium channels, which is also suggested as the most likely cause for pericyte dilation. Pericytes express a number of potassium channels including voltage-gated, inward-rectifying (K_{IR}) [19] and calcium-activated [20] channels. Activation of these channels reduces VOCC activity, thereby hyperpolarising the cell and inducing relaxation.

As well as modulating vascular tone, pericytes also play an integral role in constructing vessels; during development they are involved in vasculogenesis and post-development in angiogenesis [21]. Vasculogenesis is initiated by the clustering of primitive vascular cells which give rise to tube-like formations, thus defining the vasculature structure. When enveloped in the organ tissue, these tube-like structures, which contain endothelial cells, then recruit mural cells, i.e. pericytes, and begin organising the vasculature tree for the specific tissue in which they reside. Recruitment of pericytes by these primitive endothelial cells is not yet fully understood; however, it is suggested that there is autocrine or paracrine signalling—possibly mediated by soluble factors—as is the case for recruitment of pericytes during angiogenesis [2].

Angiogenesis describes the sprouting and extension of the existing vasculature to form new vessels. This complex process involves the detachment of pericytes from the vessel in order to allow the endothelium to form new tube-like structures. Once the new structure is in place, pericytes reattach and envelope the vessel, thus providing the extended vessel with stability. Reattachment of pericytes also encourages maturation of the vessel [1]. Throughout these processes there is constant dialogue between endothelial cells and pericytes. Firstly, during the 'sprouting' phase, endothelial cells secrete proteases which digest the basement membrane. This creates the space required for the proliferating endothelial cells. Vascular endothelial growth factor (VEGF) is thought to stimulate endothelial cells into secreting these proteases [22]. Incidentally, VEGF receptor activation will not occur if pericyte-endothelial cell communication is disrupted [23]. Upon cessation of endothelial cell proliferation, further soluble factors are secreted—this time to recruit pericytes to the newly formed vessel. Factors proposed to be involved in this process are angiopoietins (important for vessel maturation) and sphingosie-1-phosphate-1 (important for vessel stability) [24]. However, the most crucial factor in this process is PDGFR β. Indeed, mice with disrupted PDGF B—PDGFR β signalling have a distinct lack of pericytes, and as result embryo lethality is often reported due to formation of microhaemorrhages [25–27].

Pericytes also have roles outside of the vasculature. For example, CNS pericytes differentiate into macrophages and can also acquire phagocytic capabilities. These properties imply a role for pericytes in maintaining immune defence, essentially for protecting the blood-brain barrier (BBB), but in addition they also highlight the plasticity of pericytes. Renal studies have implicated pericytes as a source of myofibroblasts [28]. Furthermore, pericytes have been described as multipotent and have been shown to differentiate into adipocytes and osteoblasts. In addition, skin pericytes have been implicated in regeneration through modification of the extracellular matrix (ECM) and promotion of epidermal tissue renewal [29].

The number of pericytes along a vessel wall is thought to be determined by the functional demand of the tissue in which they reside [1, 3, 11]. Moreover, pericyte density has been shown to differ between tissues, pericyte density being greater in the kidney than in other tissues, such as the CNS and retina [1]. Interestingly, within the kidney, pericyte density also varies, with a greater density reported in the outer medulla compared with the inner medulla [3, 11]. In addition, it has previously been reported that renal pericyte density increases to meet the metabolic demands required for normal renal function [15].

5.1.2   Communication with Other Cells

Pericytes exist within close proximity of the underlying endothelium (approximately <20 nm apart), and their interaction is described as a 'peg and socket' arrangement (Fig. 1b). In addition, pericytes and endothelial cells also form gap junctions, tight junctions and adhesion plaques [2, 10]. This arrangement allows communication between pericytes and endothelial cells, other pericytes and other surrounding cell types in the tissues that they inhabit. For example, pericytes in the CNS have been shown to communicate with astrocytes, neurons, smooth muscle cells and other pericytes [5, 6, 30]. Additionally, the transmission of contractile forces from pericytes to the endothelium is considered to be attributed to gap junctions and adhesion plaques, as they contain cell adhesion molecules, fibronectin, connexins and N-cadherin [5, 22].

5.1.3   Pericytes and the Immune System

Pericytes can facilitate the trafficking of immune cells across the blood barrier into neighbouring tissues and have even been described as providing the 'highway' for immune cell migration [31]. In response to danger-associated molecular patterns (DAMPs) (see Chaps. 1, 2 and 3 for more detailed description), pericytes release chemokines and soluble mediators and express chemotactic receptors allowing them to modulate the immune response. Advanced imaging techniques have allowed pericyte-immune cell interactions to be deciphered [32]. Here, Proebstl *et al.* have shown how pericyte morphology adapts to facilitate neutrophil migration, a process that is closely controlled. Firstly, pericytes attract neutrophils via secretion of interleukin-8 (IL-8). Although IL-8 secretion may not be so crucial, neutrophils appear to be attracted specifically to pericyte gap junctions which lack the basement membrane components and therefore provide a less complex pathway for neutrophils to negate. These imaging studies have shown that the site at which neutrophils migrate is highly selective, and once the neutrophils begin to pass between pericytes, pericytes themselves undergo a conformational change to enlarge the gap and allow passage of larger numbers of neutrophils [32]. Further *in vivo* investigations have shown these morphological adaptations are in response to inflammatory stimuli, namely, tumour necrosis factor (TNF) and interleukin-1β (IL-1β) [32]. Equally, Stark *et al.* have shown that pericytes respond to a pro-inflammatory environment by mediating the passage of neutrophils and macrophages [33]. Here, the response of skin pericytes to a sterile inflammatory stimulus was evaluated. Skin pericytes were found to display a pro-inflammatory phenotype triggered by expression of adhesion molecules and specifically secretion of macrophage migration-inhibitory factor (MIF). Using intravital two-photon microscopy, pericytes were observed to elicit the chemotactic migration of interstitial neutrophils and macrophages following extravasation from postcapillary venules, evoking a pericyte-leukocyte cross talk facilitated by the intercellular adhesion molecule ICAM-1 and MIF [33]. Effectively, this unique interaction guides cells of the innate immune system to the site of injury allowing for assessment of the damaged tissue and an immediate response. Moreover, stimulation of pericytes with interferon-γ (IFN-γ) results in major histocompatibility complex II (MHC II) expression which can lead to T-cell activation. Indeed, Stark *et al.* have shown that pericytes upregulate ICAM-1 expression, which encourages T-cell activation in damaged tissues. Pericytes, specifically CNS pericytes, have been reported to behave in a phagocytic manner. A study by Balabanov *et al.* showed that CNS pericytes can phagocytose polystyrene beads and can also express macrophage antigens ED-2 and CD11b [30]. Activated pericytes also attract blood monocytes to the site of injury [33]. However, it should be noted that pericytes have a limited capacity as macrophages and it is more likely that they are responsible for maintaining blood-brain barrier (BBB) homeostasis than eliciting a full macrophage immune response. Also, to date, CNS pericytes are the only population reported to take on macrophage functions, and it is likely that this is a tissue-specific response as the CNS has a relatively low macrophage population to protect it from immune-associated damage. Recently, brain pericytes have been shown to respond to inflammatory cytokines by upregulating expression of inflammatory proteins [34]. Stimulation with TNF-α, IL-1β, IFN-γ or lipopolysaccharides (LPS) results in increased expression of cyclooxygenase-2 (COX-2). IL-1β and LPS stimulation result in increased expression of inducible nitric oxide (iNOS) and reactive oxygen and nitrogen species, whilst stimulation with IFN-γ was found to evoke expression of major histocompatibility complex II (MHC II) molecules and CD68 [34]. The pericyte response was found to be depended on the type of stimulus, concentration and duration of exposure. Taken together, these data suggest a role for brain pericytes in modulating both the innate and adaptive immune response [34], which again points to a pericyte-mediated protective mechanism in the brain and CNS.

Similarly, lung pericyte-like cells have also been shown to modulate the immune response in vitro [35]. Here, following exposure to lung bronchoalveolar lavage fluid, pericyte-like cells expressed Toll-like receptors (TLR) in addition to upregulating chemokine expression, including Cxcl2, CCl2 and IL-6. LPS-induced lung inflammation in vivo caused an increase of pericyte-like cells expressing IL-6, CXCL1, CCL2/MCP-1 and ICAM-1. Interestingly, depletion of lung pericyte-like cells resulted in a muted immune response in comparison to control following injury [35].

Taken together, these studies highlight a key role for pericytes in modulating the immune response and also highlight the importance of their barrier function. Due to their unique perivascular location, pericytes are aptly located to regulate cell migration, and their role as a barrier control unit appears to be crucial to the immune-led response and could play a pivotal role in determining the extent of tissue damage evoked by immune defences.

5.1.4 Pericytes and Pathologies

The role of pericytes in pathologies has been described in many organs, and pericyte dysfunction has been implicated in pathological conditions such as tumour angiogenesis, atherosclerosis and Alzheimer's disease [36–38]. In addition, loss of retinal pericyte function is an instrumental factor in the development of diabetic retinopathy [18, 39, 40].

Pericytes have further been implicated in the pathogenesis of renal fibrosis and progression of chronic kidney disease [41, 42]. The detachment and migration of pericytes from renal microvessels and their subsequent differentiation to myofibroblasts (defined as fibroblasts with contractile capabilities) are suggested as the mechanism by which pericytes contribute to renal fibrosis causing vessel destabilisation, rarefaction and loss of capillaries leading to an ischaemic and a pro-fibrotic environment. It is reported that this enhanced myofibroblast population can increase the production of extracellular matrix (ECM) components—a key factor in the development of interstitial fibrosis [43, 44]. Moreover genetic fate-mapping studies have implicated pericytes as the myofibroblast progenitor [28, 45]. Although, it is worth mentioning that pericytes are not recognised as being the only source of the enhanced myofibroblast population, other sources such as differentiation of resident fibroblasts [44, 46] and epithelial cells undergoing epithelial to mesenchymal transition (EMT) have also been identified as potential sources [28, 44, 46, 47]. Due to the lack of specific markers, identifying the exact source of the myofibroblast population is difficult *in vivo* or *ex vivo,* but the development of more selective markers for these cells, or more sophisticated transgenic animal models, may help to determine the role of pericytes in fibrosis.

5.1.5 Cardiac Pericytes

The cardiac pericyte (CP) population is rapidly gaining attention, particularly for their potential as novel therapeutic targets. CPs have been identified in the epicardium and myocardium in murine and human neonatal and adult hearts [48, 49]. Recently CPs have been reported to occupy 5% of the total non-myocyte cell population of the heart [50]. Similar to fibroblasts, CPs appear to be heterogeneous, with distinct populations isolated from microvessels and the adventitia [10, 51, 52]. Expansion studies have demonstrated that CPs can give rise to cardiomyocytes and smooth muscle cells, hence the current interest in determining their therapeutic value [48, 53].

To date pericytes have been shown to be beneficial to the repair processes following ischaemic injury. Injection of saphenous vein pericytes (SVPs) to the peri-infarct area resulted in improved cardiac function by reducing scar formation, cardiomyocyte apoptosis and interstitial fibrosis and stimulating angiogenesis [54]. Further investigation into the mechanism of SVP-mediated effects showed that these benefits were due to their paracrine secretion of a microRNA-132, which suppresses the differentiation of fibroblasts to myofibroblasts, thereby reducing the extent of fibrosis following injury [54, 55]. Pericytes derived from human tissues, e.g. umbilical cord and smooth muscle, have also been successfully transplanted to the murine myocardium following ischaemic injury, and these populations have also improved cardiac function [48, 55]. Transplantation of human umbilical cord pericytes to the myocardium following myocardial infarction (MI) has been shown to reduce the inflammatory response by inhibiting the migration of macrophages to the infarcted area. Further in vitro investigations have demonstrated that pericyte-conditioned media suppress the growth of macrophages under both normoxic and hypoxic conditions [55].

CPs also maintain the ability to repair cardiac function following MI. A study by Chen et al. found that a subpopulation of CPs could generate Troponin I and T- and connexin 43-positive CMs when injected into the left ventricle postischaemic injury, thus demonstrating the cardiac-specific commitment of the CP population [48]. Interestingly, CPs are the most abundant stem cell population in the heart, and unlike other stem cell populations, they do not form teratogenic tumours. This coupled with their ability to improve cardiac function makes them an optimal pool for autologous transplantation. Moreover, methods for CP isolation have been shown to be reproducible and reliable. Taken together, CPs pose an exciting avenue for the therapeutics industry to pursue.

However, it should be noted that the definition of pericytes as mesenchymal stem cells (MSCs) has been challenged. An inducible cre Tbx 18 mouse model was used to trace pericytes in different tissues (including cardiac, CNS, skin and lung) during different pathological settings (including high-fat diet and transverse aortic constriction). In each pathological environment, pericytes maintained their identity and did not significantly contribute to other cell lineages [56]. However, in terms of cardiac regeneration, the inability of resident stem cell populations to replenish cell populations post injury is largely accepted, and as such therapeutic interventions such as intra-myocardial injections of transplanted cells are routinely employed to promote the regenerative capabilities of these cell niches. Nevertheless, this study does highlight the need for caution when championing the potential *in vivo* benefit of largely *ex vivo/in vitro* models.

Additionally, it has been suggested that CPs may also potentiate ischaemic injury by preventing reflow to vessels that have been occluded [49]. The no-reflow phenomenon is well established in cerebral tissue where vessels that suffer an ischaemic insult cannot re-establish flow despite receiving adequate perfusion. In this scenario, the vessel diameter is narrowed due to swelling of endothelial cells and attachment of leukocytes to the vessel wall in response to the initial loss of perfusion. Pericytes residing on these vessels further reduce the diameter by constricting the vessel. It is possible that CPs respond in a similar manner following MI, which could potentially increase the degree of ischaemic damage [49]. Here again, CPs offer an attractive therapeutic target—encouraging dilation of pericytes could help with reperfusion of vessels and thereby limit the damage to the surrounding myocardium. Indeed, establishing reperfusion following MI is a critical step towards the repair/regeneration processes.

Pericytes have also been implicated in the progression of atherosclerosis. In response to the pro-inflammatory environment and athero-altered LDL, they accumulate lipids, and this can trigger proliferation resulting in thickening of the intima and progression to fibrotic plaques [57–59]. Pericytes can also initiate neogenesis around the developing plaques, thereby enhancing growth of the plaques [59].

5.2 Conclusion

Here we have discussed pericyte physiology from their first discovery to their latest associations in cardiac- and immune-related research. Pericytes are a diverse cell type capable of fulfilling many roles as determined by the tissue in which they reside. Indeed, their functional demand also determines their density and distribution within a tissue. Their role in angiogenesis is well established with the lack of pericyte coverage proving detrimental to the tube formation process. In addition to their crucial participation in angiogenesis, it is rapidly becoming apparent that pericytes play a pivotal role in the immune response. Largely responsible for attracting immune cells to the site of injury, they are also responsible for regulating the rate at which immune cells can migrate into the damaged tissue. Whilst investigations into the role of CPs in both homeostasis and pathological states are in their infancy, the density and distribution of CPs predispose them to having a defining role in cardiac disease. Indeed, we eagerly await the defining studies on CPs and immune responses following cardiac injury.

References

1. Bergers G, Song S. The role of pericytes in blood-vessel formation and maintenance. Neuro-Oncology. 2005;7(4):452–64. doi:10.1215/S1152851705000232.
2. Hirschi K, D'amore PA. Pericytes in the microvasculature. Cardiovasc Res. 1996;32(4):687–98.
3. Kennedy-Lydon TM, Crawford C, Wildman SP, Peppiatt-Wildman CM. Renal pericytes: regulators of medullary blood flow. Acta Physiol. 2012;207(2):212–25. doi:10.1111/apha.12026.
4. Shepro D, Morel NM. Pericyte physiology. FASEB J. 1993;7:1031.
5. Dore-Duffy P, Katychev A, Wang X, Van Buren E. CNS microvascular pericytes exhibit multipotential stem cell activity. J Cereb Blood Flow Metab. 2006;26(5):613–24. doi:10.1038/sj.jcbfm.9600272.
6. Peppiatt CM, Howarth C, Mobbs P, Attwell D. Bidirectional control of CNS capillary diameter by pericytes. Nature. 2006;443(7112):700–4. doi:10.1038/nature05193.
7. Herman IM, D'amore PA. Microvascular pericytes contain muscle and nonmuscle actins. J Cell Biol. 1985;101:43.
8. Joyce NC, Haire MF, Palade GE. Contractile proteins in pericytes. I. Immunoperoxidase localization of tropomyosin. J Cell Biol. 1985;100(5):1379–86.
9. Nehls V, Drenckhahn D. Heterogeneity of microvascular pericytes for smooth-muscle type alpha-actin. J Cell Biol. 1991;113(1):147–54.
10. Armulik A, Genové G, Betsholtz C. Pericytes: developmental, physiological, and pathological perspectives, problems, and promises. Dev Cell. 2011;21(2):193–215. doi:10.1016/j.devcel.2011.07.001.
11. Crawford C, Kennedy-Lydon T, Sprott C, Desai T. An intact kidney slice model to investigate vasa recta properties and function in situ. Nephron Physiol. 2012;120:17. doi:10.1159/000339110.
12. Crawford C, Kennedy-Lydon TM, Callaghan H, Sprott C, Simmons RL, Sawbridge L, Syme HM, Unwin RJ, Wildman SSP, Peppiatt-Wildman CM. Extracellular nucleotides affect pericyte-mediated regulation of rat in situ vasa recta diameter. Acta Physiol (Oxf). 2011;202(3):241–51. doi:10.1111/j.1748-1716.2011.02310.x.
13. Kennedy-Lydon T, Crawford C, Wildman SS, Peppiatt-Wildman CM. Nonsteroidal anti-inflammatory drugs alter vasa recta diameter via pericytes. Am J Physiol Renal Physiol. 2015;309(7):F648–57. doi:10.1152/ajprenal.00199.2015.
14. Rucker HK, Wynder HJ, Thomas WE. Cellular mechanisms of CNS pericytes. Brain Res Bull. 2000;51(5):363–9.
15. Park F, Mattson DL, Roberts LA, Cowley AW. Evidence for the presence of smooth muscle alpha-actin within pericytes of the renal medulla. Am J Phys. 1997;273(5):R1742–8.
16. Elfont RM, Sundaresan PR, Sladek CD. Adrenergic-receptors on cerebral microvessels - pericyte contribution. Am J Phys. 1989;256(1):R224–30.
17. Ferrari-Dileo G, Davis EB. Effects of cholinergic and adrenergic agonists on adenylate cyclase activity of retinal microvascular pericytes in culture. Invest Ophthalmol Vis Sci. 1992;33(1):42.
18. Sakagami K, Wu DM, Puro DG. Physiology of rat retinal pericytes: modulation of ion channel activity by serum-derived molecules. J Physiol. 1999;521(Pt 3):637–50.
19. von Beckerath N, Nees S, Neumann FJ, Krebs B, Juchem G, Schömig A. An inward rectifier and a voltage-dependent K+ current in single, cultured pericytes from bovine heart. Cardiovasc Res. 2000;46(3):569–78.
20. Berweck S, Lepple-Wienhues A, Stöss M, Wiederholt M. Large conductance calcium-activated potassium channels in cultured retinal pericytes under normal and high-glucose conditions. Arch Eur J Physiol. 1994;427(1–2):9–16.
21. Carmeliet P. Angiogenesis in life, disease and medicine. Nature. 2005;438(7070):932–6. doi:10.1038/nature04478.
22. Gerhardt H, Golding M, Fruttiger M, Ruhrberg C, Lundkvist A, Abramsson A, Jeltsch M, et al. VEGF guides angiogenic sprouting utilizing endothelial tip cell filopodia. J Cell Biol. 2003;161(6):1163–77. doi:10.1083/jcb.200302047.

23. Franco M, Roswall P, Cortez E, Hanahan D, Pietras K. Pericytes promote endothelial cell survival through induction of autocrine VEGF-A signaling and Bcl-w expression. Blood. 2011;118(10):2906–17. doi:10.1182/blood-2011-01-331694.
24. Jain RK. Molecular regulation of vessel maturation. Nat Med. 2003;9(6):685–93. doi:10.1038/nm0603-685.
25. Hellström M, Gerhardt H, Kalén M, Li X, Eriksson U, Wolburg H, Betsholtz C. Lack of pericytes leads to endothelial hyperplasia and abnormal vascular morphogenesis. J Cell Biol. 2001;153(3):543–53.
26. Levéen P, Pekny M, Gebre-Medhin S, Swolin B, Larsson E, Betsholtz C. Mice deficient for PDGF B show renal, cardiovascular, and hematological abnormalities. Genes Dev. 1994;8(16):1875–87.
27. Lindahl P, Johansson BR, Levéen P, Betsholtz C. Pericyte loss and microaneurysm formation in PDGF-B-deficient mice. Science. 1997;277(5323):242–5.
28. Humphreys BD, Lin S-L, Kobayashi A, Hudson TE, Nowlin BT, Bonventre JV, Todd Valerius M, McMahon AP, Duffield JS. Fate tracing reveals the pericyte and not epithelial origin of myofibroblasts in kidney fibrosis. Am J Pathol. 2010;176(1):85–97. doi:10.2353/ajpath.2010.090517.
29. Paquet-Fifield S, Schlüter H, Li A, Aitken T, Gangatirkar P, Blashki D, Koelmeyer R, et al. A role for pericytes as microenvironmental regulators of human skin tissue regeneration. J Clin Investig. 2009;119:2795. doi:10.1172/JCI38535DS1.
30. Balabanov R, Washington R, Wagnerova J. CNS microvascular pericytes express macrophage-like function, cell surface integrin αM, and macrophage marker ED-2. Microvascular Res. 1996;52:127.
31. Lam P-y, Huttenlocher A. Interstitial leukocyte migration in vivo. Curr Opin Cell Biol. 2013;25(5):650–8. doi:10.1016/j.ceb.2013.05.007.
32. Proebstl D, Voisin M-B, Woodfin A, Whiteford J, D'Acquisto F, Jones GE, Rowe D, Nourshargh S. Pericytes support neutrophil subendothelial cell crawling and breaching of venular walls in vivo. J Exp Med. 2012;209(6):1219–34. doi:10.1084/jem.20111622.
33. Stark K, Eckart A, Haidari S, Tirniceriu A, Lorenz M, von Brühl M-L, Gärtner F, et al. Capillary and arteriolar pericytes attract innate leukocytes exiting through venules and 'instruct' them with pattern-recognition and motility programs. Nat Immunol. 2012;14(1):41–51. doi:10.1038/ni.2477.
34. Pieper C, Marek JJ, Unterberg M, Schwerdtle T, Galla H-J. Brain capillary pericytes contribute to the immune defense in response to cytokines or LPS in vitro. Brain Res. 2014;1550(March):1–8. doi:10.1016/j.brainres.2014.01.004.
35. Hung CF, Mittelsteadt KL, Brauer R, McKinney BL, Hallstrand TS, Parks WC, Chen P, et al. Lung pericyte-like cells are functional immune sentinel cells. Am J Physiol Lung Cell Mol Physiol. 2017; doi:10.1152/ajplung.00349.2016.
36. Bell RD, Winkler EA, Sagare AP, Singh I, LaRue B, Deane R, Zlokovic BV. Pericytes control key neurovascular functions and neuronal phenotype in the adult brain and during brain aging. Neuron. 2010;68(3):409–27. doi:10.1016/j.neuron.2010.09.043.
37. Benjamin LE, Golijanin D, Itin A, Pode D, Keshet E. Selective ablation of immature blood vessels in established human tumors follows vascular endothelial growth factor withdrawal. J Clin Investig. 1999;103(2):159–65. doi:10.1172/JCI5028.
38. Morikawa S, Baluk P, Kaidoh T, Haskell A, Jain RK, McDonald DM. Abnormalities in pericytes on blood vessels and endothelial sprouts in tumors. Am J Pathol. 2002;160(3):985–1000. doi:10.1016/S0002-9440(10)64920-6.
39. Cai J, Boulton M. The pathogenesis of diabetic retinopathy: old concepts and new questions. Eye (Lond). 2002;16(3):242–60. doi:10.1038/sj/eye/6700133.
40. Tu Z, Li Y, Smith DS, Sheibani N, Huang S, Kern T, Lin F. Retinal pericytes inhibit activated T cell proliferation. Invest Ophthalmol Vis Sci. 2011;52(12):9005–10. doi:10.1167/iovs.11-8008.

41. Duffield JS, Humphreys BD. Origin of new cells in the adult kidney: results from genetic labeling techniques. Kidney Int. 2011;79(5):494–501. doi:10.1038/ki.2010.338.
42. Smith SW, Chand S, Savage COS. Biology of the renal pericyte. Nephrol Dial Transplant. 2012;27(6):2149–55. doi:10.1093/ndt/gfs134.
43. Kida Y, Duffield JS. Pivotal role of pericytes in kidney fibrosis. Clin Exp Pharmacol Physiol. 2011;38(7):467–73. doi:10.1111/j.1440-1681.2011.05531.x.
44. Liu Y. Cellular and molecular mechanisms of renal fibrosis. Nat Rev Nephrol. 2011;7(12):684–96. doi:10.1038/nrneph.2011.149.
45. Lin S-L, Kisseleva T, Brenner DA, Duffield JS. Pericytes and perivascular fibroblasts are the primary source of collagen-producing cells in obstructive fibrosis of the kidney. Am J Pathol. 2008;173(6):1617–27. doi:10.2353/ajpath.2008.080433.
46. Wada T, Sakai N, Matsushima K, Kaneko S. Fibrocytes: a new insight into kidney fibrosis. Kidney Int. 2007;72(3):269–73. doi:10.1038/sj.ki.5002325.
47. Kriz W, Kaissling B, Le Hir M. Epithelial-mesenchymal transition (EMT) in kidney fibrosis: fact or fantasy? J Clin Investig. 2011;121(2):468–74. doi:10.1172/JCI44595.
48. Chen WCW, Baily JE, Corselli M, Díaz ME, Sun B, Xiang G, Gray GA, Huard J, Péault B. Human myocardial pericytes: multipotent mesodermal precursors exhibiting cardiac specificity. Stem Cells. 2015;33(2):557–73. doi:10.1002/stem.1868.
49. O'Farrell FM, Attwell D. A role for pericytes in coronary no-reflow. Nat Rev Cardiol. 2014;11(7):427–32. doi:10.1038/nrcardio.2014.58.
50. Pinto AR, Ilinykh A, Ivey MJ, Kuwabara JT, D'Antoni ML, Debuque R, Chandran A, et al. Revisiting cardiac cellular composition. Circ Res. 2016;118(3):400–9. doi:10.1161/CIRCRESAHA.115.307778.
51. Birbrair A, Tan Z, Files DC, Mannava S, Smith T, Wang Z-M, Messi ML, Mintz A, Delbono O. Type-1 pericytes accumulate after tissue injury and produce collagen in an organ-dependent manner. Stem Cell Res Ther. 2014;5(6):122. doi:10.1186/scrt512.
52. Corselli M, Chen C-W, Sun B, Solomon Y, Peter Rubin J, Péault B. The tunica adventitia of human arteries and veins as a source of mesenchymal stem cells. Stem Cells Dev. 2012;21(8):1299–308. doi:10.1089/scd.2011.0200.
53. Avolio E, Rodriguez-Arabaolaza I, Spencer HL, Riu F, Mangialardi G, Slater SC, Rowlinson J, et al. Expansion and characterization of neonatal cardiac pericytes provides a novel cellular option for tissue engineering in congenital heart disease. J Am Heart Assoc. 2015;4(6):e002043. doi:10.1161/JAHA.115.002043.
54. Katare RG, Madeddu P. Pericytes from human veins for treatment of myocardial ischemia. Trends Cardiovasc Med. 2013;23:66. doi:10.1016/j.tcm.2012.09.002.
55. Chen C-W, Okada M, Proto JD, Gao X, Sekiya N, Beckman SA, Corselli M, et al. Human pericytes for ischemic heart repair. Stem Cells. 2013;31(2):305–16. doi:10.1002/stem.1285.
56. Guimarães-Camboa N, Cattaneo P, Sun Y, Moore-Morris T, Yusu G, Dalton ND, Rockenstein E, et al. Pericytes of multiple organs do not behave as mesenchymal stem cells in vivo. Cell Stem Cell. 2017;20:345. doi:10.1016/j.stem.2016.12.006.
57. Boström K, Watson KE, Horn S, Wortham C. Bone morphogenetic protein expression in human atherosclerotic lesions. J Clin Investig. 1993;91:1800.
58. Orekhov AN, Andreeva ER, Andrianova IV, Bobryshev YV. Peculiarities of cell composition and cell proliferation in different type atherosclerotic lesions in carotid and coronary arteries. Atherosclerosis. 2010;212(2):436–43. doi:10.1016/j.atherosclerosis.2010.07.009.
59. Orekhov AN, Bobryshev YV, Chistiakov DA. The complexity of cell composition of the intima of large arteries: focus on pericyte-like cells. Cardiovasc Res. 2014;103(4):438–51. doi:10.1093/cvr/cvu168.

Chapter 6
The Role of Cardiac Tissue Macrophages in Homeostasis and Disease

Alexei Ilinykh and Alexander R. Pinto

List of Abbreviations

BrdU	Bromodeoxyuridine
Ccr	C–C chemokine receptor
CD	Cluster of differentiation
CDC	Cardiosphere-derived cell
Chi3l3	Chitinase 3-like 3
CSF-1	Colony-stimulating factor-1
Csf1r	Colony-stimulating factor 1 receptor
cTM	Cardiac tissue macrophage
Cx_3cr1	C-X3-C chemokine receptor 1
Cxcl	Chemokine (C-X-C motif) ligand
DAMPs	Damage-associated molecular patterns
DAPI	4′,6-Diamidino-2-phenylindole
EMP	Erythromyeloid progenitor
GFP	Green fluorescent protein
HSC	Hematopoietic stem cell

A. Ilinykh
Australian Regenerative Medicine Institute, Monash University, Melbourne, VIC, Australia

A.R. Pinto (✉)
Australian Regenerative Medicine Institute, Monash University, Melbourne, VIC, Australia

The Jackson Laboratory, 600 Main Street, Bar Harbor, ME, USA
e-mail: alex.pinto@jax.org

© Springer International Publishing AG 2017
S. Sattler, T. Kennedy-Lydon (eds.), *The Immunology of Cardiovascular Homeostasis and Pathology*, Advances in Experimental Medicine and Biology 1003, DOI 10.1007/978-3-319-57613-8_6

IGF-1   Insulin-like growth factor-1
IL   Interleukin
IRF5   Interferon regulatory factor 5
Ly6C   Lymphocyte antigen 6 complex, locus C
Ly6G   Lymphocyte antigen 6 complex, locus G
Lyve-1   Lymphatic vessel endothelial hyaluronan receptor-1
MHCII   Major histocompatibility complex type class II
MI   Myocardial infarction
MIF   Migration inhibitory factor
Mrc1   Mannose receptor, C type 1
MSC   Mesenchymal stem cell
NO   Nitric oxide
PAMPs   Pathogen-associated molecular patterns
PDGF   Platelet-derived growth factor
Retnla   Resistin-like alpha
TGFβ   Transforming growth factor β
TNFα   Tumor necrosis factor α
VEGF   Vascular endothelial growth factor
WT1   Wilms' tumor 1

6.1 Identifying the Cardiac Tissue Macrophage

How cTMs are identified is an important starting point to understand cTM biology. Broadly speaking, cTMs are cardiac resident leukocytes that specialize in phagocytosis [1]. The principal tool for identifying and characterizing cTMs has been by flow cytometry. Here, the cell isolation protocols, antibody panels, and gating strategies have varied widely among studies characterizing cTMs (summarized in Table 6.1). The first systematic characterization of cTMs was conducted by analyzing GFP-expressing cells in hearts of adult $Cx_3cr1^{GFP/+}$ reporter mice [2]. These mice have been widely utilized to identify macrophages and dendritic cells in a number of tissues [7], and, accordingly, we and others have found that in the heart Cx_3cr1 is exclusively expressed in myeloid cells [2, 3]. Furthermore, this early characterization identified GFP+ cells of $Cx_3cr1^{GFP/+}$ mouse hearts as expressing canonical macrophage markers such as F4/80, MHCII, and CD14 [2]. In addition, gene expression profiling by gene arrays identified these cells as resembling alternatively activated macrophages with high expression of IL-10, IGF-1, Mrc1, and intermediate expression of Ly6C/G (GR-1).

Table 6.1 Classification of cTMs by flow cytometry

Publication	Number of subsets	Phenotypes of macrophage subsets
Pinto et al. [2]	1 (total cTM population)	*CD45, CD11b, GFP (Cx₃cr1ᴳᶠᴾ)*
Pinto et al. [3]	3	*CD45⁺CD11b⁺GFPʰⁱMrc1⁻ (Cx₃cr1ᴳᶠᴾ)* *CD45⁺CD11b⁺GFPʰⁱMrc1⁺* *CD45⁺CD11b⁺GFPˡᵒMrc1⁺*
Heidt et al. [4]	1 (total cTM population)	*CD45ʰⁱCD11b⁺F4/80ʰⁱLy6Cˡᵒ*
Epelman et al. [5]	3	*CD45⁺CD11b⁺F4/80⁺Auto⁺Ly6c⁻MHCIIʰⁱ* *CD45⁺CD11b⁺F4/80⁺Auto⁺Ly6c⁻MHCIIˡᵒ* *CD45⁺CD11b⁺F4/80⁺Auto⁺Ly6c⁺MHCII⁺ᐟ⁻* *CD45⁺CD11b⁺F4/80⁺Auto⁻Ly6c⁺MHCII⁻(monocyte)*
Molawi et al. [6]	4	*CD11b⁺Ly6cˡᵒCD11cˡᵒᐟⁱⁿᵗCD64⁺CD14⁺GFP⁻MHCII⁻ (Cx₃cr1ᴳᶠᴾ)* *CD11b⁺Ly6cˡᵒCD11cˡᵒᐟⁱⁿᵗCD64⁺CD14⁺GFP⁻MHCII⁺* *CD11b⁺Ly6cˡᵒCD11cˡᵒᐟⁱⁿᵗCD64⁺CD14⁺GFP⁺MHCII⁺* *CD11b⁺Ly6cˡᵒCD11cˡᵒᐟⁱⁿᵗCD64⁺CD14⁺GFP⁺MHCII⁻*

Notes: (1) Populations identified as monocytes or granulocytes excluded
(2) All studies gated upon dye exclusion for viability and forward and side scatter for identifying viable single cells
(3) Variable markers of subsets indicated by bolded text

It is likely that the paucity of genetic tools, such as the $Cx_3cr1^{GFP/+}$ reporter, is a major reason why detailed examination of cTM biology only began relatively recently. However, after identifying cTMs as a major cardiac cell population [2, 8], many research groups have examined cTMs using a diverse range of markers. A common strategy for flow cytometric analysis of cTMs is to first narrow analyses on leukocyte and myeloid cell populations. This is easily achieved using the common leukocyte marker CD45 and/or the common myeloid marker CD11b. However, from this point onward, substantial differences in gating strategies exist for classifying cTM populations between research groups (Table 6.1). These include the use of surface antigens such as F4/80, CD64, or GFP (in $Cx_3cr1^{GFP/+}$ mice) as identifiers of tissue macrophages within CD45⁺ and/or CD11b⁺ populations. These disparities have generated variation in identifying cTM subsets and interpretation of cTM phenotype, origins, turnover, and heterogeneity (discussed further below).

In addition to flow cytometry, we and others have also utilized immunohistochemical analyses to identify cTMs in adult and developing cardiac tissue [2, 3, 9, 10]. Transgenic mouse lines such as the $Cx_3cr1^{GFP/+}$ and $Csf1r^{GFP}$ reporters [11] and $Csf1r$ inducible lineage tracers [9, 10, 12, 13] have been useful in these contexts in addition to markers such as Mrc1 [3] (Fig. 6.1).

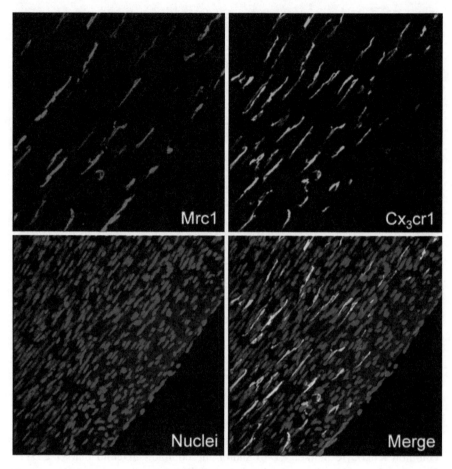

Fig. 6.1 Cardiac tissue macrophages (cTMs) in the adult murine heart. Confocal micrograph maximum projection view of a $Cx_3cr1^{GFP/+}$ mouse heart section stained for tissue macrophage marker Mrc1, GFP (Cx_3cr1), and DAPI (nuclei)

6.2 cTM Origins and Population Maintenance

How cTMs colonize the heart and how their numbers are maintained vary depending on the developmental stage of the heart. Two major mechanisms have been identified for macrophage colonization of the heart: (1) by non-hematopoietic stem cell (HSC) precursors from the yolk sac and (2) by HSC-derived populations from the fetal liver or bone marrow that colonize the heart via monocyte intermediates. During development, cTMs are detectable within the embryonic heart at ~E10.5 [5, 9]. Fate mapping studies using Csf1r^{MeriCreMer} and Cx$_3$cr1^{CreERT2} mice, following tamoxifen administration at E8.5 or E9.0, respectively, indicate that a fraction (<10%) of cTMs at 6–10 weeks of age originate from yolk-sac macrophages or erythromyeloid progenitors (EMPs) [5, 6]. These findings are consistent with observations made in other tissues of early macrophage colonization by EMP-derived cells [13, 14] and indicate that cTMs display extensive ontogenetic heterogeneity with embryonic monocytes making a large contribution to this population of cells. However, whether embryonic monocytes are derived via HSC-dependent or HSC-independent means is a topic of controversy following the development of a Kit^{MerCreMer} fate mapping strain, suggesting that the majority of tissue-resident macrophages are derived from fetal HSCs [15]. The development of novel genetic lineage tracers and clonal *in vivo* assays will help resolve the ongoing debate.

In the adult, the major source of cTMs colonizing the heart is circulating HSC-derived monocytes [4–6]. There are discordant findings regarding the extent to which monocytes contribute to the cTM population and of their importance under homeostatic conditions. A broadly utilized approach to address this question has been the use of parabiotic mouse pairs. Here, genetically distinguishable mouse pairs (with either GFP or genetically distinguishable alleles for surface markers such CD45.1 and CD45.2) are surgically fused to establish a shared circulatory system [16]. Indeed, mouse parabiosis has been instrumental for identifying monocyte-mediated turnover of tissue macrophages in the brain, lungs, peritoneum, and heart [17, 18]. Using this approach, estimations of monocyte contribution to the cTM pool have varied substantially, ranging from 2.7% after 6 weeks of parabiotic pairing [4] to approximately 12%* after a 2-week pairing [5] (*estimation from published data). Accordingly, bone marrow transplantation experiments have also shown that circulating monocytes contribute to the cTM population of cells and this was subsequently corroborated by analyzing $Ccr2^{-/-}$ mice, which have reduced circulating monocytes [6, 19]. However, analyses of monocyte contribution after bone marrow transplantation have varied greatly with estimations ranging from 10% to as high as 90%, 18 or 8 weeks (respectively) after adoptive transfer [4, 6]. Further work is required to reconcile these sets of data and to determine whether cTM subsets are able to maintain themselves without monocyte input in the steady state. As aforementioned, a major explanation for the disparate findings may be differences in experimental setup between the studies that include classification of cTMs and timing of experimental endpoints.

Following embryo- or monocyte-derived cell engraftment, cTM proliferation is a key mechanism of population maintenance. DNA labeling and immunohistochemical experiments indicate that cTMs proliferate from embryogenesis through to senescence [3–6] with estimated cTM turnover of 8–12 weeks [20]. Indeed, cTMs form the greatest proportion of all dividing cells in the adult mouse heart, particularly in the juvenile (<10 weeks old) myocardium [3]. Bromodeoxyuridine (BrdU) labeling experiments within a short temporal window of 2–4 h indicate that ~0.5–8% of cTMs are in S-phase in the steady state [4–6] with proliferation decreasing with age [3, 6] and increasing upon disruption of homeostasis [5]. Furthermore, it is apparent that the proliferative capacity of cTM subsets differs. We have found that Mrc1$^+$Cx$_3$cr1^{hi} subsets are the most proliferative [3], while others have found (using different subset designations) that MHCII^{lo}Ly6C$^-$ or Cx$_3$cr1$^+$MHCII$^-$ subsets are the most proliferative [5, 6].

While these populations are defined using different markers, it is likely that they identify the same group of macrophages. Collectively, it is clear that cTM proliferation is a major mechanism of population maintenance.

6.3   cTM Phenotype

In addition to their seemingly high proliferative capacity, cTMs are also phenotypically distinct to other tissue macrophages. Initial analyses of Cx_3cr1^+ cTM populations identified them as exhibiting an alternatively activated macrophage phenotype, with potential anti-inflammatory, angiogenic, and tissue salutary roles [2]. These findings were based on surface marker profiles (Cx_3cr1^{hi}, $Ly6C^{lo}$, $Mrc1^+$, for instance) and gene expression analyses which identified high expression of genes such as Lyve-1, IGF-1, Retnla, Chi3l3, and others as a key component of the cTM gene signature. While subsequent studies have confirmed that the majority of cTMs conform to this phenotype, at least at the surface marker level, there is limited functional evidence regarding their potential salutary roles in tissue homeostasis. However, surface marker expression, gene expression analyses, and *in vitro* experiments of cTM subsets suggest that phenotypically diverse cTMs may undertake disparate functions in myocardial homeostasis, development, and aging.

cTMs, like their counterparts in other tissues, are able to protect the tissue from invading pathogens and undertake tissue maintenance and sentinel roles such as macropinocytosis, phagocytosis, and activation of adaptive immunity [2–5]. Interestingly, these functional properties differ between various cTM subsets. For example, $MHCII^{hi}Ccr2^-$ cTMs were more efficient at stimulating T cell responses *in vitro* compared to $MHCII^{lo}Ccr2^-$ cTMs [5]. Furthermore, we found that $Mrc1^+$ cTM subsets, stained for MHCII, CD64, and CD14, undertake extensive macropinocytosis, whereas $Mrc1^-$ cTMs do not [3]. Macropinocytosis is a major mechanism by which macrophages sample the local microenvironment to sense damage-associated molecular patterns (DAMPs) and pathogen-associated molecular patterns (PAMPs); therefore, it is important for the role of cTMs as sentinels of tissue damage and foreign pathogens [21]. In contrast, we have found that $Mrc1^-$ cTMs undertake greater levels of phagocytosis compared to $Mrc1^+$ cTMs indicating divergent capacities for efferocytosis [3]. These findings are in line with those of other studies [5] and suggest that cTM subsets differ in their contribution to tissue maintenance and surveillance for pathogenic elements.

In addition to tissue maintenance and sentinel roles, cTMs are likely involved in a range of other tissue processes [22]. These include the well-established roles of macrophages in angiogenesis by paracrine mechanisms [22, 23] or by direct cell-to-cell contact [24]. Accordingly, recent studies have demonstrated that perturbation of macrophages affects the development of the nascent coronary vasculature [9]. The absence of macrophages at E16.5 in *Csf1 op/op* mice [25], which lack CSF-1, leads to impairment of coronary vessel branching and development [9]. Moreover, *in vitro* experiments using conditioned media from cultured embryonic cTMs indicate that different cTM subsets (Ccr2$^-$ versus Ccr2$^+$) may secrete disparate factors that promote or inhibit endothelial cell mobilization and aggregation [9, 26].

These findings point to potentially diverse functions of cTMs during development and injury response. However, it remains to be formerly examined whether impairment of cardiac vasculature development or other parameters is due to loss of macrophages in the heart or extra-cardiac tissues. Indeed, macrophages are involved in the development and function of the majority of tissues in the body [22, 27]. Furthermore, while it is clear that cTM subsets behave distinctly in an *in vitro* context [9, 26], whether the *in vitro* paracrine signaling effects are recapitulated *in vivo* remains to be demonstrated. Finally, the interaction of cTMs with other cardiac cell populations in development and in an injury context is unclear. Therefore, further research is required to better understand the functional role of cTMs in development, homeostasis, and injury responses, in an organ-specific manner. This demands, however, the development of novel genetic tools to manipulate cTMs.

6.4   Cellular Localization

Heterogeneity of cTMs also extends to their spatial distribution. The adult mammalian heart wall is comprised of three layers: the epicardium, myocardium, and endocardium. The epicardium is the outmost layer of the heart and is comprised of a single-cell layer. The myocardium is the muscular portion of the heart comprising cardiomyocytes and associated support cells (stroma). The endocardium is the innermost layer of the heart, lining the ventricular chamber. In the adult mouse heart, the cellular distribution of cTMs among these layers is distinct. Immunohistochemical experiments conducted on *Cx$_3$cr1$^{GFP/+}$* mice show that in juvenile mice (4 weeks old) cTMs lining or in contact with the epicardium are Cx$_3$cr1$^+$ [3]. However, in an age-dependent manner, the proportion of Cx$_3$cr1$^+$ cTMs in contact with the epicardium decreases. In 30-week-old mice, cTMs in contact with or lining the epicardium are exclusively Cx$_3$cr1$^-$ [3]. These observations may have implications for cardiac development and injury responses, especially given that the epicardium is a putative progenitor niche of the mouse heart and modulation of epicardial signaling can affect tissue repair [22].

Similarly, distinct cTM localization patterns have also been observed during embryonic development. Here, the interaction of cTMs with the epicardium has been identified as a point of cardiac colonization by cTMs as early as E12.5 [9, 10]. Ablation of the fetal epicardium by knockout of Wilms' tumor 1 (WT1) gene, which is important for epicardial development, or using a diphtheria toxin approach (WT1^{CreERT2}; Rosa26^{DTA}), results in impaired yolk-sac macrophage recruitment and loss of yolk-sac-derived cTMs [10]. Furthermore, Ccr2$^+$ monocyte-derived embryonic macrophages do not seed the epicardium but rather accumulate exclusively within the endocardial trabeculae from E14.5 [9]. Given that these two ontogenetically and transcriptionally distinct sources of embryonic macrophages colonize different areas of the heart, it would be fascinating to determine whether the same cellular distribution of cells occurs in the adult myocardium and how it may affect cellular function.

6.5   Factors Affecting cTM Phenotype

Some outstanding questions regarding cTMs include how their phenotypes are established and maintained in the heart and what influence does cTM ontology have on cTM phenotype. Observations from fate mapping experiments indicate that early embryo-derived macrophages are not restricted to any one specific cTM phenotype observed in adult hearts [5, 6]. Moreover, monocyte-derived cTMs can also comprise an array of cTM subsets [6]. What cell-intrinsic or cell-extrinsic factors direct ontogenetically distinct cells toward a specific cTM phenotype remains to be resolved.

No formal experiments have been conducted to identify factors regulating cTM phenotype or its maintenance, although experiments conducted in other tissues indicate that the local microenvironment may play an important role [28–30]. For example, TGFβ1 and retinoic acid are important for microglia and peritoneal macrophage development and phenotype, respectively [31–33]. Indeed, the tissue milieu tunes the activity of the transcription factors PU.1 and Gata6, both key determinants of macrophage lineage and phenotype [29, 33, 34]. Accordingly, relocation of ontogenetically distinct macrophages derived from yolk sac, fetal liver, or bone marrow (but not from other mature organ sources) into an empty alveolar niche alters the gene expression signature of extraneous cells to match local macrophage phenotype and function [30]. These observations point to the importance of the organ-specific microenvironment for programming tissue macrophage phenotype and prompt further research to identify environmental and cell-intrinsic factors governing the distinct cTM signature [2].

6.6   Role of cTMs in Ischemic Disease

While macrophages are a major injury-sensing cell type, our understanding of the role of cTMs in ischemic injury or tissue damage is somewhat limited. Studies examining macrophages in models of cardiac injury indicate that cTMs may have a broad range of functions in injury response initiation and resolution.

From a cellular perspective, the cardiac injury response involves an orchestrated mobilization of a broad range of cell types. Following cellular necrosis in the ischemic myocardium, the release of intracellular contents into the extracellular environment as well as the degradation of the extracellular matrix leads to the production of DAMPs which are recognized by cardiac cells including cTMs, fibroblasts, platelets, and endothelial cells [35, 36]. These cells release cytokines that initiate an inflammatory cascade and infiltration of circulating leukocytes into the injured tissue (reviewed in [37]). Within the first few hours after injury, the earliest major population of leukocytes to enter the lesion are neutrophils which follow gradients of chemokines and DAMPs [38, 39]. Neutrophils participate in multiple activities including phagocytosis of cellular debris and signaling that promote further leuko-cyte recruitment. However, some neutrophil functions may also exacerbate cardio-myocyte death by release of reactive oxygen species, proteases, and inflammatory cytokines [40, 41]. Within the first few days after injury, monocytes from the bone marrow and spleen enter the lesion to form the next wave of infiltrating leukocytes [42–44]. The earliest predominant monocyte-derived macrophage population (often termed "classically activated" or "M1" for simplicity [1, 45, 46]) has a pro-inflammatory phenotype, releasing inflammatory cytokines such as IL-1β, TNFα, nitric oxide (NO), and IL-6 [26, 47–49]. Like neutrophils, these macrophages undertake extensive phagocytosis and may also contribute to tissue damage by secreting proteolytic enzymes and recruiting infiltrating immune cells into the heart [50, 51]. Approximately 5 days after injury, pro-inflammatory macrophages are replaced by those with an anti-inflammatory phenotype (commonly termed "alter-natively activated" or "M2" macrophages [1, 45–47]). These macrophages release anti-inflammatory (IL-10 [2, 49, 52]), pro-angiogenic (IGF-1 [2, 9], PDGFα/β [9], VEGFA [9, 49, 52]), and pro-fibrotic (TGFβ1 [49], fibronectin [2, 52]) factors that help repair the necrotic lesion, re-establish vascular supply, and mechanically strengthen the heart. Accordingly, targeted depletion of anti-inflammatory macro-phages after cardiac injury impairs fibroblast activation, reduces collagen deposi-tion, increases incidence of cardiac rupture [52], and is associated with increased infarct area and inflammation [53].

While waves of monocytes and macrophages responding to injury have been characterized, little is known regarding how resident cTMs influence these popula-tions or other cell types responding to cardiac stress. Indeed, many cTMs die imme-diately after cardiac injury, and approximately 1 day after MI, resident cTM levels become negligible in comparison to the levels of infiltrating Ly6C^{hi} monocytes [4, 52]. Nevertheless, resident cTMs can proliferate upon disruption of homeostasis [4, 5]. Therefore, it remains a distinct possibility that resident cTMs play a role in car-diac repair that is different to the role played by monocyte-derived macrophages that infiltrate the injured cardiac tissue.

6.7 Targeting Macrophages for Treatment of Ischemic Injury

It remains to be tested whether cTMs can be targeted after cardiac injury to promote cardiac tissue repair in a clinical setting. Therapeutic depletion, amplification, or modulation of macrophages, however, may not be trivial considering the integral role of macrophages in the development and resolution of the injury response (reviewed in [54]). For example, local and infiltrating macrophages are necessary to efficiently clear infarct debris and to allow the reparative processes to begin. At the same time, elevated inflammation and monocyte infiltration in the initial phases after cardiac injury may exacerbate the injury even further [47, 55]. Therefore, novel therapeutic approaches to treat ischemic heart disease that target cTMs must constrain the detrimental functions of macrophages while conserving those that are beneficial. Targeting specific cTM subsets and/or ontogenetically distinct sources of cTMs may achieve this outcome in the future.

Indeed, reducing monocyte-derived cTM numbers at the onset of cardiac injury can limit inflammation and ameliorate cardiac healing in animal models of cardiac injury. For example, both antibody-mediated inhibition and genetic deletion of Ccr2 result in reduced expression of inflammatory cytokines, reduced infarct size, and improved heart function [26, 56–58]. Genetic deletion of MCP-1 (the ligand of Ccr2) attenuates left ventricle dysfunction after ischemia reperfusion injury [51, 59]. Disruption of other chemokine signaling pathways such as the Cxcl6-Cxcr6 axis [60], the Ccl2/Ccl3/Ccl4/Ccl5-Ccr5 axis [61], and the macrophage migration inhibitory factor (MIF)-Cxcr2/Cxcr4 [62] axis has also proved to be cardioprotective. Furthermore, targeted knockdown of interferon regulatory factor 5 (IRF5), a transcription factor that induces pro-inflammatory gene expression [63] in macrophages, using siRNA-loaded nanoparticles alters the inflammatory milieu and tissue repair [64].

Finally, administrating protein-based or cell-based therapeutics that alter the balance of cTM subsets from pro-inflammatory (e.g. Ccr2$^+$Ly6C^{hi}) to anti-inflammatory (e.g. Ly6C^{lo}Mrc1$^+$) or their gene expression profiles has shown promise in preclinical animal models. For example, peritoneal administration of IL-4 prior to myocardial infarction (MI) induction improves heart function and is associated with increased numbers of anti-inflammatory macrophages as well as an improved prognosis of survival [52]. Similarly, transgenic overexpression of insulin-like growth factor-1 (IGF-1) in cardiomyocytes improves heart function [65, 66], reduces the number of monocytes, and increases the number of anti-inflammatory macrophages post MI [67]. Furthermore, intramyocardial injection of cardiosphere-derived cells (CDCs) or mesenchymal stem cells (MSCs) after cardiac injury results in reduced infarct mass and is associated with alteration of macrophage inflammatory gene profiles [68, 69]. Here, the salutary effects of the cell therapy is reversed after monocyte/macrophage depletion suggesting that macrophage signaling and function are integral to the beneficial effects of these cellular strategies [68, 69].

6.8 Concluding Remarks

The development of novel reporter and lineage tracing tools in recent years has roused interest toward cTM biology and provided novel insights into cTM phenotype, origin, and population maintenance. Our current understanding of cTM function both under homeostasis and in disease is rudimentary at best, and further research is required before we can exploit these remarkable cells for therapeutic purposes. Some of the fundamental questions regarding cTMs that remain to be answered include: (1) what factors govern cTM phenotype and turnover?, (2) how do cTMs participate in cardiac injury responses?, and (3) how do cTMs interact with other cells in the complex cellular ecosystem of the heart? Answering these questions and others is bound to yield exciting new findings regarding cTM biology and their potential roles in cardiac development, homeostasis, and disease.

References

1. Guilliams M, Ginhoux F, Jakubzick C, Naik SH, Onai N, Schraml BU, et al. Dendritic cells, monocytes and macrophages: a unified nomenclature based on ontogeny. Nat Rev Immunol. 2014;14(8):571–8.
2. Pinto A, Paolicelli R, Salimova E, Gospocic J, Slonimsky E, Bilbao-Cortes D, et al. An abundant tissue macrophage population in the adult murine heart with a distinct alternatively-activated macrophage profile. PLoS One. 2012;7(5):e36814.
3. Pinto AR, Godwin JW, Chandran A, Hersey L, Ilinykh A, Debuque R, et al. Age-related changes in tissue macrophages precede cardiac functional impairment. Aging (Albany). 2014;6:399–413.
4. Heidt T, Courties G, Dutta P, Sager H, Sebas M, Iwamoto Y, et al. Differential contribution of monocytes to heart macrophages in steady-state and after myocardial infarction. Circ Res. 2014;115:284–95.
5. Epelman S, Lavine K, Beaudin A, Sojka D, Carrero J, Calderon B, et al. Embryonic and adult-derived resident cardiac macrophages are maintained through distinct mechanisms at steady state and during inflammation. Immunity. 2014;40(1):91–104.
6. Molawi K, Wolf Y, Kandalla PK, Favret J, Hagemeyer N, Frenzel K, et al. Progressive replacement of embryo-derived cardiac macrophages with age. J Exp Med. 2014;211(11):2151–8.
7. Jung S, Aliberti J, Graemmel P, Sunshine MJ, Kreutzberg GW, Sher A, et al. Analysis of fractalkine receptor CX(3)CR1 function by targeted deletion and green fluorescent protein reporter gene insertion. Mol Cell Biol. 2000;20(11):4106–14.
8. Pinto AR, Ilinykh A, Ivey MJ, Kuwabara JT, D'Antoni ML, Debuque R, et al. Revisiting cardiac cellular composition. Circ Res. 2016;118(3):400–9.
9. Leid JM, Carrelha J, Boukarabila H, Epelman S, Jacobsen SE, Lavine KJ. Primitive embryonic macrophages are required for coronary development and maturation. Circ Res. 2016;118:1488–511.
10. Stevens SM, Gise A, VanDusen N, Zhou B, Pu WT. Epicardium is required for cardiac seeding by yolk sac macrophages, precursors of resident macrophages of the adult heart. Dev Biol. 2016;413(2):153–9.
11. Sasmono RT, Oceandy D, Pollard JW, Tong W, Pavli P, Wainwright BJ, et al. A macrophage colony-stimulating factor receptor-green fluorescent protein transgene is expressed throughout the mononuclear phagocyte system of the mouse. Blood. 2003;101(3):1155–63.
12. Schulz C, Gomez Perdiguero E, Chorro L, Szabo-Rogers H, Cagnard N, Kierdorf K, et al. A lineage of myeloid cells independent of Myb and hematopoietic stem cells. Science. 2012;336(6077):86–90.
13. Gomez Perdiguero E, Klapproth K, Schulz C, Busch K, Azzoni E, Crozet L, et al. Tissue-resident macrophages originate from yolk-sac-derived erythro-myeloid progenitors. Nature. 2015;518(7540):547–51.
14. Hoeffel G, Chen J, Lavin Y, Low D, Almeida FF, See P, et al. C-Myb(+) erythro-myeloid progenitor-derived fetal monocytes give rise to adult tissue-resident macrophages. Immunity. 2015;42(4):665–78.
15. Sheng J, Ruedl C, Karjalainen K. Most tissue-resident macrophages except microglia are derived from fetal hematopoietic stem cells. Immunity. 2015;43(2):382–93.

16. Conboy MJ, Conboy IM, Rando TA. Heterochronic parabiosis: historical perspective and methodological considerations for studies of aging and longevity. Aging Cell. 2013;12(3):525–30.
17. Yona S, Kim KW, Wolf Y, Mildner A, Varol D, Breker M, et al. Fate mapping reveals origins and dynamics of monocytes and tissue macrophages under homeostasis. Immunity. 2013;38(1):79–91.
18. Hashimoto D, Chow A, Noizat C, Teo P, Beasley MB, Leboeuf M, et al. Tissue-resident macrophages self-maintain locally throughout adult life with minimal contribution from circulating monocytes. Immunity. 2013;38(4):792–804.
19. Serbina NV, Pamer EG. Monocyte emigration from bone marrow during bacterial infection requires signals mediated by chemokine receptor CCR2. Nat Immunol. 2006;7(3):311–7.
20. Ginhoux F, Guilliams M. Tissue-resident macrophage ontogeny and homeostasis. Immunity. 2016;44(3):439–49.
21. Lim JP, Gleeson PA. Macropinocytosis: an endocytic pathway for internalising large gulps. Immunol Cell Biol. 2011;89(8):836–43.
22. Pinto AR, Godwin JW, Rosenthal NA. Macrophages in cardiac homeostasis, injury responses and progenitor cell mobilisation. Stem Cell Res. 2014;13(3 Pt B):705–14.
23. Sunderkotter C, Steinbrink K, Goebeler M, Bhardwaj R, Sorg C. Macrophages and angiogenesis. J Leukoc Biol. 1994;55(3):410–22.
24. Fantin A, Vieira JM, Gestri G, Denti L, Schwarz Q, Prykhozhij S, et al. Tissue macrophages act as cellular chaperones for vascular anastomosis downstream of VEGF-mediated endothelial tip cell induction. Blood. 2010;116(5):829–40.
25. Yoshida H, Hayashi S, Kunisada T, Ogawa M, Nishikawa S, Okamura H, et al. The murine mutation osteopetrosis is in the coding region of the macrophage colony stimulating factor gene. Nature. 1990;345(6274):442–4.
26. Lavine KJ, Epelman S, Uchida K, Weber KJ, Nichols CG, Schilling JD, et al. Distinct macrophage lineages contribute to disparate patterns of cardiac recovery and remodeling in the neonatal and adult heart. Proc Natl Acad Sci U S A. 2014;111(45):16029–34.
27. Varol C, Mildner A, Jung S. Macrophages: development and tissue specialization. Annu Rev Immunol. 2015;33:643–75.
28. Lavin Y, Winter D, Blecher-Gonen R, David E, Keren-Shaul H, Merad M, et al. Tissue-resident macrophage enhancer landscapes are shaped by the local microenvironment. Cell. 2014;159(6):1312–26.
29. Gosselin D, Link VM, Romanoski CE, Fonseca GJ, Eichenfield DZ, Spann NJ, et al. Environment drives selection and function of enhancers controlling tissue-specific macrophage identities. Cell. 2014;159(6):1327–40.
30. van de Laar L, Saelens W, De Prijck S, Martens L, Scott CL, Van Isterdael G, et al. Yolk sac macrophages, fetal liver, and adult monocytes can colonize an empty niche and develop into functional tissue-resident macrophages. Immunity. 2016;44:755–68.
31. Butovsky O, Jedrychowski MP, Moore CS, Cialic R, Lanser AJ, Gabriely G, et al. Identification of a unique TGF-beta-dependent molecular and functional signature in microglia. Nat Neurosci. 2014;17(1):131–43.
32. Makwana M, Jones LL, Cuthill D, Heuer H, Bohatschek M, Hristova M, et al. Endogenous transforming growth factor beta 1 suppresses inflammation and promotes survival in adult CNS. J Neurosci. 2007;27(42):11201–13.
33. Okabe Y, Medzhitov R. Tissue-specific signals control reversible program of localization and functional polarization of macrophages. Cell. 2014;157(4):832–44.
34. Rosas M, Davies LC, Giles PJ, Liao CT, Kharfan B, Stone TC, et al. The transcription factor Gata6 links tissue macrophage phenotype and proliferative renewal. Science. 2014;344(6184):645–8.
35. van Hout GP, Arslan F, Pasterkamp G, Hoefer IE. Targeting danger-associated molecular patterns after myocardial infarction. Expert Opin Ther Targets. 2016;20(2):223–39.
36. Zhang W, Lavine KJ, Epelman S, Evans SA, Weinheimer CJ, Barger PM, et al. Necrotic myocardial cells release damage-associated molecular patterns that provoke fibroblast

activation in vitro and trigger myocardial inflammation and fibrosis in vivo. J Am Heart Assoc. 2015;4(6):e001993.

37. Liu J, Wang H, Li J. Inflammation and inflammatory cells in myocardial infarction and reperfusion injury: a double-edged sword. Clin Med Insights Cardiol. 2016;10:79–84.

38. Ivey CL, Williams FM, Collins PD, Jose PJ, Williams TJ. Neutrophil chemoattractants generated in two phases during reperfusion of ischemic myocardium in the rabbit. Evidence for a role for C5a and interleukin-8. J Clin Invest. 1995;95(6):2720–8.

39. Vinten-Johansen J. Involvement of neutrophils in the pathogenesis of lethal myocardial reperfusion injury. Cardiovasc Res. 2004;61(3):481–97.

40. Duilio C, Ambrosio G, Kuppusamy P, DiPaula A, Becker LC, Zweier JL. Neutrophils are primary source of O2 radicals during reperfusion after prolonged myocardial ischemia. Am J Physiol Heart Circ Physiol. 2001;280(6):H2649–57.

41. Ma Y, Yabluchanskiy A, Lindsey ML. Neutrophil roles in left ventricular remodeling following myocardial infarction. Fibrogenesis Tissue Repair. 2013;6(1):11.

42. Dutta P, Sager HB, Stengel KR, Naxerova K, Courties G, Saez B, et al. Myocardial infarction activates CCR2(+) hematopoietic stem and progenitor cells. Cell Stem Cell. 2015;16(5):477–87.

43. Swirski FK, Nahrendorf M, Etzrodt M, Wildgruber M, Cortez-Retamozo V, Panizzi P, et al. Identification of splenic reservoir monocytes and their deployment to inflammatory sites. Science. 2009;325(5940):612–6.

44. Leuschner F, Panizzi P, Chico-Calero I, Lee WW, Ueno T, Cortez-Retamozo V, et al. Angiotensin-converting enzyme inhibition prevents the release of monocytes from their splenic reservoir in mice with myocardial infarction. Circ Res. 2010;107(11):1364–73.

45. Mantovani A, Sica A, Sozzani S, Allavena P, Vecchi A, Locati M. The chemokine system in diverse forms of macrophage activation and polarization. Trends Immunol. 2004;25(12):677–86.

46. Sica A, Mantovani A. Macrophage plasticity and polarization: in vivo veritas. J Clin Invest. 2012;122(3):787–95.

47. Nahrendorf M, Swirski FK, Aikawa E, Stangenberg L, Wurdinger T, Figueiredo JL, et al. The healing myocardium sequentially mobilizes two monocyte subsets with divergent and complementary functions. J Exp Med. 2007;204(12):3037–47.

48. Murray PJ, Wynn TA. Obstacles and opportunities for understanding macrophage polarization. J Leukoc Biol. 2011;89(4):557–63.

49. Hilgendorf I, Gerhardt LM, Tan TC, Winter C, Holderried TA, Chousterman BG, et al. Ly-6Chigh monocytes depend on Nr4a1 to balance both inflammatory and reparative phases in the infarcted myocardium. Circ Res. 2014;114(10):1611–22.

50. Leuschner F, Dutta P, Gorbatov R, Novobrantseva TI, Donahoe JS, Courties G, et al. Therapeutic siRNA silencing in inflammatory monocytes in mice. Nat Biotechnol. 2011;29(11):1005–10.

51. Dewald O, Zymek P, Winkelmann K, Koerting A, Ren G, Abou-Khamis T, et al. CCL2/monocyte chemoattractant protein-1 regulates inflammatory responses critical to healing myocardial infarcts. Circ Res. 2005;96(8):881–9.

52. Shiraishi M, Shintani Y, Shintani Y, Ishida H, Saba R, Yamaguchi A, et al. Alternatively activated macrophages determine repair of the infarcted adult murine heart. J Clin Invest. 2016;126:2151–66.

53. Leblond AL, Klinkert K, Martin K, Turner EC, Kumar AH, Browne T, et al. Systemic and cardiac depletion of M2 macrophage through CSF-1R signaling inhibition alters cardiac function post myocardial infarction. PLoS One. 2015;10(9):e0137515.

54. Nahrendorf M, Pittet MJ, Swirski FK. Monocytes: protagonists of infarct inflammation and repair after myocardial infarction. Circulation. 2010;121(22):2437–45.

55. Hulsmans M, Sam F, Nahrendorf M. Monocyte and macrophage contributions to cardiac remodeling. J Mol Cell Cardiol. 2016;93:149–55.

56. Kaikita K, Hayasaki T, Okuma T, Kuziel WA, Ogawa H, Takeya M. Targeted deletion of CC chemokine receptor 2 attenuates left ventricular remodeling after experimental myocardial infarction. Am J Pathol. 2004;165(2):439–47.

57. Hayasaki T, Kaikita K, Okuma T, Yamamoto E, Kuziel WA, Ogawa H, et al. CC chemokine receptor-2 deficiency attenuates oxidative stress and infarct size caused by myocardial ischemia-reperfusion in mice. Circ J. 2006;70(3):342–51.
58. Majmudar MD, Keliher EJ, Heidt T, Leuschner F, Truelove J, Sena BF, et al. Monocyte-directed RNAi targeting CCR2 improves infarct healing in atherosclerosis-prone mice. Circulation. 2013;127(20):2038–46.
59. Frangogiannis NG, Dewald O, Xia Y, Ren G, Haudek S, Leucker T, et al. Critical role of monocyte chemoattractant protein-1/CC chemokine ligand 2 in the pathogenesis of ischemic cardiomyopathy. Circulation. 2007;115(5):584–92.
60. Zhao G, Wang S, Wang Z, Sun A, Yang X, Qiu Z, et al. CXCR6 deficiency ameliorated myocardial ischemia/reperfusion injury by inhibiting infiltration of monocytes and IFN-gamma-dependent autophagy. Int J Cardiol. 2013;168(2):853–62.
61. Zamilpa R, Kanakia R, Cigarroa J, Dai Q, Escobar GP, Martinez H, et al. CC chemokine receptor 5 deletion impairs macrophage activation and induces adverse remodeling following myocardial infarction. Am J Physiol Heart Circ Physiol. 2011;300(4):H1418–26.
62. Gao XM, Liu Y, White D, Su Y, Drew BG, Bruce CR, et al. Deletion of macrophage migration inhibitory factor protects the heart from severe ischemia-reperfusion injury: a predominant role of anti-inflammation. J Mol Cell Cardiol. 2011;50(6):991–9.
63. Krausgruber T, Blazek K, Smallie T, Alzabin S, Lockstone H, Sahgal N, et al. IRF5 promotes inflammatory macrophage polarization and TH1-TH17 responses. Nat Immunol. 2011;12(3):231–8.
64. Courties G, Heidt T, Sebas M, Iwamoto Y, Jeon D, Truelove J, et al. In vivo silencing of the transcription factor IRF5 reprograms the macrophage phenotype and improves infarct healing. J Am Coll Cardiol. 2014;63(15):1556–66.
65. Santini M, Tsao L, Monassier L, Theodoropoulos C, Carter J, Lara-Pezzi E, et al. Enhancing repair of the mammalian heart. Circ Res. 2007;100(12):1732–40.
66. Li B, Setoguchi M, Wang X, Andreoli A, Leri A, Malhotra A, et al. Insulin-like growth factor-1 attenuates the detrimental impact of nonocclusive coronary artery constriction on the heart. Circ Res. 1999;84(9):1007–19.
67. Gallego-Colon E, Sampson RD, Sattler S, Schneider MD, Rosenthal N, Tonkin J. Cardiac-restricted IGF-1Ea overexpression reduces the early accumulation of inflammatory myeloid cells and mediates expression of extracellular matrix remodelling genes after myocardial infarction. Mediat Inflamm. 2015;2015:484357.
68. de Couto G, Liu W, Tseliou E, Sun B, Makkar N, Kanazawa H, et al. Macrophages mediate cardioprotective cellular postconditioning in acute myocardial infarction. J Clin Invest. 2015;125(8):3147–62.
69. Ben-Mordechai T, Holbova R, Landa-Rouben N, Harel-Adar T, Feinberg MS, Abd Elrahman I, et al. Macrophage subpopulations are essential for infarct repair with and without stem cell therapy. J Am Coll Cardiol. 2013;62(20):1890–901.

Part III
The Immune System in Cardiovascular Pathology

Chapter 7
Atherosclerosis

Mohammed Shamim Rahman and Kevin Woollard

Abbreviations

ABCA1	ATP-binding cassette transporter-A1
ABCG1	ATP-binding cassette transporter-G1
BMI	Body mass index
CNS	Central nervous system
CRP	C-reactive protein
CVD	Cardiovascular disease
DC	Dendritic cell
Foxp3	Forkhead box P3
HDL	High-density lipoprotein
ICAM-1	Intracellular adhesion molecule-1
IHD	Ischaemic heart disease
IL-6	Interleukin-6
LDL	Low-density lipoprotein
LPS	Lipopolysaccharide
MAPK	Mitogen-activated protein kinase
mRNA	Messenger RNA
NK	Natural killer
PAD	Peripheral arterial disease
SBP	Systolic blood pressure

M.S. Rahman • K. Woollard (✉)
Division of Immunology and Inflammation, Department of Medicine, Imperial College London, London, UK
e-mail: k.woollard@imperial.ac.uk

© Springer International Publishing AG 2017
S. Sattler, T. Kennedy-Lydon (eds.), *The Immunology of Cardiovascular Homeostasis and Pathology*, Advances in Experimental Medicine and Biology 1003, DOI 10.1007/978-3-319-57613-8_7

T2DM   Type-2 diabetes mellitus
TLR   Toll-like receptor
TNF   Tumour necrosis factor
Treg   Regulatory T cell
VCAM-1   Vascular adhesion molecule-1
VLDL   Very low-density lipoprotein

7.1   Cardiovascular System

Cardiovascular disease (CVD) remains the leading cause of death worldwide [1, 2]. Atherosclerosis, the build-up of plaques within blood vessels resulting in restriction of flow and potential risk of rupture, contributes to the development of heart attack (myocardial infarction) and stroke. Angina pectoris, a diagnosis that correlates pain in the chest with reduced blood flow to the heart muscle, is also predominantly caused by atherosclerosis, a key burden of morbidity particularly in the developed world, affecting 19 males and 14 women in every 100,000 of the population in Western Europe [1]. The risk of developing ischaemic heart disease (IHD) and stroke both increases with age [3], and there is a slightly higher risk of developing heart attack, stroke or suffering from angina in men [2–4]. Another important contribution to CVD is peripheral arterial disease (PAD), which, although a rare cause of mortality, contributes significantly to the burden of morbidity globally [5]. Our focus in this chapter however will be the role of immunity on atherosclerotic-mediated heart attack and stroke as it is in these areas where much work has been conducted.

So-called modifiable risk factors for CVD have been identified over many years, resulting from analyses at both a populational and epidemiological level as well as characterisation of risk factors from bench side analysis of genetic mutations to link cause and effect.

Cigarette smoking has been identified as a key risk factor for CVD. This was particularly noted during the twentieth century following a sharp rise in the incidence of smoking followed, several years later, by a noticeable increase in the incidence of both lung cancers and death from CVD. Smoking has consistently shown to increase the risk of death from IHD and stroke in longitudinal follow-up studies [6, 7]. The effects of tobacco smoke inhalation on the immune system have been considered for some time [8]. Smoking is thought primarily to modulate immune responses through the lung, where innate immune cells such as alveolar macrophages and monocytes respond to environmental pathogens in order to prevent foreign material and pathogens from reaching alveoli. Smoking increases macrophage number and their production of lysozymes and secretion of elastase [9]. Although macrophages isolated from smokers produce higher levels of oxygen-free radicals, they are less able to deal with bacterial pathogens when compared with non-smokers [10] suggesting functional impairment [11]. These immunomodulatory effects are not limited to macrophages as alterations in effector function of natural killer (NK) cells [12] and lymphocytes [8]. Immunoglobulin levels are lower in smokers [12]; however autoantibodies are higher [13], perhaps providing an explanation as to the higher incidence of some autoimmune conditions in smokers. The mechanisms of this remain unclear due to the complex composition of cigarette smoke; however tar and nicotine are implied as major contributors to this effect [14].

Essential hypertension is defined as an elevated systolic blood pressure (SBP) above 120 mmHg and diastolic blood pressure above 70–80 mmHg which has been linked to accelerated CVD [15, 16]. Elevations in SBP form a linear relationship with an increasing incidence of ischaemic heart disease and stroke when adjusted for age [17]. Certainly in the West, it is accepted that blood pressure increases with age. Dietary salt intake is linked to a rise in blood pressure [18] as is body habitus recorded as body mass index (BMI) [19]. Experimental animal models and observations in hypertensive humans have linked alterations in immunity and inflammation with hypertension [20–24]; however, despite these data, no convincing pathophysiological link has been accepted [25]. The focus of research has been concentrated on the interaction of immunity with the renal, specifically renin-angiotensin, system in animal work [26–28]. Nevertheless, data has certainly suggested an altered cellular phenotype in hypertensive patients. Monocytes have been shown to be preactivated when stimulated in vitro with toll-like receptor (TLR)-4 agonist lipopolysaccharide (LPS) altering secretion of tumour necrosis factor-α (TNF-α) and interleukin-1β (IL-1β) at both protein and transcription (mRNA) level [23]. Increased macrophage and T-cell infiltration into the kidneys is seen in a variety of experimental animal models of renal disease [29–31]. Correlating these findings in experimental models to human disease however requires further work and understanding. Excellent reviews and updates are available in the journal *Hypertension* where the role and interplay between immunity, inflammation and hypertension are reviewed [25, 32–34].

Cholesterol has been strongly implicated in the development of CVD. This association can be traced back to over 100 years ago, starting with the discovery that human atherosclerotic plaques contain cholesterol. This was followed by discoveries that a high-cholesterol diet can cause atherosclerosis in rabbits and that a feedback inhibition loop for cholesterol synthesis exists leading to the discovery of a mutation in humans resulting in defective cholesterol transport who were at a high risk of premature death from CVD [35].

The terms 'good' and 'bad' cholesterol refer to different lipoproteins that transport cholesterol in the blood. This is however an oversimplification of the complexity and differences in attributable risk for these circulating transport proteins. Apolipoproteins produced by enterocytes or hepatocytes with help from hydrophilic phospholipids package hydrophobic lipids such as cholesterol, cholesterol esters and triglycerides to make them available for transport, energy delivery or storage.

The link between total cholesterol levels and the incidence of cardiovascular disease was first suggested in the 1950s [36] followed by the discovery of low-density lipoprotein (LDL) as a risk factor for CVD in 1955 [37]. The discovery of its receptor in 1973 by Brown and Goldstein [38] leads to the award of the Nobel Prize. This is further discussed in the section titled 'Lipoproteins' in more detail below.

The presence of **diabetes mellitus** is associated with a twofold increased risk of ischaemic heart disease and stroke as well as PAD [39–41]. Indeed, this risk extends to those with elevated blood glucose levels, often termed 'prediabetes' when fasting glucose levels greater than 6 mmol/L were considered [39]. Acute hyperglycaemia correlates with morbidity and mortality in critically and non-critically ill patients [42] prompting investigation into potential modulation of immune response. It has been shown to increase monocyte expression of Mac-1 (CD11b) [43] as well as to increase plasma levels of E-selectin, intercellular adhesion molecule-1 (ICAM-1) and vascular cell adhesion molecule-1 (VCAM-1), implicated in leukocyte adhesion to the vascular wall [44–47]. Hyperglycaemia has been shown to inhibit neutrophil migration and phagocytosis as well as their ability to produce superoxides for microbe killing [48] and can modulate the cytokine system and complement cascade [49].

Diabetes mellitus is a condition defined by chronically elevated blood glucose levels [50] with type-2 diabetes mellitus (T2DM) associated with a number of metabolic abnormalities. Diabetic patients are at an increased risk of infection [51], particularly susceptible to those of bacterial origin [52]. Studies have identified defects in humoral and cellular innate immunity [53] with defects in monocyte chemotactic and phagocytic profiles [54]. A link between T2DM and obesity has been observed for some time [55–57], sharing the common trait of insulin resistance [58] though a firm mechanism to support obesity as a cause of T2DM is yet to be established.

Obesity has been described as a global epidemic [59] and is associated with an increase in mortality [60]. Low-grade inflammation is a feature of obesity, with increased circulating levels of TNF-α, IL-6 and CRP [61–65]. Visceral adipose tissue is thought to be a driver of inflammation as well as being a driver of insulin resistance [66]. Accumulation of both innate and adaptive immune cells including macrophages [67–69], T cells [70, 71], B cells [72], NK cells [73] and neutrophils [74] with a 'pro-inflammatory' phenotype along with a reduction in 'anti-inflammatory' immune cells (regulatory T cells, M2-like macrophages and eosinophils) has been shown [66].

Combining the evidence presented above, it is reasonable then to extrapolate that the presence of hypertension, dyslipidaemia, dysglycaemia and obesity (specifically centripetal), otherwise termed the '**metabolic syndrome**', will exert effects on immune cells. In the USA, nearly a quarter of all adults are suspected to suffer from metabolic syndrome and are a predictor of CVD [75]. Activation of the innate immune system is implicated in the development of metabolic syndrome characteristics [76–79].

7.2   Cardiovascular Homeostasis

The cardiovascular system is subject to regulation, through an integrated network of stimuli. Cardiac output is determined by heart rate and stroke volume, which in turn are subject to autonomic, mechanoreceptor, renal, cerebral and endocrine input. Cerebral influence on the cardiovascular system includes regulation via the hypothalamus, utilising the sympathetic and parasympathetic nervous system to influence heart rate and blood pressure as well as regulation by humoral factors, such as adrenaline (epinephrine) and noradrenaline effects on vasculature and cholinergic effects on skeletal and cardiac muscle. Neurological chemoreceptors can detect changes in partial pressures of oxygen and carbon dioxide in the circulation causing vasodilation or vasoconstriction to alter mean arterial pressure.

In this section, we discuss further mechanisms of cardiovascular regulation and the susceptibility for disease when imbalance occurs.

7.2.1 Lipoproteins

As described above, much evidence from genetic and clinical trials (predominantly trials where statins have been used to lower cholesterol) now points towards the link between cholesterol and cardiovascular disease. In particular changes in low-density lipoprotein (LDL) cholesterol successfully lowered with statin therapy have demonstrated significant reductions in mortality from myocardial infarction and reduction in ischaemic stroke [80–91]. Other lipoproteins involved in the regulation and transport of cholesterol and dietary lipid and their relative contributions to the burden of CVD are discussed here.

7.2.2 LDL Cholesterol

Mounting clinical evidence has implicated elevated total cholesterol levels in early CVD [92], whilst a reduction in heart attack and the need for revascularisation therapies and stroke have been shown when therapies successfully lowering LDL cholesterol levels are employed [91, 93]. Twenty-one trials comparing statin therapy to control in the meta-analysis by the Cholesterol Treatment Trialists' (CTT) Collaboration [91] showed a reduction of LDL-C by 1.0 mmol/L equated to a reduction in heart attacks by nearly 25% (RR 0.76, 95% CI 0.73–0.79). Interest in the oxidised form of LDL in the context of atherosclerosis was developed following observations that macrophages readily accumulated cholesterol esters in vitro [94, 95], and this led to the concept that modification of LDL is felt to play a key role in atherogenesis [94, 96, 97]. The role of oxidised LDL in CVD has since gained considerable momentum as has their interplay with macrophages and the formation of cholesterol-loaded macrophage foam cells [98–103]. Oxidised LDL has been shown in vitro to have a pro-inflammatory effect on monocytes [104–106], driving polarisation to macrophages [107] and enhancing anti-microbial response [108]. It has recently been shown that circulating monocytes can, in certain conditions, such as postprandial lipaemia or exposure to non-HDL lipoproteins, also accumulate intracellular neutral lipid [109–111]. The biological relevance or fate of these so-called foamy monocytes however remains unclear. Circulating levels of oxidised LDL may also be increased in CVD [100, 112], the relevance of which remains to be fully explored.

7.2.3   HDL Cholesterol

Other forms of cholesterol include high-density lipoprotein (HDL) which has been negatively correlated with an increased risk of CVD [92, 113, 114]. The mechanism by which HDL is thought to exert cardioprotective effects includes the ability to remove cholesterol from cells, a process known as 'reverse cholesterol transport', and therefore may do this from lipid-laden foam cells [115]. HDL promotes cellular cholesterol efflux mediated by interaction through ATP-binding cassette transporters (ABCA1, ABCG1) [116, 117].

Beyond this, HDL has also been shown to exert anti-inflammatory effects by lowering expression of endothelial expression of VCAM-1, increased production of endothelial nitric oxide synthase (eNOS), reduction in monocyte expression of CD11b and migration [118] and also by downregulating TLR-dependent pro-inflammatory cytokine production in macrophages [119].

However the relationship has come under question recently, following the use of Mendelian randomisation in patients who had loss of function single nucleotide polymorphisms (SNP) associated with elevated plasma HDL levels, these patients did not have a reduction of CV events [120, 121]. These findings have been further supported by a failure of clinical trials to correlate raising HDL levels with reduced CV events [122–124], suggesting that HDL function rather than simply plasma level may be important.

7.2.4   Other Non-HDL Cholesterols

Chylomicrons represent the largest portion of dietary lipid under transport. Packaged together in the enterocyte, they consist predominantly of fatty acids esterified for transport as triglycerides, phospholipids, cholesterol and cholesterol esters [125–127]. Following the transfer out of fatty acids to either muscle or adipose tissue, these particles are now termed chylomicron remnants and are cleared by the liver. Very low-density lipoprotein (VLDL) is responsible for the transport of cholesterol and a significant proportion of triglyceride following clearance of dietary lipid by the liver. Work performed in our group has demonstrated that monocyte subsets differentially accumulate neutral lipid in response to VLDL incubation and that this can impair normal cytoskeletal activity and monocyte migration towards an inflammatory stimulus [111] and may also increase endothelial adhesion, although this remains an inconsistent finding [128].

Early hypotheses suggested these remnants and indeed the small cholesterol component are in fact contributors to atherosclerotic CVD [129], and interest in this hypothesis has recently been renewed, advocating measurement of non-fasting triglycerides as an independent predictor of CV events [130, 131]. The role of the dietary source of triglycerides, importantly whether from saturated fat-rich diets, has recently been an issue of debate. Meta-analyses have called into question the role of dietary guidelines that advocate 'low-fat' diets suggesting in fact that the link between saturated fat and CVD is not as clear as once thought [132–134], whilst support remains however for increased intake of polyunsaturated [132] and mono-unsaturated fat-rich diets [135, 136].

Other lipid- and lipoprotein-associated CVD risk markers have not been further discussed here due to the scope of the chapter, but mutations in the lipoprotein (a) gene ought to also be considered.

7.2.5 Central Nervous System

Beyond the role of circulating mediators, it is now known that the cardiovascular system is subject to regulation from the central nervous system (CNS) and mechanosensors.

Integrins, for instance, play a key role as mechanosensors in cardiac myocytes [137] and may respond to mechanical load in inducing hypertrophy. β1 integrin has been shown to play a role in combining mechanical stretch in activation of mitogen-activated protein kinases (MAPK) and Rho GTPases [138–140]. β1 integrin is also known to interact with angiotensin II, a peptide hormone that forms part of the renal-angiotensin feedback loop and can stimulate myocardial contraction [141]. This complex field of research is further elaborated in the excellent review by Dostal et al. [142].

CNS regulation of the cardiovascular system is primarily through autonomic nervous system alterations of sympathetic and parasympathetic tone. Indeed, this is particularly relevant in the context of heart failure [143, 144] and cardiac arrhythmias [145] and was thought of as a potential therapeutic target for resistant hypertension [146], though recent results have allayed early optimism in this [147].

The notion that psychological stress can influence the immune system has been considered for some time [148] and evaluated in a variety of ways, where the type of stress has differed (acute or chronic), sequence of stressful events and the different evaluative markers used to identify an effect on immunity (cell number, cytokine release or a functional assay) [149]. The impact of chronic stress and activation of the sympathetic-adrenal-medullary axis on haematopoiesis has been studied in both humans and mouse models of atherosclerosis demonstrating an increase in monocyte and neutrophil count [150]. In these studies, monocytes increase in number in the peripheral blood [151], and as further elaborated below, their subsets adopt a specific response to acute myocardial infarction that are thought to play an important role in inflammation following the ischaemic insult but may also play an important role in tissue repair [152]. Mobilisation from the splenic reservoir [153, 154] and bone marrow [155] contributes to recruitment into infarcted myocardium [156] and may contribute to further risk of atherosclerosis and re-infarction [157].

7.3 Immunity in Cardiovascular Homeostasis

Here we will mainly discuss the role played by cells of the innate immune system on cardiovascular homeostasis and atherosclerosis. We discuss monocytes and macrophages and to a lesser extent dendritic cells and granulocytes. We will finish by briefly discussing the role played by lymphocytes.

7.3.1 Monocytes

Monocytes are effector cells of the innate immune system. Their involvement in atherogenesis has been suggested for some time [158, 159]. Although previously considered simply senescent cells destined to terminally differentiate into macrophages following activation and invasion of tissue in response to inflammatory cues, it is now recognised that they may play a much wider role in the immune response. For instance, it is now recognised that they exist in subsets in humans (with murine homologs that have also been studied extensively) [160, 161]. They can be described based upon their relative expression of antigenic markers such as LPS receptor CD14 and Fcγ-receptor CD16, further described below.

7.3.1.1 Monocytes as Heterogeneous Subsets

In mammals, monocytes can be differentiated into at least two subsets, which can be described as 'classical' and 'non-classical' monocytes. Classical monocytes are the most numerate, comprising approximately 80% of the circulating number, and are $CD14^{high}CD16^{low}$, whilst non-classical monocytes, the converse, $CD14^{dim}CD16^{high}$. A third population of monocytes, termed 'intermediate' monocytes, is $CD14^{high}CD16^{high}$, demonstrating a phenotype somewhere in between the other two, responding strongly to bacterial signals whilst in some also potent viral responses [160]. For instance, classical monocytes demonstrate a rapid and potent cytokine response to bacterial stimuli via TLR-4, whilst non-classical monocytes respond preferentially to viral stimuli via TLR-7 and TLR-8. The relevance of defining and describing monocytes in terms of these subsets is that they may play distinct roles in the context of atherogenesis [161]. Non-classical cells have been described as 'patrolling', with evidence they can crawl against the microcirculatory stream, expressing differential levels of chemokine receptors [162, 163] such as fractalkine receptor, CX3 chemokine receptor (CX3CR1) expression [160], implicated in atherogenesis through murine knockout models [164].

In mouse models, murine homologs to human monocytes have been identified [160]. Classical monocytes are closest to $Gr1/Ly6C^{high}$ monocytes, whilst non-classical cells align with $Gr1/Ly6C^{low}$ cells. No discernible intermediate homologs are identified, although human intermediate monocytes align functionally with murine classical cells [160, 165] and transcriptionally with non-classical $CD16^{high}$ human monocytes [166].

Classical monocytes are preferentially recruited to early atherosclerotic plaques [163, 167]. In the mouse, $Gr1/Ly6C^{high}$ populations may give rise to their $Gr1/Ly6C^{low}$ counterparts through interconversion in the blood; however this has not been confirmed by human data [168]. Origins of monocyte heterogeneity remain to be discovered. Heterogeneity may exist due to maturation over time and interconversion between subsets ($Gr1/Ly6C^{high}$ to $Gr1/Ly6C^{low}$) or NR4A1-dependent maturation of individual progenitor cells within the bone marrow subsequently giving rise to heterogeneous subsets or in fact that differentiation is dependent on the local microenvironment and that this promotes differential expression of surface markers and functional phenotype, as shown in macrophage populations [169]. Further differences in subsets and their potential recruitment to areas of vascular endothelium at risk of atherosclerosis in terms of expression of selectins [170–172], integrins [109, 110, 173, 174] and other chemokine receptors are further elaborated in this review [161]. Monocytes do not necessarily extravasate and terminally differentiate into macrophages or dendritic cells and can in fact emigrate from tissue or apoptose [175]. Finally, it should be noted that most of our understanding of monocyte subset biology comes from murine work and that the human model is less well understood.

7.3.2 Macrophages

7.3.2.1 Derived from Circulating Monocytes or Tissue-Resident Precursors?

Macrophages had for some time been considered solely as cells terminally differentiated from activated circulating blood monocytes [155]; however this dogma has recently been questioned. Indeed, it is now recognised that most tissues of the body contain resident macrophages, some of which potentially predate the arrival of progenitors from the blood in embryological development [168, 176–179]. It is now accepted that most tissue contains resident macrophages that can self-renew independent of blood monocytes [168]. However some tissue macrophages do require continuous turnover from monocytes, the gut being a good example [180]. Resident tissue macrophages are thought to arise from early yolk sac-derived progenitor cells, bypassing monocytes, or from foetal liver monocytes that themselves have derived from erythro-myeloid progenitors (c-Myb$^+$ cells) generated in the yolk sac and dorsal aortic endothelial cells [181, 182]. Perhaps more relevant to CVD, tissue-resident macrophages that reside in the adventitia of the arterial wall derive from CX_3CR1^+ erythro-myeloid progenitors from the yolk sac and foetal liver monocytes, with subsequent influx of circulating blood monocytes in the postnatal phase accompanied by transient expression of surface receptors associated with adhesion and recruitment of circulating leukocytes [183].

Regardless of origin, tissue specificity most likely dictates tissue macrophage functionality and a spectrum of phenotypes may facilitate tissue-specific functions, including atherosclerosis—although that has yet to be well established experimentally [169].

7.3.2.2 Role in Atherogenesis

The retention of apolipoprotein B-rich particles by within areas of the vascular network susceptible to atherosclerosis and subsequent engulfment by macrophages can be identified as an important early step in the development of atherosclerotic plaque [184]. Much of the work in identifying these steps have been deduced from murine work, where accelerated atherosclerotic models [185–187] are generated from *Ldlr*

[185, 188] and *Apoe* [189, 190] knockout mice. Monocyte extravasation into the vascular wall [191] as well as the response of tissue-resident macrophages to modified lipoproteins can stimulate both a cytokine response contributing to further leukocyte recruitment and the generation of lipid-laden foam cells, described as macrophages. The role of inflammation and its regulation in atherogenesis and plaque progression, however, is poorly understood [192], and the previous hypothesis of cholesterol uptake by macrophage foam cells causing resultant inflammation has recently been questioned [193]. It is suspected that lipid clearance, through scavenger receptor-mediated endocytosis [194–196], begins as a physiological response of benefit that, following continued exposure to cholesterol without a suitable negative feedback loop, becomes dysregulated with resulting alteration of normal macrophage response [165]. Macrophage foam cells have reduced capacity to emigrate from plaque, thereby contributing to an ongoing inflammatory response, with resulting continued recruitment of other immune cells into the plaque [197]. This hypothesis of atherogenesis includes the role played by oxidation of pro-atherogenic lipoproteins [198] and interaction with proteoglycans [199, 200] in helping to retain them within plaque [200]. Dying macrophages deposit engulfed lipid into the plaque, resulting in a necrotic core that creates an unstable atherosclerotic plaque, implicated in heart attack and stroke, although the process of death may well be a far more complex and regulated sequence of events [201].

Unlike in early atherosclerotic lesions, where mouse models suggest a reliance on monocyte recruitment [202–205], mature plaque macrophage replenishment within the vessel wall is primarily through self-renewal [206, 207]. A more recent concept is the role of intraplaque haemorrhage [208] and the role played by macrophages that deal with iron overload. Macrophages have previously been referred to as either 'M1' or 'M2' in an attempt to characterise their presumed responses to inflammatory cues; however this bipolar concept, predominantly described through in vitro and murine gene knockout data, may have oversimplified the true nature of physiological differentiation in vivo where a more complex milieu contributes to final macrophage phenotype [209, 210]. Intraplaque haemorrhage is described as an important aspect of plaque progression and a possible driver of ongoing inflammatory cell influx [211]. A Mhem macrophage phenotype is described as protective and deactivated, countering the inflammatory drive of iron overload supporting a M1-type response [211–214].

7.3.3   Dendritic Cells

Like macrophages, dendritic cells (DC) can be defined by their origin with some originating from common precursors in the bone marrow, precursors in the blood or circulating monocytes that differentiate into DCs in the peripheral tissue or atherosclerotic plaque [163]. Whilst recognised as antigen-presenting cells, they also play an important role in promoting tolerance to self-antigens in part through their induction of regulatory T cells [215]. In mouse models, resident DCs that encounter free cholesterol in the arterial adventitia can accumulate lipid [216]. We will not be elaborating on their role further in this chapter; however a more in-depth description of their potential role in atherosclerosis can be found in the review by Cybulsky et al. [217].

7.3.4 Neutrophils

The most abundant leukocyte in human peripheral blood, neutrophils, is a pro-inflammatory phagocyte and one of the first responders to sites of inflammation, particularly in response to bacterial infection. They rapidly release proteolytic enzymes in order to traverse through extracellular matrix to these sites and further-more degranulate, and this release plays a role in further recruitment and activation of other innate immune cells [218]. The potential role played by neutrophils in both early and late atherosclerotic plaque generation and destabilisation is from data largely extrapolated from mouse models of CVD, and, thus, translation to human mechanistic hypothesis remains to be elucidated.

Neutrophils are implicated in atherogenesis through their presence in plaque. Staining for surface markers Ly6G and MPO in murine plaque [219] and for CD177 and CD66b in human carotid [220] and acute coronary lesions [221] helps identify their presence here. Furthermore, identification of degranulation proteins in plaque [222–225] and neutrophil accumulation in early lesions in knockout mice [219] in addition to the role of neutrophil granule effects on vascular permeability [226, 227], their potential ability to recruit monocytes to atherosclerotic plaque [228, 229] and possible activation and foam cell formation in macrophages [230] lends weight to their role as important facets to the process of atherosclerosis. Their ability to secrete proteases and transmigrate through extracellular matrix is proposed as a possible model for alteration of atherosclerotic plaque caps [231], the fragility of which is linked to acute arterial thrombosis seen in acute myocardial infarction [232].

7.3.5 Lymphocytes

Whilst macrophages may well account for the majority of inflammatory cells within human atherosclerotic plaques [233, 234], lymphocytes have been found in lesions although less abundantly. T cells constitute approximately 10% of cells in human atherosclerotic plaque with 70% of them CD4+ and the remainder CD8+ [235]. In hypercholesterolaemic knockout mice lacking both B and T cells, the atheroscle-rotic effect was reduced to a degree [236–238]. Conversely, a particular subset of T cells known as regulatory T cells (Tregs) are positive for forkhead box P3 (Foxp3+) and are immunosuppressive cells and may provide an anti-inflammatory role in ath-erosclerotic plaque formation [239]. The role of B cells in atherosclerosis remains elusive and poorly understood. Whilst some mouse work suggests that B cells play a potentially protective role [240–243], some conflicting reports point perhaps to a more subset-specific role as either pro- or anti-atherogenic [244, 245]. The review by Hedrick (ATVB, 2015) [246] summarises in greater detail the potential role played by lymphocytes and NK cells in atherosclerosis.

7.4 Summary and Conclusions

In summary we have discussed the pathophysiology of CVD, including established risk factors increasing the risk of premature atherosclerosis; the homeostatic processes involved in the regulation of the cardiovascular system, elaborating on cholesterol transport; and the role of lipoproteins in atherogenesis and reverse cholesterol transport. We have also briefly discussed the role of the CNS and the influence this can exert on both cardiovascular homeostasis and on immunity. The role of the innate immune system (monocytes and macrophages) has also been explored in relation to atherosclerotic plaque as well as the role of DCs and neutrophils. Finally, for completeness, we have included a paragraph on the emerging role seen for lymphocytes in atherosclerotic CVD.

In conclusion, the importance of delving further into the individual contributions made by immune cells to atherosclerotic CVD is that they may provide therapeutic targets for treatment of established disease and, perhaps, more pertinently the potential for prevention. Understanding in greater detail the role played by monocytes and macrophages, for instance, in the propagation of atherosclerotic plaque, may provide the ability to develop future therapies that target very specific processes in order to remove or inhibit key steps leading to the establishment of the unstable plaque.

References

1. WHO. Global status report on noncommunicable diseases 2010. In: Alwan A, editor. Apps. Who. Int. Geneva; 2010. pp. 1–176.
2. GBD 2013 Mortality and Causes of Death Collaborators. Global, regional, and national age-sex specific all-cause and cause-specific mortality for 240 causes of death, 1990–2013: a systematic analysis for the global burden of disease study 2013. Lancet. 2015;385:117–71.
3. Rothwell PM, Coull AJ, Silver LE, Fairhead JF, Giles MF, Lovelock CE, et al. Population-based study of event-rate, incidence, case fatality, and mortality for all acute vascular events in all arterial territories (Oxford vascular study). Lancet. 2005;366:1773–83.
4. Townsend N, Wickramasinghe K, Bhatnagar P. Coronary heart disease statistics. A compendium of health statistics. London: British Heart Foundation; 2012.
5. Fowkes FGR, Rudan D, Rudan I, Aboyans V, Denenberg JO, McDermott MM, et al. Comparison of global estimates of prevalence and risk factors for peripheral artery disease in 2000 and 2010: a systematic review and analysis. Lancet. 2013;382:1329–40.
6. Doll R, Peto R, Boreham J, Sutherland I. Mortality in relation to smoking: 50 years' observations on male British doctors. BMJ. 2004;328:1519–0.

7. Thun MJ, Myers DG, Day-Lally C. Age and the exposure-response relationships between cigarette smoking and premature death in cancer prevention study II. ... D: Changes in .... 1997.

8. Holt PG, Keast D. Environmentally induced changes in immunological function: acute and chronic effects of inhalation of tobacco smoke and other atmospheric contaminants in man and experimental animals. Bacteriol Rev. 1977;41:205–16.

9. Reynolds HY. Bronchoalveolar lavage. Am Rev Respir Dis. 1987;135:250–63.

10. King TE, Savici D, Campbell PA. Phagocytosis and killing of *Listeria monocytogenes* by alveolar macrophages: smokers versus nonsmokers. J Infect Dis. 1988;158:1309–16.

11. McCrea KA, Ensor JE, Nall K, Bleecker ER, Hasday JD. Altered cytokine regulation in the lungs of cigarette smokers. Am J Respir Crit Care Med. 1994;150:696–703.

12. Ferson M, Edwards A, Lind A, Milton GW, Hersey P. Low natural killer-cell activity and immunoglobulin levels associated with smoking in human subjects. Int J Cancer. 1979;23:603–9.

13. Mathews JD, Whittingham S, Hooper BM, Mackay IR, Stenhouse NS. Association of auto-antibodies with smoking, cardiovascular morbidity, and death in the Busselton population. Lancet. 1973;2:754–8.

14. Sopori M. Effects of cigarette smoke on the immune system. Nat Rev Immunol. 2002;2:372–7.

15. Rutan GH, Kuller LH, Neaton JD, Wentworth DN, McDonald RH, Smith WM. Mortality associated with diastolic hypertension and isolated systolic hypertension among men screened for the multiple risk factor intervention trial. Circulation. 1988;77:504–14.

16. MacMahon S, Peto R, Cutler J, Collins R, Sorlie P, Neaton J, et al. Blood pressure, stroke, and coronary heart disease. Part 1, prolonged differences in blood pressure: prospective observational studies corrected for the regression dilution bias. Lancet. 1990;335:765–74.

17. Lewington S, Clarke R, Qizilbash N, Peto R, Collins R, Prospective Studies Collaboration. Age-specific relevance of usual blood pressure to vascular mortality: a meta-analysis of individual data for one million adults in 61 prospective studies. Lancet. 2002;360:1903–13.

18. O'Donnell M, Mente A, Rangarajan S, McQueen MJ, Wang X, Liu L, et al. Urinary sodium and potassium excretion, mortality, and cardiovascular events. N Engl J Med. 2014;371:612–23.

19. Chen Z, Smith M, Du H, Guo Y, Clarke R, Bian Z, et al. Blood pressure in relation to general and central adiposity among 500,000 adult Chinese men and women. Int J Epidemiol. 2015;44:1305–19.

20. Bautista LE, Vera LM, Arenas IA, Gamarra G. Independent association between inflammatory markers (C-reactive protein, interleukin-6, and TNF-l[alpha]l) and essential hypertension. J Hum Hypertens. 2005;19:149–54.

21. Chae CU, Lee RT, Rifai N, Ridker PM. Blood pressure and inflammation in apparently healthy men. Hypertension. 2001;38:399–403.

22. Laviades C, Varo N, Díez J. Transforming growth factor Beta in hypertensives with cardiorenal damage. Hypertension. 2000;36:517–22.

23. Dörffel Y, Lätsch C, Stuhlmüller B, Schreiber S, Scholze S, Burmester GR, et al. Preactivated peripheral blood monocytes in patients with essential hypertension. Hypertension. 1999;34:113–7.

24. Frossard PM, Gupta A, Pravica V, Perrey C, Hutchinson IV, Lukic ML. A study of five human cytokine genes in human essential hypertension. Mol Immunol. 2002;38:969–76.

25. Harrison DG, Guzik TJ, Lob HE, Madhur MS. Inflammation, immunity, and hypertension. Hypertension. 2011;57(2):132–40.

26. Muller DN, Dechend R, Mervaala EM, Park JK, Schmidt F, Fiebeler A, et al. NF-kappaB inhibition ameliorates angiotensin II-induced inflammatory damage in rats. Hypertension. 2000;35:193–201.

27. Shagdarsuren E, Wellner M, Braesen J-H, Park J-K, Fiebeler A, Henke N, et al. Complement activation in angiotensin II-induced organ damage. Circ Res. 2005;97:716–24.

28. Müller DN, Shagdarsuren E, Park J-K, Dechend R, Mervaala E, Hampich F, et al. Immunosuppressive treatment protects against angiotensin II-induced renal damage. Am J Pathol. 2002;161:1679–93.

29. Wu K-IS, Schmid-Schönbein GW. Nuclear factor kappa B and matrix metalloprotein-ase induced receptor cleavage in the spontaneously hypertensive rat. Hypertension. 2011;57:261–8.
30. Tostes RCA, Touyz RM, He G, Chen X, Schiffrin EL. Contribution of endothelin-1 to renal activator protein-1 activation and macrophage infiltration in aldosterone-induced hyperten-sion. Clin Sci (Lond). 2002;103(Suppl 48):25S–30S.
31. Jennings BL, Anderson LJ, Estes AM, Yaghini FA, Fang XR, Porter J, et al. Cytochrome P450 1B1 contributes to renal dysfunction and damage caused by angiotensin II in mice. Hypertension. 2012;59:348–54.
32. Zubcevic J, Waki H, Raizada MK, Paton JFR. Autonomic-immune-vascular interaction: an emerging concept for neurogenic hypertension. Hypertension. 2011;57:1026–33.
33. Abboud FM, Harwani SC, Chapleau MW. Autonomic neural regulation of the immune system: implications for hypertension and cardiovascular disease. Hypertension. 2012;59:755–62.
34. Ryan MJ. An update on immune system activation in the pathogenesis of hypertension. Hypertension. 2013;62:226–30.
35. Goldstein JL, Brown MS. A century of cholesterol and coronaries: from plaques to genes to statins. Cell. 2015;161:161–72.
36. Gertler MM, White PD. Coronary heart disease in young adults. A multi-disciplinary study. Science. 1954;120:1–2.
37. Gofman JW, Delalla O, Glazier F, Freeman NK, Lindgren FT, Nichols AV, et al. The serum lipoprotein transport system in health, metabolic disorders, atherosclerosis and coronary heart disease. J Clin Lipidol. 2007;1:104–41.
38. Brown MS, Goldstein JL. Familial hypercholesterolemia: defective binding of lipoproteins to cultured fibroblasts associated with impaired regulation of 3-hydroxy-3-methylglutaryl coenzyme A reductase activity. Proc Natl Acad Sci U S A. 1974;71:788–92.
39. Emerging Risk Factors Collaboration, Sarwar N, Gao P, SRK S, Gobin R, Kaptoge S, et al. Diabetes mellitus, fasting blood glucose concentration, and risk of vascular disease: a col-laborative meta-analysis of 102 prospective studies. Lancet. 2010;375:2215–22.
40. Emerging Risk Factors Collaboration, SRK S, Kaptoge S, Thompson A, Di Angelantonio E, Gao P, et al. Diabetes mellitus, fasting glucose, and risk of cause-specific death. N Engl J Med. 2011;364:829–41.
41. Joosten MM, Pai JK, Bertoia ML, Rimm EB, Spiegelman D, Mittleman MA, et al. Associations between conventional cardiovascular risk factors and risk of peripheral artery disease in men. JAMA. 2012;308:1660–7.
42. Umpierrez GE, Isaacs SD, Bazargan N, You X, Thaler LM, Kitabchi AE. Hyperglycemia: an independent marker of in-hospital mortality in patients with undiagnosed diabetes. J Clin Endocrinol Metab. 2002;87:978–82.
43. Sampson MJ, Davies IR, Brown JC, Ivory K, Hughes DA. Monocyte and neutrophil adhesion molecule expression during acute hyperglycemia and after antioxidant treatment in type 2 diabetes and control patients. Arterioscler Thromb Vasc Biol. 2002;22:1187–93.
44. Ceriello A, Falleti E, Motz E, Taboga C, Tonutti L, Ezsol Z, et al. Hyperglycemia-induced circulating ICAM-1 increase in diabetes mellitus: the possible role of oxidative stress. Horm Metab Res. 1998;30:146–9.
45. Chen NG, Azhar S, Abbasi F, Carantoni M, Reaven GM. The relationship between plasma glucose and insulin responses to oral glucose, LDL oxidation, and soluble intercellular adhe-sion molecule-1 in healthy volunteers. Atherosclerosis. 2000;152:203–8.
46. Marfella R, Esposito K, Giunta R, Coppola G, De Angelis L, Farzati B, et al. Circulating adhesion molecules in humans: role of hyperglycemia and hyperinsulinemia. Circulation. 2000;101:2247–51.
47. Ceriello A, Quagliaro L, Piconi L, Assaloni R, Da Ros R, Maier A, et al. Effect of postprandial hypertriglyceridemia and hyperglycemia on circulating adhesion molecules and oxidative stress generation and the possible role of simvastatin treatment. Diabetes. 2004;53:701–10.
48. Jafar N, Edriss H, Nugent K. The effect of short-term hyperglycemia on the innate immune system. Am J Med Sci. 2016;351:201–11.

49. Turina M, Fry DE, Polk HC. Acute hyperglycemia and the innate immune system: clinical, cellular, and molecular aspects. Crit Care Med. 2005;33:1624–33.
50. WHO. Definition and Diagnosis of Diabetes Mellitus and Intermediate Hyperglycemia. Bull. World Health Organ. Geneva: WHO Press; 2006 pp. 1–50.
51. Deresinski S. Infections in the diabetic patient: Strategies for the clinician. Infect. Dis. Rep. 1995;1:1–12.
52. Carton JA, Maradona JA, Nuño FJ, Fernandez-Alvarez R, Pérez-Gonzalez F, Asensi V. Diabetes mellitus and bacteraemia: a comparative study between diabetic and non-diabetic patients. Eur J Med. 1992;1:281–7.
53. Geerlings SE, Hoepelman AI. Immune dysfunction in patients with diabetes mellitus (DM). FEMS Immunol Med Microbiol. 1999;26:259–65.
54. Katz S, Klein B, Elian I, Fishman P, Djaldetti M. Phagocytotic activity of monocytes from diabetic patients. Diabetes Care. 1983;6:479–82.
55. West KM. Epidemiology of diabetes and its vascular lesions. New York: Elsevier North-Holland Inc; 1978. p. 234–48.
56. Barrett-Connor E. Epidemiology, obesity, and non-insulin-dependent diabetes mellitus. Epidemiol Rev. 1989;11:172–81.
57. Ford ES, Williamson DF, Liu S. Weight change and diabetes incidence: findings from a national cohort of US adults. Am J Epidemiol. 1997;146:214–22.
58. Reaven GM. Role of insulin resistance in human disease. Diabetes. 1988;37:1595–607.
59. WHO. Waist circumference and waist-hip ratio: report of a WHO expert consultation, Geneva, 8–11 December 2008. Geneva, CH: World Health Organization; 2014. pp. 23–6.
60. Flegal KM, Kit BK, Orpana H, Graubard BI. Association of all-cause mortality with over-weight and obesity using standard body mass index categories: a systematic review and meta-analysis. JAMA. 2013;309:71–82.
61. Hotamisligil GS, Shargill NS, Spiegelman BM. Adipose expression of tumor necrosis factor-alpha: direct role in obesity-linked insulin resistance. Science. 1993;259:87–91.
62. Olefsky JM, Glass CK. Macrophages, inflammation, and insulin resistance. Annu Rev. 2010;72:219–46. doi:10.1146/annurev-physiol-021909-135846.
63. Park HS, Park JY, Yu R. Relationship of obesity and visceral adiposity with serum concentrations of CRP, TNF-alpha and IL-6. Diabetes Res Clin Pract. 2005;69:29–35.
64. Festa A, D'Agostino R, Williams K, Karter AJ, Mayer-Davis EJ, Tracy RP, et al. The relation of body fat mass and distribution to markers of chronic inflammation. Int J Obes Relat Metab Disord. 2001;25:1407–15.
65. Bulló M, García-Lorda P, Megias I, Salas-Salvadó J. Systemic inflammation, adipose tissue tumor necrosis factor, and leptin expression. Obes Res. 2003;11:525–31.
66. Winer DA, Luck H, Tsai S, Winer S. The intestinal immune system in obesity and insulin resistance. CMET. 2016;23:413–26.
67. Xu H, Barnes GT, Yang Q, Tan G, Yang D, Chou CJ, et al. Chronic inflammation in fat plays a crucial role in the development of obesity-related insulin resistance. J Clin Invest. 2003;112:1821–30.
68. Lumeng CN, Bodzin JL, Saltiel AR. Obesity induces a phenotypic switch in adipose tissue macrophage polarization. J Clin Invest. 2007;117:175–84.
69. Weisberg SP, McCann D, Desai M, Rosenbaum M, Leibel RL, Ferrante AW. Obesity is associated with macrophage accumulation in adipose tissue. J Clin Invest. 2003;112:1796–808.
70. Winer S, Chan Y, Paltser G, Truong D, Tsui H, Bahrami J, et al. Normalization of obesity-associated insulin resistance through immunotherapy. Nat Med. 2009;15:921–9.
71. Nishimura S, Manabe I, Nagasaki M, Eto K, Yamashita H, Ohsugi M, et al. CD8+ effector T cells contribute to macrophage recruitment and adipose tissue inflammation in obesity. Nat Med. 2009;15:914–20.
72. Winer DA, Winer S, Shen L, Wadia PP, Yantha J, Paltser G, et al. B cells promote insulin resistance through modulation of T cells and production of pathogenic IgG antibodies. Nat Med. 2011;17:610–7.

73. Wensveen FM, Jelenčić V, Valentić S, Šestan M, Wensveen TT, Theurich S, et al. NK cells link obesity-induced adipose stress to inflammation and insulin resistance. Nat Immunol. 2015;16:376–85.

74. Talukdar S, Oh DY, Bandyopadhyay G, Li D, Xu J, McNelis J, et al. Neutrophils mediate insulin resistance in mice fed a high-fat diet through secreted elastase. Nat Med. 2012;18:1407–12.

75. Malik S, Wong ND, Franklin SS, Kamath TV, L'Italien GJ, Pio JR, et al. Impact of the metabolic syndrome on mortality from coronary heart disease, cardiovascular disease, and all causes in United States adults. Circulation. 2004;110:1245–50.

76. Qatanani M, Lazar MA. Mechanisms of obesity-associated insulin resistance: many choices on the menu. Genes Dev. 2007;21:1443–55.

77. Odegaard JI, Chawla A. Mechanisms of macrophage activation in obesity-induced insulin resistance. Nat Clin Pract Endocrinol Metab. 2008;4:619–26.

78. Tobias P, Curtiss LK. Thematic review series: the immune system and atherogenesis. Paying the price for pathogen protection: toll receptors in atherogenesis. J Lipid Res. 2005;46:404–11.

79. Harrison DG, Guzik TJ, Goronzy J, Weyand C. Is hypertension an immunologic disease? Curr Cardiol Rep. 2008;10:464–9.

80. Scandinavian Simvastatin Survival Study Group. Randomised trial of cholesterol lowering in 4444 patients with coronary heart disease: the Scandinavian simvastatin survival study (4S). Lancet. 1994;344:1383–9.

81. Nicholls SJ, Ballantyne CM, Barter PJ, Chapman MJ, Erbel RM, Libby P, et al. Effect of two intensive statin regimens on progression of coronary disease. N Engl J Med. 2011;365:2078–87.

82. Cannon CP, Braunwald E, McCabe CH, Rader DJ, Rouleau JL, Belder R, et al. Intensive versus moderate lipid lowering with statins after acute coronary syndromes. N Engl J Med. 2004;350:1495–504.

83. Heart Protection Study Collaborative Group. MRC/BHF heart protection study of cholesterol lowering with simvastatin in 20,536 high-risk individuals: a randomised placebo-controlled trial. Lancet. 2002;360:7–22.

84. The Long-Term Intervention with Pravastatin in Ischaemic Disease (LIPID) Study Group. Prevention of cardiovascular events and death with pravastatin in patients with coronary heart disease and a broad range of initial cholesterol levels. N Engl J Med. 1998;339:1349–57.

85. Downs JR, Clearfield M, Weis S, Whitney E, Shapiro DR, Beere PA, et al. Primary prevention of acute coronary events with lovastatin in men and women with average cholesterol levels: results of AFCAPS/TexCAPS. JAMA. 1998;279:1615–22.

86. Sacks FM, Pfeffer MA, Moye LA, Rouleau JL, Rutherford JD, Cole TG, et al. The effect of pravastatin on coronary events after myocardial infarction in patients with average cholesterol levels. Cholesterol and recurrent events trial investigators. N Engl J Med. 1996;335:1001–9.

87. Shepherd J, Cobbe SM, Ford I, Isles CG, Lorimer AR, MacFarlane PW, et al. Prevention of coronary heart disease with pravastatin in men with hypercholesterolemia. West of Scotland coronary prevention study group. N Engl J Med. 1995;333:1301–7.

88. Pedersen TR, Faergeman O, Kastelein JJP, Olsson AG, Tikkanen MJ, Holme I, et al. High-dose atorvastatin vs usual-dose simvastatin for secondary prevention after myocardial infarction: the IDEAL study: a randomized controlled trial. JAMA. 2005;294:2437–45.

89. LaRosa JC, Grundy SM, Waters DD, Shear C, Barter P, Fruchart J-C, et al. Intensive lipid lowering with atorvastatin in patients with stable coronary disease. N Engl J Med. 2005;352:1425–35.

90. Ridker PM, Danielson E, Fonseca FAH, Genest J, Gotto AM, Kastelein JJP, et al. Rosuvastatin to prevent vascular events in men and women with elevated C-reactive protein. N Engl J Med. 2008;359:2195–207.

91. Cholesterol Treatment Trialists' (CTT) Collaboration, Baigent C, Blackwell L, Emberson J, Holland LE, Reith C, et al. Efficacy and safety of more intensive lowering of LDL cholesterol: a meta-analysis of data from 170,000 participants in 26 randomised trials. Lancet 2010; 376:1670–1681.

92. Prospective Studies Collaboration, Lewington S, Whitlock G, Clarke R, Sherliker P, Emberson J, et al. Blood cholesterol and vascular mortality by age, sex, and blood pressure: a meta-analysis of individual data from 61 prospective studies with 55,000 vascular deaths. Lancet. 2007;370:1829–39.
93. Stamler J, Vaccaro O, Neaton JD, Wentworth D, The Multiple Risk Factor Intervention Trial Research Group. Diabetes, other risk factors, and 12-Yr cardiovascular mortality for men screened in the multiple risk factor intervention trial. Diabetes Care. 1993;16:434–44.
94. Quinn MT, Parthasarathy S, Fong LG, Steinberg D. Oxidatively modified low density lipoproteins: a potential role in recruitment and retention of monocyte/macrophages during atherogenesis. Proc Natl Acad Sci U S A. 1987;84:2995–8.
95. Parthasarathy S, Quinn MT, Steinberg D. Is oxidized low density lipoprotein involved in the recruitment and retention of monocyte/macrophages in the artery wall during the initiation of atherosclerosis? Basic Life Sci. 1988;49:375–80.
96. Steinbrecher UP, Parthasarathy S, Leake DS, Witztum JL, Steinberg D. Modification of low density lipoprotein by endothelial cells involves lipid peroxidation and degradation of low density lipoprotein phospholipids. Proc Natl Acad Sci U S A. 1984;81:3883–7.
97. Steinberg D, Parthasarathy S, Carew TE, Khoo JC, Witztum JL. Beyond cholesterol. Modifications of low-density lipoprotein that increase its atherogenicity. N Engl J Med. 1989;320:915–24.
98. Carpenter KL, Wilkins GM, Fussell B, Ballantine JA, Taylor SE, Mitchinson MJ, et al. Production of oxidized lipids during modification of low-density lipoprotein by macrophages or copper. Biochem J. 1994;304(Pt 2):625–33.
99. Folcik VA, Nivar-Aristy RA, Krajewski LP, Cathcart MK. Lipoxygenase contributes to the oxidation of lipids in human atherosclerotic plaques. J Clin Invest. 1995;96:504–10.
100. Berliner J, Leitinger N, Watson A, Huber J, Fogelman A, Navab M. Oxidized lipids in atherogenesis: formation, destruction and action. Thromb Haemost. 1997;78:195–9.
101. Parthasarathy S, Santanam N, Ramachandran S, Meilhac O. Potential role of oxidized lipids and lipoproteins in antioxidant defense. Free Radic Res. 2000;33:197–215.
102. Navab M, Hama SY, Reddy ST, Ng CJ, Van Lenten BJ, Laks H, et al. Oxidized lipids as mediators of coronary heart disease. Curr Opin Lipidol. 2002;13:363–72.
103. Birukov KG. Oxidized lipids: the two faces of vascular inflammation. Curr Atheroscler Rep. 2006;8:223–31.
104. Jovinge S, Ares MP, Kallin B, Nilsson J. Human monocytes/macrophages release TNF-alpha in response to Ox-LDL. Arterioscler Thromb Vasc Biol. 1996;16:1573–9.
105. Terkeltaub R, Banka CL, Solan J, Santoro D, Brand K, Curtiss LK. Oxidized LDL induces monocytic cell expression of interleukin-8, a chemokine with T-lymphocyte chemotactic activity. Arterioscler Thromb. 1994;14:47–53.
106. Bekkering S, Quintin J, Joosten LAB, van der Meer JWM, Netea MG, Riksen NP. Oxidized low-density lipoprotein induces long-term proinflammatory cytokine production and foam cell formation via epigenetic reprogramming of monocytes. Arterioscler Thromb Vasc Biol. 2014;34:1731–8.
107. Fuhrman B, Partoush A, Volkova N, Aviram M. Ox-LDL induces monocyte-to-macrophage differentiation in vivo: possible role for the macrophage colony stimulating factor receptor (M-CSF-R). Atherosclerosis. 2008;196:598–607.
108. Brand K, Banka CL, Mackman N, Terkeltaub RA, Fan ST, Curtiss LK. Oxidized LDL enhances lipopolysaccharide-induced tissue factor expression in human adherent monocytes. Arterioscler Thromb. 1994;14:790–7.
109. Foster GA, Xu L, Chidambaram AA, Soderberg SR, Armstrong EJ, Wu H, et al. CD11c/CD18 signals very late antigen-4 activation to initiate foamy monocyte recruitment during the onset of hypercholesterolemia. J Immunol. 2015;195(11):5380–92.
110. Gower RM, Wu H, Foster GA, Devaraj S, Jialal I, Ballantyne CM, et al. CD11c/CD18 expression is upregulated on blood monocytes during hypertriglyceridemia and enhances adhesion to vascular cell adhesion molecule-1. Arterioscler Thromb Vasc Biol. 2011; 31:160–6.

111. Jackson WD, Weinrich TW, Woollard KJ. Very-low and low-density lipoproteins induce neutral lipid accumulation and impair migration in monocyte subsets. Nature Publishing Group; 2016; pp. 1–12.
112. Berliner JA, Heinecke JW. The role of oxidized lipoproteins in atherogenesis. Free Radic Biol Med. 1996;20:707–27.
113. Gordon T, Castelli WP, Hjortland MC, Kannel WB, Dawber TR. High density lipoprotein as a protective factor against coronary heart disease. The Framingham study. Am J Med. 1977;62:707–14.
114. Emerging Risk Factors Collaboration, Di Angelantonio E, Sarwar N, Perry P, Kaptoge S, Ray KK, et al. Major lipids, apolipoproteins, and risk of vascular disease. JAMA. 2009;302:1993–2000.
115. Mineo C, Shaul PW. Novel biological functions of high-density lipoprotein cholesterol. Circ Res. 2012;111:1079–90.
116. Baldán A, Bojanic DD, Edwards PA. The ABCs of sterol transport. J Lipid Res. 2009;50(Suppl):S80–5.
117. Yvan-Charvet L, Wang N, Tall AR. Role of HDL, ABCA1, and ABCG1 transporters in cholesterol efflux and immune responses. Arterioscler Thromb Vasc Biol. 2010;30:139–43.
118. Barter PJ, Nicholls S, Rye K-A, Anantharamaiah GM, Navab M, Fogelman AM. Antiinflammatory properties of HDL. Circ Res. 2004;95:764–72.
119. De Nardo D, Labzin LI, Kono H, Seki R, Schmidt SV, Beyer M, et al. High-density lipoprotein mediates anti-inflammatory reprogramming of macrophages via the transcriptional regulator ATF3. Nat Immunol. 2014;15:152–60.
120. Voight BF, Peloso GM, Orho-Melander M, Frikke-Schmidt R, Barbalic M, Jensen MK, et al. Plasma HDL cholesterol and risk of myocardial infarction: a mendelian randomisation study. Lancet. 2012;380:572–80.
121. Zanoni P, Khetarpal SA, Larach DB, Hancock-Cerutti WF, Millar JS, Cuchel M, et al. Rare variant in scavenger receptor BI raises HDL cholesterol and increases risk of coronary heart disease. Science. 2016;351:1166–71.
122. Barter PJ, Caulfield M, Eriksson M, Grundy SM, Kastelein JJP, Komajda M, et al. Effects of torcetrapib in patients at high risk for coronary events. N Engl J Med. 2007;357:2109–22.
123. AIM-HIGH Investigators, Boden WE, Probstfield JL, Anderson T, Chaitman BR, Desvignes-Nickens P, et al. Niacin in patients with low HDL cholesterol levels receiving intensive statin therapy. N Engl J Med. 2011;365:2255–67.
124. Schwartz GG, Olsson AG, Ballantyne CM, Barter PJ, Holme IM, Kallend D, et al. Rationale and design of the dal-OUTCOMES trial: efficacy and safety of dalcetrapib in patients with recent acute coronary syndrome. Am Heart J. 2009;158:896–901.e3.
125. Lambert JE, Parks EJ. Postprandial metabolism of meal triglyceride in humans. BBA Mol Cell Biol Lipids. 2012;1821:721–6.
126. Redgrave TG. Chylomicron metabolism. Biochem Soc Trans. 2004;32:79–82.
127. López-Miranda J, Marín C. Chapter 17: dietary, physiological, and genetic impacts on postprandial lipid metabolism. Fat Detect Taste Texture Post Ingestive Effects. 2010:1–59.
128. Hartigh den LJ, Altman R, Norman JE, Rutledge JC. Postprandial VLDL lipolysis products increase monocyte adhesion and lipid droplet formation via activation of ERK2 and NFκB. Am J Physiol Heart Circ Physiol. 2014;306:H109–20.
129. Zilversmit DB. Atherogenesis: a postprandial phenomenon. Circulation. 1979;60:473–85.
130. Nordestgaard BG, Benn M, Schnohr P, Tybjærg-Hansen A. Nonfasting triglycerides and risk of myocardial infarction, ischemic heart disease, and death in men and women. JAMA. 2007;298:299–308.
131. Nordestgaard BG, Varbo A. Triglycerides and cardiovascular disease. Lancet. 2014;384:626–35.
132. Chowdhury R, Warnakula S, Kunutsor S, Crowe F, Ward HA, Johnson L, et al. Association of dietary, circulating, and supplement fatty acids with coronary risk: a systematic review and meta-analysis. Ann Intern Med. 2014;160:398–406.
133. Harcombe Z, Baker JS, Cooper SM, Davies B, Sculthorpe N, DiNicolantonio JJ, et al. Evidence from randomised controlled trials did not support the introduction of dietary fat guidelines in 1977 and 1983: a systematic review and meta-analysis. Open Heart. 2015;2:e000196.

134. de Souza RJ, Mente A, Maroleanu A, Cozma AI, Ha V, Kishibe T, et al. Intake of saturated and trans unsaturated fatty acids and risk of all cause mortality, cardiovascular disease, and type 2 diabetes: systematic review and meta-analysis of observational studies. BMJ. 2015;351:h3978–16.
135. Siri-Tarino PW, Sun Q, FB H, Krauss RM. Meta-analysis of prospective cohort studies evaluating the association of saturated fat with cardiovascular disease. Am J Clin Nutr. 2010;91:535–46.
136. Estruch R, Ros E, Salas-Salvadó J, Covas M-I, Corella D, Arós F, et al. Primary prevention of cardiovascular disease with a Mediterranean diet. N Engl J Med. 2013;368:1279–90.
137. Li R, Wu Y, Manso AM, Gu Y, Liao P, Israeli S, et al. β1 integrin gene excision in the adult murine cardiac myocyte causes defective mechanical and signaling responses. Am J Pathol. 2012;180:952–62.
138. Lal H, Verma SK, Smith M, Guleria RS, Lu G, Foster DM, et al. Stretch-induced MAP kinase activation in cardiac myocytes: differential regulation through beta1-integrin and focal adhesion kinase. J Mol Cell Cardiol. 2007;43:137–47.
139. Lal H, Verma SK, Golden HB, Foster DM, Smith M, Dostal DE. Stretch-induced regulation of angiotensinogen gene expression in cardiac myocytes and fibroblasts: opposing roles of JNK1/2 and p38alpha MAP kinases. J Mol Cell Cardiol. 2008;45:770–8.
140. Verma SK, Lal H, Golden HB, Gerilechaogetu F, Smith M, Guleria RS, et al. Rac1 and RhoA differentially regulate angiotensinogen gene expression in stretched cardiac fibroblasts. Cardiovasc Res. 2011;90:88–96.
141. Burgess ML, Carver WE, Terracio L, Wilson SP, Wilson MA, Borg TK. Integrin-mediated collagen gel contraction by cardiac fibroblasts. Effects of angiotensin II. Circ Res. 1994;74:291–8.
142. Dostal DE, Feng H, Nizamutdinov D, Golden HB, Afroze SH, Dostal JD, et al. Mechanosensing and regulation of cardiac function. J Clin Exp Cardiolog. 2014;5:314.
143. Olshansky B, Sabbah HN, Hauptman PJ, Colucci WS. Parasympathetic nervous system and heart failure: pathophysiology and potential implications for therapy. Circulation. 2008;118:863–71.
144. Kishi T. Heart failure as an autonomic nervous system dysfunction. J Cardiol. 2012;59:117–22.
145. Shen MJ, Zipes DP. Role of the autonomic nervous system in modulating cardiac arrhythmias. Circ Res. 2014;114:1004–21.
146. Esler MD, Krum H, Schlaich M, Schmieder RE, Böhm M, Sobotka PA, et al. Renal sympathetic denervation for treatment of drug-resistant hypertension: one-year results from the Symplicity HTN-2 randomized, controlled trial. Circulation. 2012;126:2976–82.
147. Bhatt DL, Kandzari DE, O'Neill WW, D'Agostino R, Flack JM, Katzen BT, et al. A controlled trial of renal denervation for resistant hypertension. N Engl J Med. 2014;370:1393–401.
148. Khansari DN, Murgo AJ, Faith RE. Effects of stress on the immune system. Immunol Today. 1990;11(5):170.
149. Segerstrom SC, Miller GE. Psychological stress and the human immune system: a meta-analytic study of 30 years of inquiry. Psychol Bull. 2004;130:601–30.
150. Heidt T, Sager HB, Courties G, Dutta P, Iwamoto Y, Zaltsman A, et al. Chronic variable stress activates hematopoietic stem cells. Nat Med. 2014;20:754–8.
151. Nahrendorf M, Swirski FK, Aikawa E, Stangenberg L, Wurdinger T, Figueiredo J-L, et al. The healing myocardium sequentially mobilizes two monocyte subsets with divergent and complementary functions. J Exp Med. 2007;204:3037–47.
152. Nahrendorf M, Pittet MJ, Swirski FK. Monocytes: protagonists of infarct inflammation and repair after myocardial infarction. Circulation. 2010;121:2437–45.
153. Swirski FK, Nahrendorf M, Etzrodt M, Wildgruber M, Cortez-Retamozo V, Panizzi P, et al. Identification of splenic reservoir monocytes and their deployment to inflammatory sites. Science. 2009;325:612–6.
154. Emami H, Singh P, MacNabb M, Vucic E, Lavender Z, Rudd JHF, et al. Splenic metabolic activity predicts risk of future cardiovascular events: demonstration of a cardiosplenic axis in humans. JACC Cardiovasc Imaging. 2015;8:121–30.
155. van Furth R, Cohn ZA. The origin and kinetics of mononuclear phagocytes. J Exp Med. 1968;128:415–35.

156. Tsujioka H, Imanishi T, Ikejima H, Kuroi A, Takarada S, Tanimoto T, et al. Impact of heterogeneity of human peripheral blood monocyte subsets on myocardial salvage in patients with primary acute myocardial infarction. J Am Coll Cardiol. 2009;54:130–8.
157. Dutta P, Courties G, Wei Y, Leuschner F, Gorbatov R, Robbins CS, et al. Myocardial infarction accelerates atherosclerosis. Nature. 2012;487:325–9.
158. Gerrity RG. The role of the monocyte in atherogenesis: I. Transition of blood-borne monocytes into foam cells in fatty lesions. Am J Pathol. 1981;103:181–90.
159. Gerrity RG. The role of the monocyte in atherogenesis: II. Migration of foam cells from atherosclerotic lesions. Am J Pathol. 1981;103:191–200.
160. Cros J, Cagnard N, Woollard KJ, Patey N, Zhang S-Y, Senechal B, et al. Human CD14dim monocytes patrol and sense nucleic acids and viruses via TLR7 and TLR8 receptors. Immunity. 2010;33:375–86.
161. Woollard KJ, Geissmann F. Monocytes in atherosclerosis: subsets and functions. Nat Rev Cardiol. 2010:1–10.
162. Combadière C, Potteaux S, Rodero M, Simon T, Pezard A, Esposito B, et al. Combined inhibition of CCL2, CX3CR1, and CCR5 abrogates Ly6C(hi) and Ly6C(lo) monocytosis and almost abolishes atherosclerosis in hypercholesterolemic mice. Circulation. 2008;117:1649–57.
163. Tacke F, Alvarez D, Kaplan TJ, Jakubzick C, Spanbroek R, Llodra J, et al. Monocyte subsets differentially employ CCR2, CCR5, and CX3CR1 to accumulate within atherosclerotic plaques. J Clin Invest. 2007;117:185–94.
164. Lesnik P, Haskell CA, Charo IF. Decreased atherosclerosis in CX3CR1−/− mice reveals a role for fractalkine in atherogenesis. J Clin Invest. 2003;111:333–40.
165. Moore KJ, Sheedy FJ, Fisher EA. Macrophages in atherosclerosis: a dynamic balance. Nat Rev Immunol. 2013;13:709–21.
166. Wong KL, Tai JJ-Y, Wong W-C, Han H, Sem X, Yeap W-H, et al. Gene expression profiling reveals the defining features of the classical, intermediate, and nonclassical human monocyte subsets. Blood. 2011;118:e16–31.
167. Swirski FK, Libby P, Aikawa E, Alcaide P, Luscinskas FW, Weissleder R, et al. Ly-6Chi monocytes dominate hypercholesterolemia-associated monocytosis and give rise to macrophages in atheromata. J Clin Invest. 2007;117:195–205.
168. Yona S, Kim K-W, Wolf Y, Mildner A, Varol D, Breker M, et al. Fate mapping reveals origins and dynamics of monocytes and tissue macrophages under homeostasis. Immunity. 2013;38:79–91.
169. Ginhoux F, Jung S. Monocytes and macrophages: developmental pathways and tissue homeostasis. Nat Rev Immunol. 2014;14:392–404.
170. Palframan RT, Jung S, Cheng G, Weninger W, Luo Y, Dorf M, et al. Inflammatory chemokine transport and presentation in HEV a remote control mechanism for monocyte recruitment to lymph nodes in inflamed tissues. J Exp Med. 2001;194:1361–74.
171. Luscinskas FW, Ding H, Tan P, Cumming D, Tedder TF, Gerritsen ME. L- and P-selectins, but not CD49d (VLA-4) integrins, mediate monocyte initial attachment to TNF-alpha-activated vascular endothelium under flow in vitro. J Immunol. 1996;157:326–35.
172. An G, Wang H, Tang R, Yago T, McDaniel JM, McGee S, et al. P-selectin glycoprotein ligand-1 is highly expressed on Ly-6Chi monocytes and a major determinant for Ly-6Chi monocyte recruitment to sites of atherosclerosis in mice. Circulation. 2008;117:3227–37.
173. Geissmann F, Jung S, Littman DR. Blood monocytes consist of two principal subsets with distinct migratory properties. Immunity. 2003;19:71–82.
174. Grage-Griebenow E, Flad HD, Ernst M. Heterogeneity of human peripheral blood monocyte subsets. J Leukoc Biol. 2001;69:11–20.
175. Jakubzick C, Gautier EL, Gibbings SL, Sojka DK, Schlitzer A, Johnson TE, et al. Minimal differentiation of classical monocytes as they survey steady-state tissues and transport antigen to lymph nodes. Immunity. 2013;39:599–610.
176. Ginhoux F, Greter M, Leboeuf M, Nandi S, See P, Gokhan S, et al. Fate mapping analysis reveals that adult microglia derive from primitive macrophages. Science. 2010;330:841–5.

177. Schulz C, Gomez Perdiguero E, Chorro L, Szabo-Rogers H, Cagnard N, Kierdorf K, et al. A lineage of myeloid cells independent of Myb and hematopoietic stem cells. Science. 2012;336:86–90.

178. Hoeffel G, Wang Y, Greter M, See P, Teo P, Malleret B, et al. Adult Langerhans cells derive predominantly from embryonic fetal liver monocytes with a minor contribution of yolk sac-derived macrophages. J Exp Med. 2012;209:1167–81.

179. Epelman S, Lavine KJ, Beaudin AE, Sojka DK, Carrero JA, Calderon B, et al. Embryonic and adult-derived resident cardiac macrophages are maintained through distinct mechanisms at steady state and during inflammation. Immunity. 2014;40:91–104.

180. Bain CC, Bravo-Blas A, Scott CL, Gomez Perdiguero E, Geissmann F, Henri S, et al. Constant replenishment from circulating monocytes maintains the macrophage pool in the intestine of adult mice. Nat Immunol. 2014;15:929–37.

181. Hoeffel G, Chen J, Lavin Y, Low D, Almeida FF, See P, et al. C-Myb(+) erythro-myeloid progenitor-derived fetal monocytes give rise to adult tissue-resident macrophages. Immunity. 2015;42:665–78.

182. Gomez Perdiguero E, Klapproth K, Schulz C, Busch K, Azzoni E, Crozet L, et al. Tissue-resident macrophages originate from yolk-sac-derived erythro-myeloid progenitors. Nature. 2015;518:547–51.

183. Ensan S, Li A, Besla R, Degousee N, Cosme J, Roufaiel M, et al. Self-renewing resident arterial macrophages arise from embryonic CX3CR1(+) precursors and circulating monocytes immediately after birth. Nat Immunol. 2016;17:159–68.

184. Moore KJ, Tabas I. Macrophages in the pathogenesis of atherosclerosis. Cell. 2011;145:341–55.

185. Ishibashi S, Goldstein JL, Brown MS, Herz J, Burns DK. Massive xanthomatosis and atherosclerosis in cholesterol-fed low density lipoprotein receptor-negative mice. J Clin Invest. 1994;93:1885–93.

186. Nakashima Y, Plump AS, Raines EW, Breslow JL, Ross R. ApoE-deficient mice develop lesions of all phases of atherosclerosis throughout the arterial tree. Arterioscler Thromb Vasc Biol. 1994;14:133–40.

187. Reddick RL, Zhang SH, Maeda N. Atherosclerosis in mice lacking apo E. Evaluation of lesional development and progression. Arterioscler Thromb. 1994;14:141–7.

188. Ishibashi S, Brown MS, Goldstein JL, Gerard RD, Hammer RE, Herz J. Hypercholesterolemia in low density lipoprotein receptor knockout mice and its reversal by adenovirus-mediated gene delivery. J Clin Invest. 1993;92:883–93.

189. Plump AS, Smith JD, Hayek T, Aalto-Setälä K, Walsh A, Verstuyft JG, et al. Severe hypercholesterolemia and atherosclerosis in apolipoprotein E-deficient mice created by homologous recombination in ES cells. Cell. 1992;71:343–53.

190. Zhang FX, Kirschning CJ, Mancinelli R, Xu XP, Jin Y, Faure E, et al. Bacterial lipopolysaccharide activates nuclear factor-kappaB through interleukin-1 signaling mediators in cultured human dermal endothelial cells and mononuclear phagocytes. J Biol Chem. 1999;274: 7611–4.

191. Woollard KJ. Immunological aspects of atherosclerosis. Clin Sci. 2013;125:221–35.

192. Randolph GJ. Mechanisms that regulate macrophage burden in atherosclerosis. Circ Res. 2014;114:1757–71.

193. Spann NJ, Garmire LX, McDonald JG, Myers DS, Milne SB, Shibata N, et al. Regulated accumulation of desmosterol integrates macrophage lipid metabolism and inflammatory responses. Cell. 2012;151:138–52.

194. Horiuchi S, Sakamoto Y, Sakai M. Scavenger receptors for oxidized and glycated proteins. Amino Acids. 2003;25:283–92.

195. Hazen SL. Oxidized phospholipids as endogenous pattern recognition ligands in innate immunity. J Biol Chem. 2008;283:15527–31.

196. Park YM, Febbraio M, Silverstein RL. CD36 modulates migration of mouse and human macrophages in response to oxidized LDL and may contribute to macrophage trapping in the arterial intima. J Clin Invest. 2009;119:136–45.

197. Randolph GJ. Emigration of monocyte-derived cells to lymph nodes during resolution of inflammation and its failure in atherosclerosis. Curr Opin Lipidol. 2008;19:462–8.
198. Williams KJ, Tabas I. The response-to-retention hypothesis of early atherogenesis. Arterioscler Thromb Vasc Biol. 1995;15:551–61.
199. Tabas I. Nonoxidative modifications of lipoproteins in atherogenesis. Annu Rev Nutr. 1999;19:123–39.
200. Skålén K, Gustafsson M, Rydberg EK, Hultén LM, Wiklund O, Innerarity TL, et al. Subendothelial retention of atherogenic lipoproteins in early atherosclerosis. Nature. 2002;417:750–4.
201. Libby P, Clinton SK. Cytokines as mediators of vascular pathology. Nouv Rev Fr Hematol. 1992;34(Suppl):S47–53.
202. Munro JM, Cotran RS. The pathogenesis of atherosclerosis: atherogenesis and inflammation. Lab Investig. 1988;58:249–61.
203. Ross R. Atherosclerosis – an inflammatory disease. N Engl J Med. 1999;340:115–26.
204. Libby P, Ridker PM, Maseri A. Inflammation and atherosclerosis. Circulation. 2002;105:1135–43.
205. de Villiers WJ, Smith JD, Miyata M, Dansky HM, Darley E, Gordon S. Macrophage phenotype in mice deficient in both macrophage-colony-stimulating factor (op) and apolipoprotein E. Arterioscler Thromb Vasc Biol. 1998;18:631–40.
206. Robbins CS, Hilgendorf I, Weber GF, Theurl I, Iwamoto Y, Figueiredo J-L, et al. Local proliferation dominates lesional macrophage accumulation in atherosclerosis. Nat Med. 2013;19:1166–72.
207. Zhu S-N, Chen M, Jongstra-Bilen J, Cybulsky MI. GM-CSF regulates intimal cell proliferation in nascent atherosclerotic lesions. J Exp Med. 2009;206:2141–9.
208. Rosenfeld ME, Polinsky P, Virmani R, Kauser K, Rubanyi G, Schwartz SM. Advanced atherosclerotic lesions in the innominate artery of the ApoE knockout mouse. Arterioscler Thromb Vasc Biol. 2000;20:2587–92.
209. Martinez FO, Gordon S. The M1 and M2 paradigm of macrophage activation: time for reassessment. F1000Prime Rep. 2014;6:13.
210. Libby P, Ridker PM, Hansson GK. Progress and challenges in translating the biology of atherosclerosis. Nature. 2011;473:317–25.
211. Boyle JJ. Heme and haemoglobin direct macrophage Mhem phenotype and counter foam cell formation in areas of intraplaque haemorrhage. Curr Opin Lipidol. 2012;
212. Boyle JJ, Johns M, Kampfer T, Nguyen AT, Game L, Schaer DJ, et al. Activating transcription factor 1 directs Mhem atheroprotective macrophages through coordinated iron handling and foam cell protection. Circ Res. 2012;110:20–33.
213. Finn AV, Nakano M, Polavarapu R, Karmali V, Saeed O, Zhao X, et al. Hemoglobin directs macrophage differentiation and prevents foam cell formation in human atherosclerotic plaques. J Am Coll Cardiol. 2012;59:166–77.
214. Boyle JJ, Harrington HA, Piper E, Elderfield K, Stark J, Landis RC, et al. Coronary intraplaque hemorrhage evokes a novel atheroprotective macrophage phenotype. Am J Pathol. 2009;174:1097–108.
215. Steinman RM. Decisions about dendritic cells: past, present, and future. Annu Rev Immunol. 2012;30:1–22.
216. Paulson KE, Zhu S-N, Chen M, Nurmohamed S, Jongstra-Bilen J, Cybulsky MI. Resident intimal dendritic cells accumulate lipid and contribute to the initiation of atherosclerosis. Circ Res. 2010;106:383–90.
217. Cybulsky MI, Cheong C, Robbins CS. Macrophages and dendritic cells partners in atherogenesis. Circ Res. 2016;118:637–52.
218. Soehnlein O, Weber C, Lindbom L. Neutrophil granule proteins tune monocytic cell function. Trends Immunol. 2009;30:538–46.
219. van Leeuwen M, Gijbels MJJ, Duijvestijn A, Smook M, van de Gaar MJ, Heeringa P, et al. Accumulation of myeloperoxidase-positive neutrophils in atherosclerotic lesions in LDLR−/− mice. Arterioscler Thromb Vasc Biol. 2008;28:84–9.

220. Ionita MG, van den Borne P, Catanzariti LM, Moll FL, de Vries J-PPM, Pasterkamp G, et al. High neutrophil numbers in human carotid atherosclerotic plaques are associated with characteristics of rupture-prone lesions. Arterioscler Thromb Vasc Biol. 2010;30:1842–8.

221. Naruko T, Ueda M, Haze K, van der Wal AC, van der Loos CM, Itoh A, et al. Neutrophil infiltration of culprit lesions in acute coronary syndromes. Circulation. 2002;106: 2894–900.

222. Lee TD, Gonzalez ML, Kumar P, Chary-Reddy S, Grammas P, Pereira HA. CAP37, a novel inflammatory mediator. Am J Pathol. 2002;160:841–8.

223. Edfeldt K, Agerberth B, Rottenberg ME, Gudmundsson GH, Wang X-B, Mandal K, et al. Involvement of the antimicrobial peptide LL-37 in human atherosclerosis. Arterioscler Thromb Vasc Biol. 2006;26:1551–7.

224. Barnathan ES, Raghunath PN, Tomaszewski JE, Ganz T, Cines DB, Higazi A a-R. Immunohistochemical localization of defensin in human coronary vessels. Am J Pathol. 1997;150:1009–20.

225. Hemdahl A-L, Gabrielsen A, Zhu C, Eriksson P, Hedin U, Kastrup J, et al. Expression of neutrophil gelatinase-associated lipocalin in atherosclerosis and myocardial infarction. Arterioscler Thromb Vasc Biol. 2006;26:136–42.

226. Wedmore CV, Williams TJ. Control of vascular permeability by polymorphonuclear leukocytes in inflammation. Nature. 1981;289:646–50.

227. Soehnlein O, Xie X, Ulbrich H, Kenne E, Rotzius P, Flodgaard H, et al. Neutrophil-derived heparin-binding protein (HBP/CAP37) deposited on endothelium enhances monocyte arrest under flow conditions. J Immunol. 2005;174:6399–405.

228. Soehnlein O, Zernecke A, Eriksson EE, Rothfuchs AG, Pham CT, Herwald H, et al. Neutrophil secretion products pave the way for inflammatory monocytes. Blood. 2008;112:1461–71.

229. Chertov O, Ueda H, Xu LL, Tani K, Murphy WJ, Wang JM, et al. Identification of human neutrophil-derived cathepsin G and azurocidin/CAP37 as chemoattractants for mononuclear cells and neutrophils. J Exp Med. 1997;186:739–47.

230. Gombart AF, Krug U, O'Kelly J, An E, Vegesna V, Koeffler HP. Aberrant expression of neutrophil and macrophage-related genes in a murine model for human neutrophil-specific granule deficiency. J Leukoc Biol. 2005;78:1153–65.

231. Leclercq A, Houard X, Philippe M, Ollivier V, Sebbag U, Meilhac O, et al. Involvement of intraplaque hemorrhage in atherothrombosis evolution via neutrophil protease enrichment. J Leukoc Biol. 2007;82:1420–9.

232. Stone GW, Maehara A, Lansky AJ, de Bruyne B, Cristea E, Mintz GS, et al. A prospective natural-history study of coronary atherosclerosis. N Engl J Med. 2011;364:226–35.

233. Libby P. Inflammation in atherosclerosis. Arterioscler Thromb Vasc Biol. 2012;32:2045–51.

234. Aubry M-C, Riehle DL, Edwards WD, Maradit-Kremers H, Roger VL, Sebo TJ, et al. B-lymphocytes in plaque and adventitia of coronary arteries in two patients with rheumatoid arthritis and coronary atherosclerosis. Cardiovasc Pathol. 2004;13:233–6.

235. Jonasson L, Holm J, Skalli O, Bondjers G, Hansson GK. Regional accumulations of T cells, macrophages, and smooth muscle cells in the human atherosclerotic plaque. Arteriosclerosis. 1986;6:131–8.

236. Reardon CA, Blachowicz L, White T, Cabana V, Wang Y, Lukens J, et al. Effect of immune deficiency on lipoproteins and atherosclerosis in male apolipoprotein E-deficient mice. Arterioscler Thromb Vasc Biol. 2001;21(6):1011.

237. Dansky HM, Charlton SA. T and B lymphocytes play a minor role in atherosclerotic plaque formation in the apolipoprotein E-deficient mouse. Proc Natl Acad Sci U S A. 1997;94(9):4642–6.

238. Zhou X, Nicoletti A, Elhage R, Hansson GK. Transfer of CD4(+) T cells aggravates atherosclerosis in immunodeficient apolipoprotein E knockout mice. Circulation. 2000;102:2919–22.

239. Ketelhuth DFJ, Hansson GK. Adaptive response of T and B cells in atherosclerosis. Circ Res. 2016;118:668–78.

240. Caligiuri G, Nicoletti A, Poirier B, Hansson GK. Protective immunity against atherosclerosis carried by B cells of hypercholesterolemic mice. J Clin Invest. 2002;109:745–53.

241. Major AS, Fazio S, Linton MF. B-lymphocyte deficiency increases atherosclerosis in LDL receptor-null mice. Arterioscler Thromb Vasc Biol. 2002;22:1892–8.
242. Kyaw T, Tay C, Krishnamurthi S, Kanellakis P. B1a B lymphocytes are atheroprotective by secreting natural IgM that increases IgM deposits and reduces necrotic cores in atherosclerotic lesions. Circulation. 2011;109(8):830–40.
243. Rosenfeld SM, Perry HM, Gonen A, Prohaska TA, Srikakulapu P, Grewal S, et al. B-1b cells secrete atheroprotective IgM and attenuate atherosclerosis. Circ Res. 2015;117:e28–39.
244. Kyaw T, Tay C, Khan A, Dumouchel V, Cao A, To K, et al. Conventional B2 B cell depletion ameliorates whereas its adoptive transfer aggravates atherosclerosis. J Immunol. 2010;185:4410–9.
245. Clement M, Guedj K, Andreata F, Morvan M, Bey L, Khallou-Laschet J, et al. Control of the T follicular helper-germinal center B-cell axis by CD8+ regulatory T cells limits atherosclerosis and tertiary lymphoid organ development. Circulation. 2015;131:560–70.
246. Hedrick CC. Lymphocytes in atherosclerosis. Arterioscler Thromb Vasc Biol. 2015;35:253–7.

Chapter 8
Immune-Mediated Heart Disease

Elena Generali, Marco Folci, Carlo Selmi, and Piersandro Riboldi

8.1 Introduction

Autoimmune diseases represent a broad range of related disorders affecting nearly 5% of the European population [1]. These conditions are cumulatively characterized by more or less defined clinical pictures sometimes overlapping within the same patient. These include connective tissue diseases such as systemic lupus erythematosus (SLE), systemic sclerosis (SSc), mixed connective tissue disease (MCTD), Sjögren's syndrome (SS), rheumatoid arthritis (RA), myositis, and antiphospholipid syndrome (APS). The common pathogenic mark is the breakdown of tolerance against self-peptide antigens which derives from a failure of peripheral tolerance under genetic predisposing factors and environmental triggering agents [2, 3]. One of the most threatening complications is the cardiovascular (CV) involvement, which represents a significant cause of morbidity and mortality [4–10].

E. Generali
Rheumatology and Clinical Immunology, Humanitas Research Hospital,
Rozzano, Milan, Italy

M. Folci • P. Riboldi (✉)
Allergy, Clinical Immunology and Rheumatology Unit, IRCCS Istituto Auxologico Italiano,
Milan, Italy
e-mail: p.riboldi@auxologico.it

C. Selmi
Rheumatology and Clinical Immunology, Humanitas Research Hospital,
Rozzano, Milan, Italy

BIOMETRA Department, University of Milan, Milan, Italy

© Springer International Publishing AG 2017
S. Sattler, T. Kennedy-Lydon (eds.), *The Immunology of Cardiovascular Homeostasis and Pathology*, Advances in Experimental Medicine and Biology 1003, DOI 10.1007/978-3-319-57613-8_8

8.1.1   Mechanisms of CV Damage

The hypothesized pathogenesis encompasses different mechanisms, but only some of these have been clarified, especially in their cellular and biochemical pathways, but ultimately remaining elusive. The heart can be primarily involved by the localization of an autoimmune process or can be indirectly damaged by chronic inflammation, by other injured organs, and by drugs used to manage the primary disease. In the case of a primary involvement, the impairment of different cardiac structures derives from the inflammatory infiltrate, the deposition of immune complexes, leading to the activation of the complement cascade (Fig. 8.1). Alternatively, the cardiac function is threatened by the general inflammatory status, strictly dependent on disease activity, or the heart can be severely damaged in end stages of a systemic autoimmune process. This last condition is principally determined by the impaired function of other organs, such as the

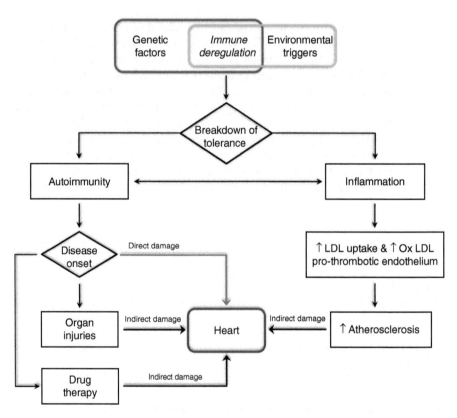

Fig. 8.1 Pathogenic mechanisms of heart damages in autoimmune diseases. *LDL* light-density lipoprotein, *oxLDLs* oxidized light-density lipoproteins

kidneys or the lungs, which compromise hemodynamic. It is now well established that atherosclerosis appears to be significantly accelerated in systemic autoimmune diseases compared to general population. This condition is one of the most powerful causes of CV diseases due to thromboembolic phenomena following plaque rupture; moreover, chronic inflammation activates the endothelial cells which express different surface molecule patterns acquiring a prothrombotic phenotype.

The mechanisms of the accelerated atherosclerosis are not well defined, but chronic inflammation has been suggested as a contributing factor with pro-inflammatory cytokines (i.e., TNFα and IL-6) leading to endothelial dysfunction and activation and subsequent rise of low-density lipoprotein (LDL) uptake and deposition under endothelial surface. Specifically, TNFα can alter the endothelial structure mediating the inflammatory vascular injury in both acute and chronic conditions, ranging from the remodeling by smooth muscle cells to a direct role in rupture of atherosclerotic plaques [11]. Similarly, IL-6 induces an overall change of surface molecules of the endothelium that develops a pro-inflammatory status. This enhances the migration of lipoproteins, especially LDLs, from bloodstream to subendothelial space at higher concentrations than the cellular metabolic needs and when in contact with high amount of free oxygen radicals produced by activated inflammatory cells undergoing oxidation (oxLDLs). High oxLDL levels stimulate macrophages through the interaction with scavenger receptors and lead to massive phagocytosis which, after a gradual engulfment of cytoplasm, generates the so-called foam cells. The reaction of the immune system against oxLDLs is of paramount importance because it represents the first pathological mechanism leading to the atheromatous plaque. OxLDLs stimulate not only innate immunity but also the adaptive compartment. Studies have demonstrated the production of antibodies against oxLDLs which seem to be related to cardiovascular events [12, 13], even though some authors have reported, conversely, a protective role [14].

Chronic inflammation stimulates the expression of adhesion molecules, such as VCAM-1, by the endothelium and smooth muscle cells. This pathological activation promotes the recruitment of leukocytes into the subendothelial space which ultimately lead to the perpetuation of inflammation [15]. T cell activation can also be involved, and activated T cells are present in atherosclerotic plaques, especially in unstable plaques accounting for the increased CV risk and higher mortality. The clinical manifestations of heart involvement can be strikingly diverse because all the anatomical heart structures can be affected simultaneously or not, with damages of various seriousness [16] (Fig. 8.2). Recognized since the beginning of the twentieth century, cardiac involvement related to autoimmunity conditions has been carefully investigated in the last decades. The following findings led to recognize new clinical entities but also to introduce different available treatments. We will focus on cardiac manifestations operating in systemic autoimmune diseases, with particular interest on pathogenic mechanisms.

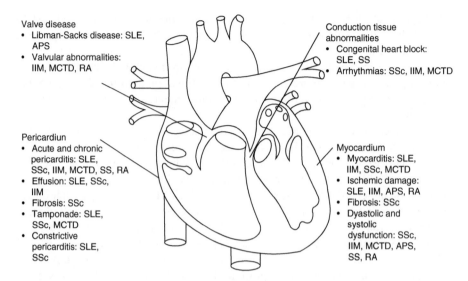

Valve disease
- Libman-Sacks disease: SLE, APS
- Valvular abnormalities: IIM, MCTD, RA

Conduction tissue abnormalities
- Congenital heart block: SLE, SS
- Arrhythmias: SSc, IIM, MCTD

Pericardiun
- Acute and chronic pericarditis: SLE, SSc, IIM, MCTD, SS, RA
- Effusion: SLE, SSc, IIM
- Fibrosis: SSc
- Tamponade: SLE, SSc, MCTD
- Constrictive pericarditis: SLE, SSc

Myocardium
- Myocarditis: SLE, IIM, SSc, MCTD
- Ischemic damage: SLE, IIM, APS, RA
- Fibrosis: SSc
- Dyastolic and systolic dysfunction: SSc, IIM, MCTD, APS, SS, RA

Fig. 8.2 Pathological involvement of the heart by different systemic autoimmune diseases. *SLE* systemic lupus erythematosus, *APS* antiphospholipid syndrome, *IIM* idiopathic inflammatory myositis, *MCTD* mixed connective tissue diseases, *RA* rheumatoid arthritis, *SSc* systemic sclerosis, *SS* Sjögren's syndrome

8.1.2   The Impact of Medical Treatments

Medications used to treat the autoimmune diseases can have, sometimes, a negative impact on cardiac function by a direct toxicity (antimalarials, nonsteroidal anti-inflammatory drugs (NSAIDs)) or worsening a pre-existing cardiac disease (Fig. 8.1). On the other hand, several drugs used in chronic inflammatory diseases represent paradigms of potential treatments for CV comorbidities, but effects are poorly defined.

First, antimalarials, such as chloroquine and hydroxychloroquine, in chronic use rarely cause conduction abnormalities, arrhythmias, and infiltrative cardiomyopathy with heart failure (HF) due to impairment of diastolic, systolic, or both cardiac functions [17, 18]. Second, biologics were ideal candidates as anti-TNFα biologics are used for RA treatment, but data from clinical trials reported no beneficial effects and a possible worsening of heart function leading to a contraindication of anti-TNFα use in patients with HF New York Heart Association (NYHA) classes III–IV (moderate and severe) [19]. To further investigate the HF risk with anti-TNFα, longer observational studies were conducted on almost all TNFα inhibitors, including etanercept, which, due to its peculiar structure, has lower avidity for TNFα compared to monoclonal antibodies, but results were inconsistent [20, 21]. Other biologics, with different mechanisms of action, have also been investigated: rituximab (anti-CD20), tocilizumab (anti-IL-6), and abatacept (anti-CTLA4) showed no overall increased CV risk in the RA population; however, no reduction of the risk of developing HF and other CV events was found in comparison with the RA population treated on standard therapy or anti-TNFα biologic agents [22]. Third, NSAIDs are frequently used in rheumatic conditions and are associated with an increased CV risk, and a recent meta-analysis of various clinical, preclinical, meta-analysis and observational studies showed that coxibs and NSAIDs increase the risk of cardiotoxicity in a dose-dependent manner. The cardiotoxicity associated with the use of NSAIDs might be due to inhibition of prostacyclin synthesis, oxidative stress, increase in blood pressure, and impaired endothelial function [23].

8.2 Systemic Lupus Erythematosus

SLE is frequently associated with CV manifestations, and all three layers of the heart (i.e., pericardium, myocardium, and endocardium) can be affected with the parietal sheet of cardiac serous being the most frequently involved, as suggested by its inclusion in the American College of Rheumatology (ACR) classification criteria [24]. The valvular apparatus, the conducting system, and the coronary vessels may be other noteworthy sites of pathological involvement in SLE.

8.2.1 Pericardium

Clinically, pericarditis manifests with variable symptoms ranging from precordial or substernal positional chest pain to dyspnea. At physical examination, patients may have fever, tachycardia, decreased heart sounds, and pericardial rubs, a specific sign which, however, is rarely hearable. The diagnosis may be sustained by an electrocardiogram (ECG) showing elevated ST segments and peaked T waves (although slight T-wave changes and transient elevation of ST segments are most characteristic) [25]. Transthoracic echocardiography and chest X-ray are the standard methods to investigate pericarditis [26, 27]. One of the most fearsome complications is cardiac tamponade, although constrictive and purulent processes are equally challenging. Pericarditis may be either characterized by an acute or chronic process which leads to the appearance of clinical symptoms in only 25% of the SLE population; however it is reported in as many as >50% of patients undergoing echocardiography or up to 62% during autoptic examination [28–39]. Pericardial involvement appears more frequently at SLE onset or during disease relapses, although it can occur at any time [40]. Common pathological findings include fibrinous or fibrous reactions, which, in chronic conditions, can lead to adhesive processes both focal and diffuse. Microscopically, the pericardium appears infiltrated by plasma cells and lymphocytes with fibroblastic proliferation, findings that are not unique for SLE and which resemble tubercular pericarditis [35]. The identification of hematoxylin bodies is a more specific finding, but particles of denatured nuclei are rarely seen [41]. Immunofluorescence may be helpful in characterizing SLE pericarditis; indeed it is possible to demonstrate a granular deposition of immunoglobulin, C1q, and C3, in the pericardial vessels, which ultimately suggests a pathogenic role of immune complexes [42].

8.2.2 Myocardium

Clinically, patients manifest with symptoms resembling ischemic heart disease such as chest pain dyspnea, tachycardia, and arrhythmias [40]. Diagnosis may be challenging, with ECG not showing any typical findings and cardiac enzymes within limits. Echocardiographic imaging cannot definitely diagnose myocarditis, but the finding of global hypokinesis or pericardial effusion, in the absence of other known causes, is strongly suggestive [43]. More recently, cardiac magnetic resonance imaging (MRI), the gold standard for measuring ventricular volumes and ejection fraction, can be used to detect acute myocarditis, myocardial fibrosis, and even subtle tissue changes [43]. Endomyocardial biopsy is the gold standard for diagnosis; however this challenging procedure can be aggravated by complications both during and after execution, and for these reasons, it should be reserved only for selected situations [6, 44]. One of the most threatening consequences of chronic myocarditis is represented by dilated cardiomyopathy, which ultimately can evolve toward HF. Myocarditis represents one of the most important manifestations of heart involvement in SLE, even if myocardial disease may be determined or worsened by other mechanisms, such as drug toxicity (i.e., antimalarials). The inflammation of the myocardium, largely ignited by immune complex deposition and complement activation, is the pathological condition determining tissue injuries. Myocarditis prevalence is reported to be as high as 80% in SLE autoptic series [30]; however, recent findings suggest a rate of 6%, probably due to the introduction of effective treatments. From a clinical standpoint, this process can be detected only in 3–15% of patients with SLE due to the paucity of symptoms [45]. Pathologically, the findings are nonspecific, with a perivascular and interstitial infiltrate of mononuclear cells, constituted by lymphocytes, plasma cells, macrophages, and myocardial fibrosis. Immunohistochemistry is helpful to identify aggregates of lymphocytes and macrophages. The presence of myocyte vacuolization at optical microscopy, defined as a dilatation of sarcoplasmic reticulum that contains laminar amorphous material, is a characteristic of antimalarial-induced cardiomyopathy, even if the detection of myeloid bodies by electron microscope is the only pathognomonic sign [35, 46].

8.2.3 Valvular Disease

From a clinical standpoint, most of the valvular findings are asymptomatic, but extended lesions which cause hemodynamic dysfunctions become clinically evident and require, in about 3–4% of cases, valve replacement [6]. Valvular involvement in SLE is one of the most important and prevalent forms of carditis, and nearly 60% of patients who undergo echocardiography manifest abnormalities, with postmortem studies showing a prevalence between 11 and 74% [47]. The most common pathological findings derive from regurgitation and stenosis even if milder defects such as thickening and vegetations can be found. Among valve alterations, the Libman-Sacks endocarditis is a histopathological picture significantly associated with SLE and APS, albeit currently is rare thanks to the better treatment of the underlying disease. The persistent inflammation of endocardium generates sterile verrucous lesions affecting all structures with a remarkable prevalence for the mitral valve [48]. Histologically, Libman-Sacks vegetations consist of platelets, fibrin, degenerating blood products, chronic fibrosis, active fibroblasts, and neovascularization. These lesions may be active or healed [35].

8.2.4 Arrhythmias

Congenital heart block (CHB) is one the most representative cardiac rhythm disturbances associated with autoimmune diseases. This condition, among endocardial fibroelastosis and dilated cardiomyopathy, is a threatening manifestation of neonatal lupus, characterized by cardiac and skin involvement in newborns from mothers with SLE or Sjögren's syndrome positive for anti-Ro/SSA and/or anti-La/SSB antibodies [49]. CHB arises by definition during uterine life or in the neonatal period (<28 days of life) [50, 51], but the entity of the problem remains elusive. Two studies, performed, respectively, in Finland and the USA on large case series, have estimated an incidence of ~1 case on 20,000 live births; but it was impossible to evaluate what is the real impact of maternal autoimmunity, given that no autoantibody status was reported [50, 51]. Nonetheless, CHB prevalence was recently determined to be less than 1% in anti-SSA-positive women [52, 53], and recurrence rate is defined at 19% [53]. The pathogenic pathway is represented by the transfer of maternal autoantibodies through the placenta into fetal bloodstream, even though the mechanism by which anti-SSA/Ro and anti-SSB/La act on the heart conduction system is not yet understood. Evidence of complete atrioventricular (AV) block in mice pups passively injected with anti-SSA/Ro 52 antibodies supports data from earlier reports [54]. Furthermore, studies in vitro demonstrate how anti-SSA/Ro IgG inhibits L-type CA2þ channel in rat and rabbit heart [55, 56]. Researches on humans have confirmed the potential role of what previously described. The presence of maternal autoantibodies in fetal circulation and the elution of anti-SSA/Ro antibodies from cardiac tissues of affected fetuses support animal models, even if the rarity of CHB and discordance rate in twins remain unsolved problems [57]. National database analyses reveal a CHB-associated mortality rate of 20% with nearly 80% of deaths occurring in the uterus [58]. The great majority of pregnancies results in live births (81%), with a prematurity rate (birth <37 weeks) of 38% [58]. CHB can present with various grades of rhythm alterations in live births, and challenge refers to therapeutic strategies because most of the babies require pacing for the first 10 days of life and about two thirds have to maintain this support for 1 year; in fact, a quarter of total deaths related to autoimmune CHB are reported during this span of life [50]. Other rare rhythm disturbances have been described in association with anti-SSA/

Ro antibodies, and the most significant include bradycardia, AV blocks of various degrees, and prolongation of the QT interval that usually resolve within the first year of life when maternal autoantibodies disappear [57].

Limited prevention strategies are available for women who are anti-SSA/SSB positive and are considered at high risk for offspring CHB as those with a previous history of neonatal lupus syndrome. Fetal monitoring with echocardiography is a safe and noninvasive method for screening CHB that offers an accurate assessment of the fetal heart rate, rhythm, and ventricular function. This procedure should be performed weekly between 16th and 24th week of gestation. At birth neonates should be observed during the first month of life [50]. If rhythm alterations are detected prenatally, therapeutic options to reduce the risk of CHB are represented by fluorinated steroids, which should diminish the inflammatory component in the fetal heart reducing tissue injury. Other strategies to treat intrauterine heart blocks include plasma exchange and/or intravenous immunoglobulin used in various combinations [59].

8.3   Systemic Sclerosis

SSc is a connective tissue disorder of unknown etiology characterized by the damage and fibrosis of multiple organs. The main pathogenic treats are represented by microvascular damages but also dysregulation of innate and adaptive immunity which lead to fibrosis in multiple organs. The prevalence ranges from 7 to 700 cases per million depending on geographic regions, ethnic differences, and gender; in fact women are more frequently affected than men [60, 61]. SSc can be classified into limited and diffuse variant, according to the extension of skin fibrosis [62]. Patients can develop heterogeneous clinical manifestations on the basis of variable involvement of different organs. Heart damage can derive from indirect chronic injuries which are principally dependent on lung and kidney pathology. Pulmonary arterial hypertension (PAH) and interstitial lung disease (ILD) are the main causes of right ventricular dysfunction. These conditions determine a persistent increased outflow resistance which causes right ventricular remodeling. The myocardial response to this chronic excessive work brings the heart to adopt counterproductive mechanisms, such as hypertrophy, generating various grades of HF. The kidney involvement is represented by scleroderma renal crisis, a rare (4–6%) but life-threatening manifestation, defined by malignant hypertension and acute renal failure which can be sometimes associated with congestive HF [63].

Primary cardiac involvement represents a frequent cause of morbidity and mortality in limited and diffuse SSc, as demonstrated by several studies [64, 65]. All heart structures can be affected, resulting in different impairments, which are often subclinical [66]. The overall hazard of early disease is higher in diffuse pattern, especially during the first year after the onset of the disease [67], and in patients with anti-RNA polymerases (I–III) and anti-fibrillarin antibodies [68]

Table 8.1 Systemic sclerosis clinical phenotype and specific autoantibodies

Autoantibody	Frequency (lcSSc/dcSSc, %)	Clinical association
ANA	95 (both)	–
ACA	60–80/2–5	Pulmonary arterial hypertension, digital ulceration
Anti-SCL70	10–15/20–40	Progressive skin thickening, scleroderma renal crisis, pulmonary fibrosis
Anti-U1-RNP	5–10/n.a.	Severe GI involvement
Anti-U3-RNP (anti-fibrillarin)	n.a./5–15	Severe lung disease, severe GI involvement
Anti-PM/Scl	4/n.a.	Severe GI involvement, pulmonary fibrosis, inflammatory myopathy
Anti-RNA polymerase	n.a./5–40	Rapidly progressive skin thickening, scleroderma renal crisis, decreased frequency of severe lung disease

lcSSc limited cutaneous systemic sclerosis, *dcSSc* diffuse cutaneous systemic sclerosis, *ANA* antinuclear antibodies, *ACA* anti-centromere antibodies, *n.a.* not available

(Table 8.1). The etiology of cardiac damages is likely dependent from microvascular ischemic lesions and from fibrous tissue deposition. These events could impair regional microcirculation causing areas of localized myocardial hypokinesis which could evolve toward global heart dysfunction in later stages of disease [69, 70]. Interestingly, nailfold capillaroscopy could help in identifying patients more prone to develop cardiac involvement through the identification of peripheral microangiopathy, which has been shown to correlate with internal organ involvement [71].

8.3.1 Pericardium

The clinical picture of pericardial SSc manifestations may cover a wide range of conditions, including acute or constrictive pericardial effusion and the most threatening cardiac tamponade. The pericardial involvement is relatively common in SSc, even though it is frequently asymptomatic. Autoptic studies reported pathological findings in about 78% of specimens, but only 5–16% of patients present symptoms [72]. The cause of pericardial pathology in SSc is not well understood, even if studies performed on pericardial biopsies have often found diffuse fibrosis as in other tissues [73]. Clinically, the inflammation of pericardium is associated with chest and substernal pain, dyspnea, pericardial effusion, and symptoms of HF if tamponade is present. Echocardiography with Doppler imaging is demonstrated to be a precious instrument in diagnostic process of pericardial disease; indeed, it can precociously detect effusion. Treatment is usually unnecessary, even if pericardiocentesis should be considered to discern diagnostic doubts and for patients who develop hemodynamic impairment. Constrictive pericarditis may be difficult to identify; moreover its differentiation from restrictive cardiomyopathy can be a hard challenge for the clinician, especially when both processes coexist. Two echocardiographic signs favor a diagnosis of pericardium pathology; in fact, abnormal interventricular motion and preserved mitral parameters focus the attention on the serous sack. Cardiac MRI and computed tomography (CT) may be of additional help [72]. Intrinsic myocardial disease in SSc manifests as myocardial fibrosis due to microvascular ischemia and ultimately determines left ventricular dysfunction.

8.3.2 Myocardium

Myocardial fibrosis has been reported to be an important manifestation of SSc, being found in as many as 80% of autoptic cases, because symptomatic conditions are less frequent. The pathogenic mechanisms are still matter of discussion even if several factors have been identified as possible actors in myocardial injuries which lead to fibrotic process. Some of these are strikingly dependent on recurrent vasospasms and poor vasodilator reserve which determine, respectively, recurrent ischemia-reperfusion damages and areas of focal ischemia. Histology of SSc myocardium demonstrates focal myocardial fibrosis and necrosis of the contraction bands, findings that are extremely similar to non-SSc-related ischemia-reperfusion injury. From a clinical standpoint, myocardial fibrosis becomes manifest only in late stages, when the heart stiffness is so important to produce a function deficit. The tissue alterations can impair the systolic (reduced ejection fraction) or diastolic (preserved ejection fraction) function, leading to various degrees of heart chamber dysfunction. Right ventricular dysfunction has been frequently described in SSc, independently of PAH. The main clinical sign is a reduced right ventricle ejection fraction due to myocardial fibrosis as proved by a recent study which demonstrates altered ejection fractions in about one fifth of SSc patients using cardiac MRI [74]. A clinical suspect of heart fibrosis can be solved performing cardiac MRI, even if echocardiography and natriuretic peptide levels are a useful instrument to monitor cardiac function [75].

8.3.3 Arrhythmias

Arrhythmias are common in SSc and may be considered a complication of the fibrotic process of the conduction system and myocardium. Patients will develop different symptoms such as palpitations, vertigo, dizziness, syncope, and even sudden death; for these reasons, a precocious recognition and an accurate identification are essential. Atrial and ventricular tachyarrhythmias derive from myocardial fibrosis, whereas the conduction system involvement could give rise to brady-arrhythmias [66, 76]. Supraventricular rhythm disturbances are more common and manifest in about two thirds of SSc patients, compared to other conditions which have a lower prevalence [77]. ECG represents the first diagnostic tool even if up to 50% of patients have not any alterations at rest [78]. Some studies demonstrate that ECG abnormalities are predictive of survival, although it is unclear whether these changes contribute directly to morbidity and mortality or reflect the overall disease burden [77]. Symptomatic patients, who have a normal ECG, should undergo ECG Holter monitoring to better characterize cardiac rhythm changes; moreover, treadmill exercise can be performed to identify exertional arrhythmias. Echocardiography should be performed as second-line test. Treatment of arrhythmias should be according to general guidelines [76].

Early assessment of the overall CV involvement represents a mandatory step in a proper management of SSc patients, since its development increases morbidity and mortality. A good organ involvement screening should be sought in every patient, with special attention to those who have complaints which refer to cardiac involvement.

8.4 Inflammatory Muscle Disease

Idiopathic inflammatory myositis (IIM) includes a group of diseases characterized by proximal muscle weakness due to chronic inflammation of striated muscles mirrored by elevation of serum muscle enzymes, particularly creatine kinase [79]. Heart involvement is uncommon in IIM, especially in polymyositis (PM) and dermatomyositis (DM), but represents a poor prognostic factor responsible approximately of 10–20% of deaths [80]. Cardiac abnormality prevalence ranges from 6 to 72% in PM/DM. These results are strongly dependent on selection criteria; in fact, the broad interval suggests an underestimation of the problem, as demonstrated by autoptic studies which report alterations in about 30% of cases [81]. There is no clear relationship between IIM clinical patterns and specific heart diseases [81], and most studies reveal the occurrence of several cardiac pathologies during the course of both active and under remission myositis [2], even if a recent study shows significant correlations with disease onset [82]. Clinically, about 3–6% of patients with PM/DM present with symptoms such as dyspnea, chest pain, palpitations, or less common peripheral edema and syncope [83]. All these manifestations are mainly due to end-stage heart disease which ultimately evolves toward pump failure.

8.4.1 Pericardium

Pericardial disease is generally asymptomatic and sporadic, being reported in less than 10% of patients. The most frequent finding is pericardial effusion which is often revealed by investigations made for other clinical needs [81].

8.4.2   Myocardium

Myocarditis has been linked to IIM and is found in approximately 8% of patients. Cardiac MRI is a helpful tool to detect inflammatory infiltrates in the tissue [84–87], making endomyocardial biopsy less necessary. The histopathology resembles the picture found in skeletal muscles, with focal fibrosis, vasculitis, intimal proliferation, and medial sclerosis of blood vessels [88]. Clinically, it manifests with chest pain and dyspnea [83], but it can produce advanced signs of heart failure in widespread involvement of myocardial muscle. This group of patient is related with a worse prognosis, and for this reason, it could benefit from immunosuppressant therapies, but available data are lacking [83] in spite of some case reports which show a benefit of steroid [89].

8.4.3   Conduction System

Arrhythmias are a common feature observed in IIM. The incidence of EKG alterations is reported between 25 and 85% of patients with PM/DM. Branch block and supraventricular arrhythmias are the most frequent findings which range from 13.6% to 2.4%, in prospective and retrospective cohorts, respectively [83]. Other disturbances include atrial or ventricular premature beats, tachycardia, atrial fibrillation, conduction blocks, and abnormal Q-waves as nonspecific ST-T wave changes. Histopathologically, abnormalities in the conducting system include lymphocytic infiltration, sinoatrial node fibrosis, and contraction band necrosis [81].

8.4.4   Valves, Coronary, and Heart Function

Valvular abnormalities are relatively uncommon, as clinically significant valve diseases may be observed in 7–23% of patients [90].

Coronary heart disease is reported with uncertain incidence; in fact a recent study investigating CV risk factors in IIM suggests a prevalence of 26%. Sporadic reports of inflammatory arteritis of coronaries without obstruction have been described. Vasospastic angina (Prinzmetal's angina) is occasionally reported in DM with Raynaud's phenomenon [91]. HF develops as a consequence of left ventricular diastolic dysfunction that is observed in 12–42% of cases. Traditional echocardiography associated with tissue Doppler imaging can detect this pump defect in about 14–62% of circumstances [81] and should be carefully performed in high-risk patients, such as female sex and late onset and long course of disease [92].

8.5 Mixed Connective Tissue Disease

Overlap autoimmune features of SLE, PM, SSc, and RA associated with antibodies directed toward U1 nuclear ribonucleoprotein (RNP) configure MCTD [93]. CV involvement is rather frequent in MCTD. It has been reported from 13 to 65% depending on patient selection criteria and to diagnostic procedures performed; in fact, in symptomatic patients, cardiac disease ranges from 24 to 63% [94].

8.5.1 Pericardium

Pericarditis is the most common cardiac manifestation with a prevalence of 10–40% [95], when echocardiography is used. This condition can be related to the rheumatoid arthritis-like and/or the lupus-like spectra of MCTD [94]. The treatment is based on NSAIDs or steroids (0.25–1.0 mg/kg). Rare cases of large effusion [96] which evolve toward cardiac tamponade [97] may need percutaneous and surgical drainage.

8.5.2 Myocardium

Myocarditis has been rarely reported, although it could be underestimated as demonstrated in postmortem studies. This pathological entity might be responsible for conduction abnormalities and diastolic dysfunction [94]. Symptoms include dyspnea, chest pain, arrhythmias, and elevated cardiac enzymes. When an endomyocardial biopsy is performed, the most common findings include interstitial lymphocytic infiltrate, myocardial fiber, and interstitial necrosis [98, 99].

8.5.3 Valve, Conduction System, and Heart Function

Valvular abnormalities are reported with high frequency, especially verrucous thickening alterations or mitral valve prolapse (MVP), which is detectable by echocardiography in about 12–32% of patients [100, 101]. MVP might be due to focal degeneration of the valve leaflets resulting in reduced capacity to support systolic stress, as seen in SLE [8]. Conduction disorder prevalence rates are reported as high as 20%, and the most common condition observed is a deviation of QRS axis, which is related to anterior hemiblock [102]. The presence of ST-T abnormalities is detected with prevalence around 29% on ECG [103, 104]. Diastolic dysfunction is a common defect in MCTD, and echocardiography demonstrates abnormalities of the diastolic filling indexes due to atrial contraction, such as prolongation of iso-volumetric relaxation time, reduction of peak early diastolic flow velocity, and an increase of peak late diastolic flow velocity [105, 106]. Systolic function is usually conserved. Histologically sections reveal inflammatory cell infiltrate and/or prolif-erative vasculopathy of the epicardial and intramural arteries. Autoptic studies have proven the presence of lymphocytic and polymorphonuclear infiltrates in the peri-vascular space but also intimal proliferation with an increased number of acellular elements [103].

8.6 Antiphospholipid Syndrome

APS is a rare autoimmune disease characterized by a high tendency of developing thrombotic events. It is diagnosed on the basis of defined clinical criteria and spe-cific laboratory findings [107]. The former are represented by vascular thrombosis and/or pregnancy morbidity, while the latter are elevated levels of serum antiphos-pholipid antibodies (aPL). These include lupus anticoagulant (LA), anticardiolipin (aCL), and/or anti-beta2-glycoprotein I (anti-β2GPI) antibodies. The syndrome can be a primary disorder or it can be secondary to an underlying condition, most com-monly SLE. The heart involvement is a frequent finding that is supposed to be medi-ated by direct aPL actions on cardiac structures or through vessel thrombosis which lead to myocardial ischemia.

8.6.1 Valve Involvement

Valvular damage is the most frequent cardiac manifestation of APS, being detected in one third of patients. The major alterations include vegetations or thickening of valve leaflets as Libman-Sacks endocarditis which was first described in SLE [108–110]. The pathogenic role of aPL seems to have a close link with the valvular dam-age, as supported by the evidence of deformed heart valves in patients with aPL positivity and no clinical signs or symptoms of disease [108, 111]. The prevalence of valvular defects in primary APS is reported to be between 32 and 38%, based on echocardiographic studies [112]. The most frequent altered valve is the mitral, fol-lowed by aortic; on the contrary, Libman-Sacks endocarditis involves often the tri-cuspid valve. These abnormalities are usually asymptomatic from a clinical standpoint; in fact, only 4–6% of APS patients develop severe disease that requires surgical treatment [40, 113]. The diagnosis can be made with traditional echocar-diography, even if transesophageal approach is more sensitive [114, 115]. The importance of this pathological consequence of the syndrome goes beyond heart damage; indeed, some studies prove how it may be considered as a major risk factor for cerebrovascular accidents, particularly in primary APS [116, 117]. The pathogen-esis of the valvular damage is referred to micro-injuries of some hemodynamically vulnerable sites which undergo repetitive mechanical stress [118]. These conditions should induce the exposition of negative phospholipids on both valve surface and endothelial cells of intra-valve capillaries leading to the interaction with aPL [118]. Histologically, some studies prove the coexistence of new and old lesions characterized by the presence of superficial or intravalvular fibrin deposits. This pathological feature triggers subsequent vascular proliferation, fibrosis, and calcification which lead to valve thickening, fusion of commissures, and rigidity of valvular apparatus [119]. Inflammation seems to be not a prominent feature, even in the presence of a linear subendothelial deposition of immunoglobulins and complement components [119]. The same pattern and location of staining were observed with anti-idiotypic antibody to aCL; moreover, a significant amount of IgG immunoglobulins that bound to cardiolipin was eluted from valves of patient with secondary APS [119]. Such deposits may be probably involved in the pathogenesis of valvular lesions [119].

8.6.2 Atherosclerosis

Atherosclerosis is significantly accelerated and more prevalent in patients with APS than in the general population, despite similar CV risk factors [120]. From a clinical standpoint, this process manifests with syndromes of different severity, from angina to sudden death, passing through myocardial infarction. Increasingly data demonstrate how this process is driven by direct immunological effects of aPL, especially anti-β2GPI [121], but also through autoantibodies cross-reactions and increased oxidative stress [122]. Histological studies on atherosclerotic plaques prove the contiguity of beta-2 glycoprotein I to T-CD^{4+} lymphocytes areas in the subendothelial regions [123]; moreover, in vitro experiments demonstrate how aPL accelerate plaque formation, enhance macrophage transformation in foam cells, and reduce the activity of paraoxonase which increases oxLDLs [124]. The binding of beta-2 glycoprotein I to oxLDLs generates a molecular complex that interacts with aPL leading to an increased uptake by macrophages via Fcγ receptors [125]. The proof of an increased rate of CV events in APS patients is represented by the prevalence of myocardial infarction which is 5.5% [108], 2.8% as first manifestation of the disease, compared to 1.4–3.2% of general population [126]; moreover, some studies correlate the levels of aPL with the incidence of severe CV events [127].

8.6.3 Myocardium

Chronic damages to heart tissue can manifest also with a less acute myocardial dysfunction. The pathogenesis is hypothesized to be derived from both direct antibody effects and repeated micro-embolism phenomena which ultimately impair pump function. Histologically, there is evidence of inflammation, immune deposits, and thrombosis in intramyocardial arteriolar with microinfarction of surrounding areas [122]. Cardiac MRI is the most sensible test to detect microvascular damages; in fact, a study shed on light that APS patients with low pretest probability of coronary heart diseases (CHD) have ischemic lesions in 11% of cases, while only 3.7% of the controls show the same alterations [128]. For all these reasons, the assessment of patient atherosclerotic status is crucial to estimate the overall CV risk of thromboembolic complications. Carotid intima-media thickness is considered an early marker of generalized atherosclerosis [122] and can be easily explored with echocardiography, allowing a noninvasive but accurate evaluation of the situation.

8.7 Sjögren's Syndrome

Sjögren's syndrome is an autoimmune condition characterized by a chronic inflammation of exocrine glands which leads to their functional impairment and manifests with sicca syndrome.

The extraglandular signs are represented mainly by arthritis, even though it is described a wide range of organ involvement such as pulmonary and renal abnormalities but also vascular and gastrointestinal alterations. Heart injuries are rarely reported, even though echocardiographic studies suggest that subclinical abnormalities are relatively common [8].

8.7.1 Pericardium

Data demonstrate that approximately 33% of patients affected by SS present ultrasound signs of pericarditis, but only half of them complaint some symptoms [129]. Pericardium wall thickening or echodense signals may be consequences of subclinical conditions which can be derived from either the underlying disease or other causes. Some studies suggest that pericardial inflammation may be more frequent in older patients or in those that present a shorter disease duration and ANA positivity but also high levels of orosomucoid and haptoglobin [130].

8.7.2 Heart Function

Left ventricle diastolic dysfunction is an important cause of morbidity and may be an early sign of myocardial damage in various diseases. It has been shown that it is detectable in a significant number of patients. The pathogenesis underlying this heart abnormality remains still unclear, even if it has been suggested that myocardial Raynaud's phenomenon may mediate the damage. Other mechanisms refer to stable microcircle alterations such as small intramyocardial vessel vasculitis or vasa vasorum impairment, but these conditions can be confirmed only by myocardial biopsy [130]. Only a limited number of HF cases have been reported and no histological diagnosis was made. The suspicion of autoimmune etiology was derived from the exclusion of other possible causes and from the rapid response to immunosuppressive therapy [131, 132].

8.8 Rheumatoid Arthritis

Rheumatoid arthritis (RA) is a systemic disease characterized by a chronic inflammatory condition affecting primarily the joints. Extra-articular manifestations include frequently and can directly involve several organs such as the lungs, skin, and eyes. Heart involvement is frequently found and substantially increases the risk of mortality, accounting for about a 50% excess compared to the general population [133, 134]. The pathogenesis is mainly related to the pro-inflammatory status of the patients which drive augmented oxidative stress of lipoprotein leading to accelerated atherosclerosis. For this reason, RA should be considered as a major CV risk factor. European League Against Rheumatism (EULAR) guidelines for CV risk recommend an annual assessment [135]; however it is important to note that traditional scores may underestimate the real hazard in RA patients [136].

8.8.1 Pericardium

Pericarditis is believed to be the most common cardiac manifestation of RA [137], and clinical symptoms are present in less than 5% of patients, while asymptomatic finding is seen in 20–50% by echocardiography. Pericarditis is more frequent in men, especially if autoantibodies are positive and in case of severe or active disease [138]. It can include both exudative and constrictive manifestations. Studies on pericardial fluid have demonstrated the presence of high level of proteins and lactate dehydrogenase but low levels of glucose [139]. Symptomatic patients usually manifest chest pain and dyspnea, but some of these develop nonspecific clinical pictures; therefore, echocardiography is being revealed an essential procedure to clarify undefined clinical situations detecting pericardial effusion. It is important to point out that sometimes pericarditis may develop after biologic initiation; in this case infections and tumors should be excluded, as well as SLE after anti-TNFα treatment [140].

8.8.2 Valvular Disease

Valvular heart disease is not considered a major extra-articular manifestation of RA, even if echocardiographic studies demonstrate the presence of different valve defects which affect from 24 to 39% of patients. Mitral valve, the most frequent site of pathological involvement, can be aggravated by both stenosis and regurgitation of various grades. This is the result of structure thickening generated by localized fibrosis or nodules [138].

8.8.3 Atherosclerosis

Atherosclerosis is considered as a collateral but not secondary process related to RA; in fact, chronic systemic inflammation is known to increase the CV burden inducing endothelial dysfunction that leads to accelerated atherogenesis [141, 142]. Several studies prove how inflammatory molecules, such as CRP or cytokines, are common key players in the pathogenesis of both diseases [11]. TNFα can alter the endothelial metabolism, and similarly, IL-6 induce an overall change of surface molecules of the endothelium that develops a pro-inflammatory status; moreover a study demonstrates how IL-6 overproduction reduces lipid concentrations in RA patient and enhances the expression of very low-density lipoprotein receptors in mice [143]. The link between inflammation and atherosclerosis in RA patients is further underlined by the evidence that the association between carotid plaques and inflammatory markers is independent of classical CV risk factors [144]. The major complex of histocompatibility DRB1 is significantly associated with RA susceptibility and also can potentially confer an increased risk of coronary heart disease [145]. This finding adds evidence to the not completely clarified role of adaptive immunity in the pathogenesis in atherosclerosis [145]. Nonetheless, additional factors (i.e., smoke habit, obesity, hypertension, dyslipidemia) alter the fibrinolytic pathway and coagulation status, raising the rate of plaque rupture. For these reasons, EULAR recommends using a modified Systematic Coronary Risk Evaluation (SCORE) to determine the 10-year risk of fatal CVD in RA patients [146].

8.8.4 Heart Function

Ischemic heart disease is a frequent complication in RA. The risk of acute myocardial infarction is about double compared to the general population, and the presence of unrecognized coronary heart disease is not rare in RA. Sudden death prevalence in RA patients is almost twofold than the general population [10]. HF has been reported in about 4–11% of RA cases; however, some studies demonstrate how prevalence can rise to 24% in selected RA populations which are characterized by high disease activity, glucocorticoid treatments, and positivity of rheumatoid factor [147]. HF derives from a progressively reduced organ reserve that ultimately leads to HF resulting from a detrimental remodeling of myocardial tissue driven by acute or chronic insults. The pathological injury can be the result of ischemic heart events as well as valvular disease, cardiomyopathies, and rhythm abnormalities [138]. Echocardiography and MRI are helpful to recognize potential etiologies and also to establish cardiac function, which, in RA patient, is usually depressed in its diastolic function. Studies on myocardial damage demonstrate how innate immunity cells are critical players in HF remodeling. The production of pro-inflammatory cytokines by injured tissue is the first step in the activation of acute inflammation [138] which aggravates the damage. The amplification of inflammatory pathways determines harmful effects on healthy cell metabolism by increased oxidative stress; moreover, these redundant molecular circuits recall additional immune cells in situ which worsen the process. The strong relation between inflammation and heart disease is nowadays widely proved by several data; some of these demonstrate the active roles played by TNFα and other pro-inflammatory cytokines (i.e., *IL*-6 and IL-1β) on the progression of obstructive coronary artery disease [138] and left ventricle remodeling [148–150]. Interestingly, Giles et al. have observed a robust association among myocardial dysfunction and disease activity and age but also interstitial fibrosis in RA compared to non-RA groups [151]; these findings are strengthened by histological analysis of myocardial samples which manifest higher levels of interstitial citrullination and fibrosis [151].

8.9 Conclusions

Cardiac involvement is a very common comorbidity of systemic autoimmune diseases which greatly contributes to a general deterioration of patient health status and to a higher mortality rate in comparison to general population. Traditional risk factors do not explain entirely a so significant CV risk, as reported in different case series and national databases; in fact, increasingly evidences link the mediators involved in chronic inflammation and in other immune mechanisms to the harmful action on heart tissue, as previously described. The cornerstone for a comprehensive management of autoimmune diseases lies thus in an aggressive control of disease activity associated with an accurate modification of traditional CV risk factors.

References

1. Cooper GS, Bynum ML, Somers EC. Recent insights in the epidemiology of autoimmune diseases: improved prevalence estimates and understanding of clustering of diseases. J Autoimmun. 2009;33:197–207.
2. Cavazzana I, Fredi M, Selmi C, Tincani A, Franceschini F. The clinical and histological spectrum of idiopathic inflammatory myopathies. Clin Rev Allergy Immunol. 2015;52(1):88–98.
3. Meroni PL, Penatti AE. Epigenetics and systemic lupus erythematosus: unmet needs. Clin Rev Allergy Immunol. 2015;50(3):367–76.
4. Agmon-Levin N, Selmi C. The autoimmune side of heart and lung diseases. Clin Rev Allergy Immunol. 2013;44:1–5.
5. Mason JC, Libby P. Cardiovascular disease in patients with chronic inflammation: mechanisms underlying premature cardiovascular events in rheumatologic conditions. Eur Heart J. 2015;36:482–9c.

6. Miner JJ, Kim AH. Cardiac manifestations of systemic lupus erythematosus. Rheum Dis Clin N Am. 2014;40:51–60.

7. Muangchan C, Canadian Scleroderma Research Group, Baron M, Pope J. The 15% rule in scleroderma: the frequency of severe organ complications in systemic sclerosis. A systematic review. J Rheumatol. 2013;40:1545–56.

8. Riboldi P, Gerosa M, Luzzana C, Catelli L. Cardiac involvement in systemic autoimmune diseases. Clin Rev Allergy Immunol. 2002;23:247–61.

9. Van Gelder H, Charles-Schoeman C. The heart in inflammatory myopathies. Rheum Dis Clin N Am. 2014;40:1–10.

10. Wright K, Crowson CS, Gabriel SE. Cardiovascular comorbidity in rheumatic diseases: a focus on heart failure. Heart Fail Clin. 2014;10:339–52.

11. Sattar N, McCarey DW, Capell H, McInnes IB. Explaining how "high-grade" systemic inflammation accelerates vascular risk in rheumatoid arthritis. Circulation. 2003;108:2957–63.

12. Inoue T, Uchida T, Kamishirado H, Takayanagi K, Hayashi T, Morooka S. Clinical significance of antibody against oxidized low density lipoprotein in patients with atherosclerotic coronary artery disease. J Am Coll Cardiol. 2001;37:775–9.

13. Nowak B, Szmyrka-Kaczmarek M, Durazinska A, Plaksej R, Borysewicz K, Korman L, Wiland P. Anti-ox-LDL antibodies and anti-ox-LDL-B2GPI antibodies in patients with systemic lupus erythematosus. Adv Clin Exp Med. 2012;21:331–5.

14. Karvonen J, Paivansalo M, Kesaniemi YA, Horkko S. Immunoglobulin M type of autoantibodies to oxidized low-density lipoprotein has an inverse relation to carotid artery atherosclerosis. Circulation. 2003;108:2107–12.

15. Bartoloni E, Shoenfeld Y, Gerli R. Inflammatory and autoimmune mechanisms in the induction of atherosclerotic damage in systemic rheumatic diseases: two faces of the same coin. Arthritis Care Res (Hoboken). 2011;63:178–83.

16. Hollan I, Meroni PL, Ahearn JM, Cohen Tervaert JW, Curran S, Goodyear CS, Hestad KA, Kahaleh B, Riggio M, Shields K, Wasko MC. Cardiovascular disease in autoimmune rheumatic diseases. Autoimmun Rev. 2013;12:1004–15.

17. Costedoat-Chalumeau N, Hulot JS, Amoura Z, Delcourt A, Maisonobe T, Dorent R, Bonnet N, Sable R, Lechat P, Wechsler B, Piette JC. Cardiomyopathy related to antimalarial therapy with illustrative case report. Cardiology. 2007;107:73–80.

18. White NJ. Cardiotoxicity of antimalarial drugs. Lancet Infect Dis. 2007;7:549–58.

19. Singh JA, Saag KG, Bridges SL Jr, Akl EA, Bannuru RR, Sullivan MC, Vaysbrot E, McNaughton C, Osani M, Shmerling RH, Curtis JR, Furst DE, Parks D, Kavanaugh A, O'dell J, King C, Leong A, Matteson EL, Schousboe JT, Drevlow B, Ginsberg S, Grober J, St Clair EW, Tindall E, Miller AS, McAlindon T. 2015 American College of Rheumatology guideline for the treatment of rheumatoid arthritis. Arthritis Rheumatol. 2016;68:1–26.

20. Diamantopoulos AP, Larsen AI, Omdal R. Is it safe to use TNF-alpha blockers for systemic inflammatory disease in patients with heart failure? Importance of dosage and receptor specificity. Int J Cardiol. 2013;167:1719–23.

21. Javed Q, Murtaza I. Therapeutic potential of tumour necrosis factor-alpha antagonists in patients with chronic heart failure. Heart Lung Circ. 2013;22:323–7.

22. Rubbert-Roth A. Assessing the safety of biologic agents in patients with rheumatoid arthritis. Rheumatology (Oxford). 2012;51(Suppl 5):V38–47.

23. Singh BK, Haque SE, Pillai KK. Assessment of nonsteroidal anti-inflammatory drug-induced cardiotoxicity. Expert Opin Drug Metab Toxicol. 2014;10:143–56.

24. Hochberg MC. Updating the American College of Rheumatology revised criteria for the classification of systemic lupus erythematosus. Arthritis Rheum. 1997;40:1725.

25. Yoneda S, Koyama M, Matsubara T, Toyama S. Electrocardiographic studies in acute pericarditis with specific reference to ventricular involvement of non-specific pericarditis. Acta Cardiol. 1977;32:337–52.

26. Doria A, Iaccarino L, Sarzi-Puttini P, Atzeni F, Turriel M, Petri M. Cardiac involvement in systemic lupus erythematosus. Lupus. 2005;14:683–6.
27. Turiel M, Peretti R, Sarzi-Puttini P, Atzeni F, Doria A. Cardiac imaging techniques in systemic autoimmune diseases. Lupus. 2005;14:727–31.
28. Brigden W, Bywaters EG, Lessof MH, Ross IP. The heart in systemic lupus erythematosus. Br Heart J. 1960;22:1–16.
29. Bulkley BH, Roberts WC. The heart in systemic lupus erythematosus and the changes induced in it by corticosteroid therapy. A study of 36 necropsy patients. Am J Med. 1975;58:243–64.
30. Griffith GC, Vural IL. Acute and subacute disseminated lupus erythematosus; a correlation of clinical and postmortem findings in eighteen cases. Circulation. 1951;3:492–500.
31. Gross L. The cardiac lesions in Libman-Sacks disease: with a consideration of its relationship to acute diffuse lupus erythematosus. Am J Pathol. 1940;16:375–408. 11
32. Harvey AM, Shulman LE, Tumulty PA, Conley CL, Schoenrich EH. Systemic lupus erythematosus: review of the literature and clinical analysis of 138 cases. Medicine (Baltimore). 1954;33:291–437.
33. Hejtmancik MR, Wright JC, Quint R, Jennings FL. The cardiovascular manifestations of systemic lupus erythematosus. Am Heart J. 1964;68:119–30.
34. Humphreys EM. The cardiac lesions of acute disseminated lupus erythematosus. Ann Intern Med. 1948;28:12–4.
35. Jain D, Halushka MK. Cardiac pathology of systemic lupus erythematosus. J Clin Pathol. 2009;62:584–92.
36. Jessar RA, Lamont-Havers RW, Ragan C. Natural history of lupus erythematosus disseminatus. Ann Intern Med. 1953;38:717–31.
37. Kong TQ, Kellum RE, Haserick JR. Clinical diagnosis of cardiac involvement in systemic lupus erythematosus. A correlation of clinical and autopsy findings in thirty patients. Circulation. 1962;26:7–11.
38. Panchal L, Divate S, Vaideeswar P, Pandit SP. Cardiovascular involvement in systemic lupus erythematosus: an autopsy study of 27 patients in India. J Postgrad Med. 2006;52:5–10. Discussion 10
39. Shearn MA. The heart in systemic lupus erythematosus. Am Heart J. 1959;58:452–66.
40. Tincani A, Rebaioli CB, Taglietti M, Shoenfeld Y. Heart involvement in systemic lupus erythematosus, anti-phospholipid syndrome and neonatal lupus. Rheumatology (Oxford). 2006;45(Suppl 4):iv8–13.
41. Ansari A, Larson PH, Bates HD. Cardiovascular manifestations of systemic lupus erythematosus: current perspective. Prog Cardiovasc Dis. 1985;27:421–34.
42. Bidani AK, Roberts JL, Schwartz MM, Lewis EJ. Immunopathology of cardiac lesions in fatal systemic lupus erythematosus. Am J Med. 1980;69:849–58.
43. Lin K, Lloyd-Jones DM, Li D, Liu Y, Yang J, Markl M, Carr JC. Imaging of cardiovascular complications in patients with systemic lupus erythematosus. Lupus. 2015;24:1126–34.
44. Yilmaz A, Ferreira V, Klingel K, Kandolf R, Neubauer S, Sechtem U. Role of cardiovascular magnetic resonance imaging (CMR) in the diagnosis of acute and chronic myocarditis. Heart Fail Rev. 2013;18:747–60.
45. Wijetunga M, Rockson S. Myocarditis in systemic lupus erythematosus. Am J Med. 2002;113:419–23.
46. Yogasundaram H, Putko BN, Tien J, Paterson DI, Cujec B, Ringrose J, Oudit GY. Hydroxychloroquine-induced cardiomyopathy: case report, pathophysiology, diagnosis, and treatment. Can J Cardiol. 2014;30:1706–15.
47. Moyssakis I, Tektonidou MG, Vasilliou VA, Samarkos M, Votteas V, Moutsopoulos HM. Libman-Sacks endocarditis in systemic lupus erythematosus: prevalence, associations, and evolution. Am J Med. 2007;120:636–42.
48. Roldan CA, Tolstrup K, Macias L, Qualls CR, Maynard D, Charlton G, Sibbitt WL Jr. Libman-Sacks endocarditis: detection, characterization, and clinical correlates by three-dimensional transesophageal echocardiography. J Am Soc Echocardiogr. 2015;28:770–9.

49. Brucato A, Cimaz R, Caporali R, Ramoni V, Buyon J. Pregnancy outcomes in patients with autoimmune diseases and anti-Ro/SSA antibodies. Clin Rev Allergy Immunol. 2011;40:27–41.
50. Brito-Zeron P, Izmirly PM, Ramos-Casals M, Buyon JP, Khamashta MA. The clinical spectrum of autoimmune congenital heart block. Nat Rev Rheumatol. 2015;11:301–12.
51. Landtman B, Linder E, Hjelt L, Tuuteri L. Congenital complete heart block. I. A clinical study of 27 cases. Ann Paediatr Fenn. 1964;10:99–104.
52. Costedoat-Chalumeau N, Amoura Z, Lupoglazoff JM, Huong DL, Denjoy I, Vauthier D, Sebbouh D, Fain O, Georgin-Lavialle S, Ghillani P, Musset L, Wechsler B, Duhaut P, Piette JC. Outcome of pregnancies in patients with anti-SSA/Ro antibodies: a study of 165 pregnancies, with special focus on electrocardiographic variations in the children and comparison with a control group. Arthritis Rheum. 2004;50:3187–94.
53. Izmirly PM, Costedoat-Chalumeau N, Pisoni CN, Khamashta MA, Kim MY, Saxena A, Friedman D, Llanos C, Piette JC, Buyon JP. Maternal use of hydroxychloroquine is associated with a reduced risk of recurrent anti-SSA/Ro-antibody-associated cardiac manifestations of neonatal lupus. Circulation. 2012;126:76–82.
54. Buyon JP, Clancy RM. Neonatal lupus: basic research and clinical perspectives. Rheum Dis Clin N Am. 2005;31:299–313. vii
55. Garcia S, Nascimento JH, Bonfa E, Levy R, Oliveira SF, Tavares AV, De Carvalho AC. Cellular mechanism of the conduction abnormalities induced by serum from anti-Ro/SSA-positive patients in rabbit hearts. J Clin Invest. 1994;93:718–24.
56. Xiao GQ, Hu K, Boutjdir M. Direct inhibition of expressed cardiac L- and T-type calcium channels by igg from mothers whose children have congenital heart block. Circulation. 2001;103:1599–604.
57. Tincani A, Biasini-Rebaioli C, Cattaneo R, Riboldi P. Nonorgan specific autoantibodies and heart damage. Lupus. 2005;14:656–9.
58. Brito-Zeron P, Izmirly PM, Ramos-Casals M, Buyon JP, Khamashta MA. Autoimmune congenital heart block: complex and unusual situations. Lupus. 2016;25:116–28.
59. Tonello M, Ruffatti A, Marson P, Tison T, Marozio L, Hoxha A, De Silvestro G, Punzi L. Plasma exchange effectively removes 52- and 60-kDa anti-Ro/SSA and anti-La/SSB antibodies in pregnant women with congenital heart block. Transfusion. 2015;55:1782–6.
60. Elhai M, Avouac J, Walker UA, Matucci-Cerinic M, Riemekasten G, Airo P, Hachulla E, Valentini G, Carreira PE, Cozzi F, Balbir Gurman A, Braun-Moscovici Y, Damjanov N, Ananieva LP, Scorza R, Jimenez S, Busquets J, Li M, Muller-Ladner U, Kahan A, Distler O, Allanore Y. A gender gap in primary and secondary heart dysfunctions in systemic sclerosis: a EUSTAR prospective study. Ann Rheum Dis. 2016;75:163–9.
61. Ranque B, Mouthon L. Geoepidemiology of systemic sclerosis. Autoimmun Rev. 2010;9:A311–8.
62. Van Den Hoogen F, Khanna D, Fransen J, Johnson SR, Baron M, Tyndall A, Matucci-Cerinic M, Naden RP, Medsger TA Jr, Carreira PE, Riemekasten G, Clements PJ, Denton CP, Distler O, Allanore Y, Furst DE, Gabrielli A, Mayes MD, Van Laar JM, Seibold JR, Czirjak L, Steen VD, Inanc M, Kowal-Bielecka O, Muller-Ladner U, Valentini G, Veale DJ, Vonk MC, Walker UA, Chung L, Collier DH, Csuka ME, Fessler BJ, Guiducci S, Herrick A, Hsu VM, Jimenez S, Kahaleh B, Merkel PA, Sierakowski S, Silver RM, Simms RW, Varga J, Pope JE. 2013 classification criteria for systemic sclerosis: an American College of Rheumatology/European League against rheumatism collaborative initiative. Arthritis Rheum. 2013;65:2737–47.
63. Mouthon L, Bussone G, Berezne A, Noel LH, Guillevin L. Scleroderma renal crisis. J Rheumatol. 2014;41:1040–8.
64. Elhai M, Meune C, Avouac J, Kahan A, Allanore Y. Trends in mortality in patients with systemic sclerosis over 40 years: a systematic review and meta-analysis of cohort studies. Rheumatology (Oxford). 2012;51:1017–26.
65. Ferri C, Sebastiani M, Lo Monaco A, Iudici M, Giuggioli D, Furini F, Manfredi A, Cuomo G, Spinella A, Colaci M, Govoni M, Valentini G. Systemic sclerosis evolution of disease

pathomorphosis and survival. Our experience on Italian patients' population and review of the literature. Autoimmun Rev. 2014;13:1026–34.

66. Vacca A, Meune C, Gordon J, Chung L, Proudman S, Assassi S, Nikpour M, Rodriguez-Reyna TS, Khanna D, Lafyatis R, Matucci-Cerinic M, Distler O, Allanore Y, Scleroderma Clinical Trial Consortium Cardiac Subcommittee. Cardiac arrhythmias and conduction defects in systemic sclerosis. Rheumatology (Oxford). 2014;53:1172–7.

67. Fernandez-Codina A, Simeon-Aznar CP, Pinal-Fernandez I, Rodriguez-Palomares J, Pizzi MN, Hidalgo CE, Del Castillo AG, Prado-Galbarro FJ, Sarria-Santamera A, Fonollosa-Pla V, Vilardell-Tarres M. Cardiac involvement in systemic sclerosis: differences between clinical subsets and influence on survival. Rheumatol Int. 2015;37(1):75–84.

68. Harvey GR, Butts S, Rands AL, Patel Y, McHugh NJ. Clinical and serological associations with anti-RNA polymerase antibodies in systemic sclerosis. Clin Exp Immunol. 1999;117:395–402.

69. Allanore Y, Meune C. Primary myocardial involvement in systemic sclerosis: evidence for a microvascular origin. Clin Exp Rheumatol. 2010;28:S48–53.

70. Kahan A, Allanore Y. Primary myocardial involvement in systemic sclerosis. Rheumatology (Oxford). 2006;45(Suppl 4):Iv14–7.

71. Cutolo M, Sulli A, Secchi ME, Paolino S, Pizzorni C. Nailfold capillaroscopy is useful for the diagnosis and follow-up of autoimmune rheumatic diseases. A future tool for the analysis of microvascular heart involvement? Rheumatology (Oxford). 2006;45(Suppl 4):Iv43–6.

72. Desai CS, Lee DC, Shah SJ. Systemic sclerosis and the heart: current diagnosis and management. Curr Opin Rheumatol. 2011;23:545–54.

73. Kitchongcharoenying P, Foocharoen C, Mahakkanukrauh A, Suwannaroj S, Nanagara R. Pericardial fluid profiles of pericardial effusion in systemic sclerosis patients. Asian Pac J Allergy Immunol. 2013;31:314–9.

74. Hachulla AL, Launay D, Gaxotte V, De Groote P, Lamblin N, Devos P, Hatron PY, Beregi JP, Hachulla E. Cardiac magnetic resonance imaging in systemic sclerosis: a cross-sectional observational study of 52 patients. Ann Rheum Dis. 2009;68:1878–84.

75. Allanore Y, Meune C. N-terminal pro brain natriuretic peptide: the new cornerstone of cardiovascular assessment in systemic sclerosis. Clin Exp Rheumatol. 2009;27:59–63.

76. Lambova S. Cardiac manifestations in systemic sclerosis. World J Cardiol. 2014;6:993–1005.

77. Clements PJ, Furst DE, Cabeen W, Tashkin D, Paulus HE, Roberts N. The relationship arrhythmias and conduction disturbances to other manifestations of cardiopulmonary disease in progressive systemic sclerosis (PSS). Am J Med. 1981;71:38–46.

78. Follansbee WP, Curtiss EI, Rahko PS, Medsger TA Jr, Lavine SJ, Owens GR, Steen VD. The electrocardiogram in systemic sclerosis (Scleroderma). Study of 102 consecutive cases with functional correlations and review of the literature. Am J Med. 1985;79:183–92.

79. Dalakas MC, Hohlfeld R. Polymyositis and dermatomyositis. Lancet. 2003;362:971–82.

80. Danieli MG, Gambini S, Pettinari L, Logullo F, Veronesi G, Gabrielli A. Impact of treatment on survival in polymyositis and dermatomyositis. A single-centre long-term follow-up study. Autoimmun Rev. 2014;13:1048–54.

81. Zhang L, Wang GC, Ma L, Zu N. Cardiac involvement in adult polymyositis or dermatomyositis: a systematic review. Clin Cardiol. 2012;35:686–91.

82. Diederichsen LP, Simonsen JA, Diederichsen AC, Kim WY, Hvidsten S, Hougaard M, Junker P, Lundberg IE, Petersen H, Hansen ES, Eskerud KS, Kay SD, Jacobsen S. Cardiac abnormalities assessed by non-invasive techniques in patients with newly diagnosed idiopathic inflammatory myopathies. Clin Exp Rheumatol. 2015;33:706–14.

83. Gupta R, Wayangankar SA, Targoff IN, Hennebry TA. Clinical cardiac involvement in idiopathic inflammatory myopathies: a systematic review. Int J Cardiol. 2011;148:261–70.

84. Mavrogeni S, Douskou M, Manoussakis MN. Contrast-enhanced CMR imaging reveals myocardial involvement in idiopathic inflammatory myopathy without cardiac manifestations. JACC Cardiovasc Imaging. 2011;4:1324–5.

85. Mavrogeni S, Sfikakis PP, Dimitroulas T, Kolovou G, Kitas GD. Cardiac and muscular involvement in idiopathic inflammatory myopathies: noninvasive diagnostic assessment and the role of cardiovascular and skeletal magnetic resonance imaging. Inflamm Allergy Drug Targets. 2014;13:206–16.
86. Rosenbohm A, Buckert D, Gerischer N, Walcher T, Kassubek J, Rottbauer W, Ludolph AC, Bernhardt P. Early diagnosis of cardiac involvement in idiopathic inflammatory myopathy by cardiac magnetic resonance tomography. J Neurol. 2015;262:949–56.
87. Toong C, Puranik R, Adelstein S. Use of cardiac MR imaging to evaluate the presence of myocarditis in autoimmune myositis: three cases. Rheumatol Int. 2012;32:779–82.
88. Haupt HM, Hutchins GM. The heart and cardiac conduction system in polymyositis-dermatomyositis: a clinicopathologic study of 16 autopsied patients. Am J Cardiol. 1982;50:998–1006.
89. Matsumoto K, Tanaka H, Yamana S, Kaneko A, Tsuji T, Ryo K, Sekiguchi K, Kawakami F, Kawai H, Hirata K. Successful steroid therapy for heart failure due to myocarditis associated with primary biliary cirrhosis. Can J Cardiol. 2012;28:515.e3–6.
90. Gonzalez-Lopez L, Gamez-Nava JI, Sanchez L, Rosas E, Suarez-Almazor M, Cardona-Munoz C, Ramos-Remus C. Cardiac manifestations in dermato-polymyositis. Clin Exp Rheumatol. 1996;14:373–9.
91. Bazzani C, Cavazzana I, Ceribelli A, Vizzardi E, Dei Cas L, Franceschini F. Cardiological features in idiopathic inflammatory myopathies. J Cardiovasc Med (Hagerstown). 2010;11:906–11.
92. Lu Z, Wei Q, Ning Z, Qian-Zi Z, Xiao-Ming S, Guo-Chun W. Left ventricular diastolic dysfunction—early cardiac impairment in patients with polymyositis/dermatomyositis: a tissue Doppler imaging study. J Rheumatol. 2013;40:1572–7.
93. Sharp GC, Irvin WS, Tan EM, Gould RG, Holman HR. Mixed connective tissue disease—an apparently distinct rheumatic disease syndrome associated with a specific antibody to an Extractable Nuclear Antigen (ENA). Am J Med. 1972;52:148–59.
94. Ungprasert P, Wannarong T, Panichsillapakit T, Cheungpasitporn W, Thongprayoon C, Ahmed S, Raddatz DA. Cardiac involvement in mixed connective tissue disease: a systematic review. Int J Cardiol. 2014;171:326–30.
95. Hajas A, Szodoray P, Nakken B, Gaal J, Zold E, Laczik R, Demeter N, Nagy G, Szekanecz Z, Zeher M, Szegedi G, Bodolay E. Clinical course, prognosis, and causes of death in mixed connective tissue disease. J Rheumatol. 2013;40:1134–42.
96. Kim P, Grossman JM. Treatment of mixed connective tissue disease. Rheum Dis Clin N Am. 2005;31:549–65. Viii
97. Arroyo-Avila M, Vila LM. Cardiac tamponade in a patient with mixed connective tissue disease. J Clin Rheumatol. 2015;21:42–5.
98. Hammann C, Genton CY, Delabays A, Bischoff Delaloye A, Bogousslavsky J, Spertini F. Myocarditis of mixed connective tissue disease: favourable outcome after intravenous pulsed cyclophosphamide. Clin Rheumatol. 1999;18:85–7.
99. Lash AD, Wittman AL, Quismorio FP Jr. Myocarditis in mixed connective tissue disease: clinical and pathologic study of three cases and review of the literature. Semin Arthritis Rheum. 1986;15:288–96.
100. Comens SM, Alpert MA, Sharp GC, Pressly TA, Kelly DL, Hazelwood SE, Mukerji V. Frequency of mitral valve prolapse in systemic lupus erythematosus, progressive systemic sclerosis and mixed connective tissue disease. Am J Cardiol. 1989;63:369–70.
101. Leung WH, Wong KL, Lau CP, Wong CK, Cheng CH, Tai YT. Echocardiographic identification of mitral valvular abnormalities in patients with mixed connective tissue disease. J Rheumatol. 1990;17:485–8.
102. Rebollar-Gonzalez V, Torre-Delgadillo A, Orea-Tejeda A, Ochoa-Perez V, Navarrete-Gaona R, Asensio-Lafuente E, Dorantes-Garcia J, Narvaez R, Rangel-Pena AM, Hernandez-Reyes P, Oseguera-Moguel J. Cardiac conduction disturbances in mixed connective tissue disease. Rev Investig Clin. 2001;53:330–4.

103. Alpert MA, Goldberg SH, Singsen BH, Durham JB, Sharp GC, Ahmad M, Madigan NP, Hurst DP, Sullivan WD. Cardiovascular manifestations of mixed connective tissue disease in adults. Circulation. 1983;68:1182–93.

104. Oetgen WJ, Mutter ML, Lawless OJ, Davia JE. Cardiac abnormalities in mixed connective tissue disease. Chest. 1983;83:185–8.

105. Leung WH, Wong KL, Lau CP, Wong CK, Cheng CH, Tai YT. Doppler-echo evaluation of left ventricular diastolic filling in patient with mixed connective tissue disease. Cardiology. 1990;77:93–100.

106. Vegh J, Hegedus I, Szegedi G, Zeher M, Bodolay E. Diastolic function of the heart in mixed connective tissue disease. Clin Rheumatol. 2007;26:176–81.

107. Miyakis S, Lockshin MD, Atsumi T, Branch DW, Brey RL, Cervera R, Derksen RH, Pg DEG, Koike T, Meroni PL, Reber G, Shoenfeld Y, Tincani A, Vlachoyiannopoulos PG, Krilis SA. International consensus statement on an update of the classification criteria for definite Antiphospholipid Syndrome (APS). J Thromb Haemost. 2006;4:295–306.

108. Cervera R, Piette JC, Font J, Khamashta MA, Shoenfeld Y, Camps MT, Jacobsen S, Lakos G, Tincani A, Kontopoulou-Griva I, Galeazzi M, Meroni PL, Derksen RH, De Groot PG, Gromnica-Ihle E, Baleva M, Mosca M, Bombardieri S, Houssiau F, Gris JC, Quere I, Hachulla E, Vasconcelos C, Roch B, Fernandez-Nebro A, Boffa MC, Hughes GR, Ingelmo M, Euro-Phospholipid Project G. Antiphospholipid syndrome: clinical and immunologic manifestations and patterns of disease expression in a cohort of 1,000 patients. Arthritis Rheum. 2002;46:1019–27.

109. Long BR, Leya F. The role of antiphospholipid syndrome in cardiovascular disease. Hematol Oncol Clin North Am. 2008;22:79–94. vi–vii

110. Roldan CA. Valvular and coronary heart disease in systemic inflammatory diseases: systemic disorders in heart disease. Heart. 2008;94:1089–101.

111. Hojnik M, George J, Ziporen L, Shoenfeld Y. Heart valve involvement (Libman-Sacks endo-carditis) in the antiphospholipid syndrome. Circulation. 1996;93:1579–87.

112. Vianna JL, Khamashta MA, Ordi-Ros J, Font J, Cervera R, Lopez-Soto A, Tolosa C, Franz J, Selva A, Ingelmo M, et al. Comparison of the primary and secondary antiphospholipid syndrome: a European Multicenter Study of 114 patients. Am J Med. 1994;96:3–9.

113. Nesher G, Ilany J, Rosenmann D, Abraham AS. Valvular dysfunction in antiphospholipid syndrome: prevalence, clinical features, and treatment. Semin Arthritis Rheum. 1997;27:27–35.

114. Espinola-Zavaleta N, Vargas-Barron J, Colmenares-Galvis T, Cruz-Cruz F, Romero-Cardenas A, Keirns C, Amigo MC. Echocardiographic evaluation of patients with primary antiphos-pholipid syndrome. Am Heart J. 1999;137:973–8.

115. Zavaleta NE, Montes RM, Soto ME, Vanzzini NA, Amigo MC. Primary antiphospho-lipid syndrome: a 5-year transesophageal echocardiographic followup study. J Rheumatol. 2004;31:2402–7.

116. Erdogan D, Goren MT, Diz-Kucukkaya R, Inanc M. Assessment of cardiac structure and left atrial appendage functions in primary antiphospholipid syndrome: a transesophageal echo-cardiographic study. Stroke. 2005;36:592–6.

117. Krause I, Lev S, Fraser A, Blank M, Lorber M, Stojanovich L, Rovensky J, Chapman J, Shoenfeld Y. Close association between valvular heart disease and central nervous system manifestations in the antiphospholipid syndrome. Ann Rheum Dis. 2005;64:1490–3.

118. Garcia-Torres R, Amigo MC, De La Rosa A, Moron A, Reyes PA. Valvular heart disease in primary antiphospholipid syndrome (PAPS): clinical and morphological findings. Lupus. 1996;5:56–61.

119. Ziporen L, Goldberg I, Arad M, Hojnik M, Ordi-Ros J, Afek A, Blank M, Sandbank Y, Vilardell-Tarres M, De Torres I, Weinberger A, Asherson RA, Kopolovic Y, Shoenfeld Y. Libman-Sacks endocarditis in the antiphospholipid syndrome: immunopathologic find-ings in deformed heart valves. Lupus. 1996;5:196–205.

120. Cervera R, Boffa MC, Khamashta MA, Hughes GR. The Euro-phospholipid project: epide-miology of the antiphospholipid syndrome in Europe. Lupus. 2009;18:889–93.

121. Artenjak A, Lakota K, Frank M, Cucnik S, Rozman B, Bozic B, Shoenfeld Y, Sodin-Semrl S. Antiphospholipid antibodies as non-traditional risk factors in atherosclerosis based cardiovascular diseases without overt autoimmunity. A critical updated review. Autoimmun Rev. 2012;11:873–82.
122. Denas G, Jose SP, Bracco A, Zoppellaro G, Pengo V. Antiphospholipid syndrome and the heart: a case series and literature review. Autoimmun Rev. 2015;14:214–22.
123. George J, Shoenfeld Y, Harats D. The involvement of beta2-glycoprotein I (beta2-GPI) in human and murine atherosclerosis. J Autoimmun. 1999;13:57–60.
124. Delgado Alves J, Ames PR, Donohue S, Stanyer L, Nourooz-Zadeh J, Ravirajan C, Isenberg DA. Antibodies to high-density lipoprotein and beta2-glycoprotein I are inversely correlated with paraoxonase activity in systemic lupus erythematosus and primary antiphospholipid syndrome. Arthritis Rheum. 2002;46:2686–94.
125. Matsuura E, Kobayashi K, Koike T, Shoenfeld Y. Autoantibody-mediated atherosclerosis. Autoimmun Rev. 2002;1:348–53.
126. Daly CA, De Stavola B, Sendon JL, Tavazzi L, Boersma E, Clemens F, Danchin N, Delahaye F, Gitt A, Julian D, Mulcahy D, Ruzyllo W, Thygesen K, Verheugt F, Fox KM. Predicting prognosis in stable angina—results from the Euro heart survey of stable angina: prospective observational study. BMJ. 2006;332:262–7.
127. Veres K, Lakos G, Kerenyi A, Szekanecz Z, Szegedi G, Shoenfeld Y, Soltesz P. Antiphospholipid antibodies in acute coronary syndrome. Lupus. 2004;13:423–7.
128. Mavrogeni SI, Sfikakis PP, Kitas GD, Kolovou G, Tektonidou MG. Cardiac involvement in antiphospholipid syndrome: the diagnostic role of noninvasive cardiac imaging. Semin Arthritis Rheum. 2015;45(5):611–6.
129. Rantapaa-Dahlqvist S, Backman C, Sandgren H, Ostberg Y. Echocardiographic findings in patients with primary Sjogren's syndrome. Clin Rheumatol. 1993;12:214–8.
130. Gyongyosi M, Pokorny G, Jambrik Z, Kovacs L, Kovacs A, Makula E, Csanady M. Cardiac manifestations in primary Sjogren's syndrome. Ann Rheum Dis. 1996;55:450–4.
131. Golan TD, Keren D, Elias N, Naschitz JE, Toubi E, Misselevich I, Yeshurun D. Severe reversible cardiomyopathy associated with systemic vasculitis in primary Sjogren's syndrome. Lupus. 1997;6:505–8.
132. Levin MD, Zoet-Nugteren SK, Markusse HM. Myocarditis and primary Sjogren's syndrome. Lancet. 1999;354:128–9.
133. Del Rincon ID, Williams K, Stern MP, Freeman GL, Escalante A. High incidence of cardiovascular events in a rheumatoid arthritis cohort not explained by traditional cardiac risk factors. Arthritis Rheum. 2001;44:2737–45.
134. Nurmohamed MT, Heslinga M, Kitas GD. Cardiovascular comorbidity in rheumatic diseases. Nat Rev Rheumatol. 2015;11:693–704.
135. Ikdahl E, Rollefstad S, Olsen IC, Kvien TK, Hansen IJ, Soldal DM, Haugeberg G, Semb AG. Eular task force recommendations on annual cardiovascular risk assessment for patients with rheumatoid arthritis: an audit of the success of implementation in a rheumatology outpatient clinic. Biomed Res Int. 2015;2015:515280.
136. Arts EE, Popa C, Den Broeder AA, Semb AG, Toms T, Kitas GD, Van Riel PL, Fransen J. Performance of four current risk algorithms in predicting cardiovascular events in patients with early rheumatoid arthritis. Ann Rheum Dis. 2015;74:668–74.
137. Voskuyl AE. The heart and cardiovascular manifestations in rheumatoid arthritis. Rheumatology (Oxford). 2006;45(Suppl 4):iv4–7.
138. Sen D, Gonzalez-Mayda M, Brasington RD Jr. Cardiovascular disease in rheumatoid arthritis. Rheum Dis Clin N Am. 2014;40:27–49.
139. Barcin C, Yalcinkaya E, Kabul HK. Cholesterol pericarditis associated with rheumatoid arthritis: a rare cause of pericardial effusion. Int J Cardiol. 2013;166:E56–8.
140. Ambrose NL, O'connell PG. Anti-TNF alpha therapy does not always protect rheumatoid arthritis patients against developing pericarditis. Clin Exp Rheumatol. 2007;25:660.

141. Choy E, Ganeshalingam K, Semb AG, Szekanecz Z, Nurmohamed M. Cardiovascular risk in rheumatoid arthritis: recent advances in the understanding of the pivotal role of inflammation, risk predictors and the impact of treatment. Rheumatology (Oxford). 2014;53:2143–54.
142. Maradit-Kremers H, Crowson CS, Nicola PJ, Ballman KV, Roger VL, Jacobsen SJ, Gabriel SE. Increased unrecognized coronary heart disease and sudden deaths in rheumatoid arthritis: a population-based cohort study. Arthritis Rheum. 2005;52:402–11.
143. Hashizume M, Yoshida H, Koike N, Suzuki M, Mihara M. Overproduced interleukin 6 decreases blood lipid levels via upregulation of very-low-density lipoprotein receptor. Ann Rheum Dis. 2010;69:741–6.
144. Park YB, Ahn CW, Choi HK, Lee SH, In BH, Lee HC, Nam CM, Lee SK. Atherosclerosis in rheumatoid arthritis: morphologic evidence obtained by carotid ultrasound. Arthritis Rheum. 2002;46:1714–9.
145. Paakkanen R, Lokki ML, Seppanen M, Tierala I, Nieminen MS, Sinisalo J. Proinflammatory HLA-DRB1*01-haplotype predisposes to ST-elevation myocardial infarction. Atherosclerosis. 2012;221:461–6.
146. Peters MJ, Symmons DP, McCarey D, Dijkmans BA, Nicola P, Kvien TK, McInnes IB, Haentzschel H, Gonzalez-Gay MA, Provan S, Semb A, Sidiropoulos P, Kitas G, Smulders YM, Soubrier M, Szekanecz Z, Sattar N, Nurmohamed MT. Eular evidence-based recommendations for cardiovascular risk management in patients with rheumatoid arthritis and other forms of inflammatory arthritis. Ann Rheum Dis. 2010;69:325–31.
147. Myasoedova E, Crowson CS, Nicola PJ, Maradit-Kremers H, Davis JM 3rd, Roger VL, Therneau TM, Gabriel SE. The influence of rheumatoid arthritis disease characteristics on heart failure. J Rheumatol. 2011;38:1601–6.
148. Deswal A, Petersen NJ, Feldman AM, Young JB, White BG, Mann DL. Cytokines and cytokine receptors in advanced heart failure: an analysis of the cytokine database from the Vesnarinone trial (VEST). Circulation. 2001;103:2055–9.
149. Levine B, Kalman J, Mayer L, Fillit HM, Packer M. Elevated circulating levels of tumor necrosis factor in severe chronic heart failure. N Engl J Med. 1990;323:236–41.
150. Myasoedova E, Davis JM 3rd, Crowson CS, Roger VL, Karon BL, Borgeson DD, Therneau TM, Matteson EL, Rodeheffer RJ, Gabriel SE. Brief report: rheumatoid arthritis is associated with left ventricular concentric remodeling: results of a population-based cross-sectional study. Arthritis Rheum. 2013;65:1713–8.
151. Giles JT, Fert-Bober J, Park JK, Bingham CO 3rd, Andrade F, Fox-Talbot K, Pappas D, Rosen A, Van Eyk J, Bathon JM, Halushka MK. Myocardial citrullination in rheumatoid arthritis: a correlative histopathologic study. Arthritis Res Ther. 2012;14:R39.

Chapter 9
Vasculitis in the Central Nervous System

Anastasia Bougea and Nikolaos Spantideas

9.1 Introduction

Traditionally, central nervous system (CNS) vasculitides are defined as a group of clinical and pathological entities characterized by an inflammatory cell infiltration and necrosis of blood vessel walls. Three main mechanisms of vascular injury are:

1. Cell-mediated inflammation mediated by cytotoxic CD8+ T cells which release INF-gamma, recruiting and activating macrophages.
2. Immune complex (IC)-mediated inflammation or in situ formation of immune complex within the vessel wall. Complement activation is responsible for chemotactic attraction of neutrophils. Subsequent phagocytosis and secretion of neutrophil granular products result in vascular damage.
3. Antineutrophil cytoplasmic antibody (ANCA)-mediated inflammation. ANCA-associated vasculitides include Wegener granulomatosis, microscopic polyangiitis, Churg–Strauss syndrome, and renal-limited vasculitis (Fig. 9.1).

Vasculitides may be primary, involving large, medium and small vessels, or secondary, associated with infections, malignancies, drugs, and systemic vasculitides (Table 9.1). The latter cover a wide range of multisystem inflammatory disorders involving muscles, joints, and skin, such as rheumatoid arthritis (RA), systemic

A. Bougea, MD, PhD (✉) • N. Spantideas, PhD
Department of Neurology, University of Athens Medical School,
Aeginition Hospital, Athens, Greece
e-mail: annita139@yahoo.gr

© Springer International Publishing AG 2017
S. Sattler, T. Kennedy-Lydon (eds.), *The Immunology of Cardiovascular Homeostasis and Pathology*, Advances in Experimental Medicine and Biology 1003, DOI 10.1007/978-3-319-57613-8_9

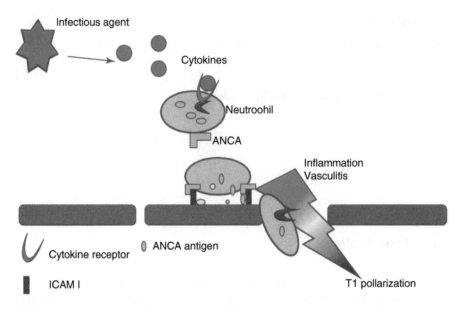

Fig. 9.1 Diagram of the cellular events of ANCA-associated small vessel vasculitis

Table 9.1 The most common classification of vasculitides adopted by the 2012 International Chapel Hill Consensus Conference on the Nomenclature of Vasculitides (CHCC2012)

Large vessel vasculitis	Takayasu arteritis, temporal arteritis
Medium vessel vasculitis	Polyarteritis nodosa
Small vessel vasculitis	Antineutrophil cytoplasmic antibody (ANCA)-associated vasculitis (AAV), microscopic polyangiitis, granulomatosis with polyangiitis (Wegener's), eosinophilic granulomatosis with polyangiitis (Churg–Strauss)
Variable vessel vasculitis	Behçet disease (BD) Cogan's syndrome
Single-organ vasculitis	Primary central nervous system vasculitis
Vasculitis associated with systemic disease	Lupus vasculitis Rheumatoid vasculitis
Vasculitis associated with probable etiology	Hydralazine-associated microscopic polyangiitis, hepatitis B virus-associated vasculitis, hepatitis C virus-associated cryoglobulinemic vasculitis

lupus erythematosus (SLE), primary Sjögren's syndrome (SS), and systemic sclerosis [1, 2]. However, due to complex spectrum of overlapping clinical manifestations, lack of efficient noninvasive diagnostic tests, and the relative rarity of their presentation, it is often difficult to recognize these disorders.

The CNS complications are likely to be fatal without judicious use of immunosuppression; thus, prompt diagnosis can avoid pervasive injury and disability. This chapter aimed to update on recent information about CNS vasculitis-related immunological mechanisms and their most common neurological complications, diagnosis, and management.

9.1.1   Large Vessel Vasculitis

9.1.1.1   Temporal Arteritis

Temporal arteritis (TA), otherwise known as giant cell arteritis, affects the temporal artery of middle-aged or elderly patients [3]. Notwithstanding its name, giant cells are not a requirement for diagnosis; histopathological findings are consistent with diffuse vascular involvement.

In TA, vasculitis is essentially a T-cell-driven process that is triggered by infectious agents. Dendritic cells present in the adventitia of vessels play the role of antigen-presenting cells (APCs) by activating CD4$^+$ T cells, such as T helper 1 (Th1) and Th17. In the next step, Th1 cells provoke vascular injury by recruiting macrophages and monocytes into the vessel niche. There is also release of cytokines – interleukin (IL)-1, IL-6, IL-17, and interferon-γ. Sustained inflammation mediated by these cells leads to extensive intimal thickening and vessel occlusion [4]. Platelet-derived growth factor and vascular endothelial growth factor take part in occlusion of the internal carotid artery lumen-occlusive arteritis in TA.

Apart from the carotid artery, this occlusive arteritis commonly involves the temporal arteries. The most common and serious complication of TA is that of unilateral or bilateral loss of vision due to ischemic optic neuropathy with an overall incidence between 6 and 70% [5]. Fundoscopic findings consist of slight pallor and edema of the optic disc, with scattered cotton-wool patches and small hemorrhages. Both visual loss and cerebral infarction have premonitory symptoms such as amaurosis fugax, diplopia, eye pain, and jaw claudication. CNS events secondary to the vertebrobasilar system involvement include ataxia, lateral medullary syndrome, hemianopsia, and hearing loss [6].

Polymyalgia rheumatica coexists in 40% of patients with temporal arteritis. Given the significant risk of vision loss, glucocorticoids should be started with no delay. However, glucocorticoids diminish T_H17 cells but cannot clear T_H1 cells from the vascular lesions. Cyclophosphamide (CYC) may effectively target IFN-γ-positive T cells representing a useful option for patients requiring prolonged medium- to high-dose GC therapy [7]. A randomized controlled trial of 44 patients showed that maintenance therapy with infliximab failed to show more efficacy in disease control than that of steroids, and it did not allow a reduction in the dose of steroids required to prevent relapse [7]. A dramatic response to low-dose corticosteroids remains a valuable tool in patients with uncertain diagnosis. Blood tests reveal lymphocytosis and an increased erythrocyte sedimentation rate, while temporal artery biopsy confirms the presence of inflammation and giant cells. IL-1 and IL-6 stimulate acute-phase protein production by hepatocytes. However, the challenge lies in recognizing atypical cases that lack the more specific manifestations. We conclude that the diagnosis of giant cell arteritis should always be considered in elderly patients with an unexplained elevation of inflammatory markers and other neglected symptoms, such as trismus, facial edema, and chronic dry cough, to avoid severe complications.

9.1.1.2 Takayasu Disease

Takayasu disease is a granulomatous vasculitis causing stenosis and aneurysmal dilatation of large arteries, such as the aorta and its major branches, in patients <40 years [8]. The pathogenesis is still unknown, but there is evidence of genetical predisposition (HLA-B52, B39). Cell-mediated immunity involves CD4+ (14% of total cells) and CD8+ (15%) T lymphocytes displaying T-cell receptor $\alpha\beta$, CD14+ macrophages (13%), CD16+ natural killer cells (20%), and CD4- and CD8- T lymphocytes displaying T-cell receptor $\gamma\delta$ (31%). Seko et al. showed an increased expression of perforin in peripheral cytoplasmic granules of natural killer cells, CD8+, and $\gamma\delta$ T lymphocytes, infiltrating cells directly onto the surface of aortic vascular cells [9]. These results suggest that perforin-mediated necrosis but not Fas/ Fas-L apoptosis may play a major role in immunopathology of vascular injury in Takayasu's arteritis.

Neurological dysfunction may be the initial manifestation, but more often, it occurs later in the disease course. Headache and dizziness are the most prevalent symptoms related to stealing phenomena due to steno-occlusive lesions. Ischemic optic neuropathy, other isolated cranial nerve palsies, and stroke have been reported due to involvement of the internal carotid artery or its branches. However, angiographic findings confirming this hypothesis have not ever been reported. Therefore, stroke might be related to carotid or vertebral arteries occlusion or to embolization into intracranial vessels, rather than to direct involvement of intracranial vessels by vasculitis. Also notable is the absence of large epidemiologic data for the incidence of strokes.

Despite the fact that no prospective controlled study has been conducted to date, antitumor necrosis factor alpha could be a good therapeutic option in Takayasu's arteritis, which was unable to achieve or maintain remission with steroids alone or cyclophosphamide or low-dose methotrexate. Recently, in rheumatic patients on TNF-α blocking agents, no response to this treatment was noted, which suggests the presence of different pathogenic mechanisms [8].

9.1.2 Medium Vessel Vasculitis

9.1.2.1 Polyarteritis Nodosa (PAN)

PAN is a primary necrotizing systemic vasculitis of medium vessels. Unlike some other vasculitides (e.g., microscopic polyarteritis, granulomatosis with polyangiitis [Wegener's]), polyarteritis nodosa is not associated with antineutrophil cytoplasmic antibodies (ANCA). In idiopathic PAN, the role of immune complexes is unclear. Vascular inflammation from HBV has been associated with immune-complex deposition. However, the presence of CD4+ in vascular lesions suggests a T-cell-mediated immunity. In addition, there is evidence of endothelial dysfunction resulting from an increase in inflammatory cytokines and adhesion molecules (intercellular adhesion molecule 1, vascular cell adhesion molecule 1, and E-selectin) [10]. The inflammatory lesions are often found at the bifurcation of vessels, as result of increased adhesion molecules deposits. Neurological manifestations are very common in PAN due to systemic necrotizing vasculitis that causes ischemia, leading to microaneurysms, thrombosis, or bleeding [1, 2, 9, 11, 12]. CNS involvement occurs relatively late in the course of the disease that may be accompanied by systemic symptoms and signs, e.g., fever, malaise, myalgias, and wasting syndrome. Patients with PAN typically demonstrate CNS neurological signs, such as personality and memory disorders, atypical persistent headaches, aphasia, hemiplegia, visual disturbance (blurred vision and hemianopia), seizures, transverse myelitis, and subarachnoid hemorrhage. Elevations in the serum levels of INF-γ and IL-2 and increased serum levels of IL-8, a potent chemoattractant and activator of neutrophils, have been found in these patients.

Corticosteroids (1 mg/kg/day) affect T-cell-mediated inflammation by the inhibition of cytokine production [10]. However, relapses are frequent in severe cases, with neurological, renal, or cardiac manifestations. Cyclophosphamide plus corticosteroids (CYC) could change to a better outcome [10, 13]. Twelve CYC pulses have been shown to be superior to six pulses in preventing relapses, although mortality rates were similar in both of them. Other immunosuppressive agents of T-cell responses such as azathioprine or methotrexate may also maintain remission.

9.1.3   Small Vessel Vasculitis

9.1.3.1   Allergic Granulomatosis (Churg–Strauss Syndrome (CSS))

CSS is an ANCA-associated systemic vasculitis occurring in patients with asthma and eosinophilia, according to the 1990 criteria, from the American College of Rheumatology [14].

CSS is a multifactorial, immune-mediated disorder triggered by exposure to allergens, with strong genetic background (HLA-DRB4). Th2 responses are prominent, with upregulation of IL-4, IL-13, and IL-5; tissue recruitment of Th2 cells is mediated by specific chemokines CCL17, most likely produced by dendritic cells. CCL17 serum levels strongly correlate with peripheral eosinophil counts. The strong Th2 immune response precipitates a B-cell response resulting in IgG4, IgE, and antineutrophil cytoplasmic antibody (ANCA) production. Increased secretion of eotaxin-3 guides eosinophils to the endothelium. Eosinophils induce an activated Th2 imbalance toward IL-25 production, thereby maintaining a vicious circle. Local degranulation of activated eosinophils finally causes damage, necrosis, and fibrosis to various tissues. In particular, myocardial injury is caused by eosinophilic cytotoxicity with marked endomyocardial fibrosis, lymphocytic infiltration, and eosinophilia. However, clinical phenotype cannot be explained only by Th2 response. Th1 and Th17 cells secrete high amounts of IL-17A resulting in extravascular eosinophilic granulomas, as the histopathological hallmark [15].

The neurological findings in allergic granulomatosis are caused by systemic necrotizing vasculitis, with eosinophil infiltrate affecting small vessels. CNS events are rare and resemble nodular polyarteritis [1, 16]. CNS involvement may include paralysis of seventh cranial nerve and phrenic nerve palsy, seizures, psychosis, and coma, but these events are much less typical. Cerebrovascular events have been reported in association with cerebral angiitis and infarcts in the subcortical white matter.

Given its ability to halt eosinophil degranulation, INF-a has been used alone or in combination with plasma exchange, CYC. Because of the potential side effects of CYC, other biologic agents such as the anti-IL-5 monoclonal antibody mepolizumab and possibly rituximab are promising treatment options. Of note, rituximab reduced eosinophil and IL-5 levels. This finding ,may suggest that B-cell depletion strongly influences T-cell function [15].

9.1.3.2 Polyangiitis Granulomatosa (Wegener Granulomatosis (WG))

WG is a systemic multi-organ disease characterized by immune small-vessel vasculitis and the presence of ANCAs. Both genetic and nongenetic factors are implicated in exposing cytoplasmic proteins in the neutrophil (e.g., proteinase 3 and lysosome-associated membrane protein 2), following likely interaction with T and B lymphocytes. Autoantibodies may also be generated to an epitope that is complementary to the autoantigen, such as antisense proteinase 3, or by molecular mimicry, such as the bacterial adhesion molecule FimH. ANCA-induced neutrophil activation also activates the alternative complement pathway. In addition to complement-mediated microvascular injury, ANCA also mediates endothelial damage by enhancing neutrophil–endothelial cell interactions and increasing neutrophil degranulation of cytotoxic agents and chemoattractants [17]. Neutrophilic microabscesses dominate the early phase of the "granuloma," a mixed infiltrate of multinucleated giant cells, neutrophils, and dendritic cells (Fig. 9.1).

Based on the 1994 Chapel Hill Consensus, the diagnosis of vasculitis requires a positive biopsy of granuloma of the involved organ [18]. Approximately 50% of patients with WG has neurological complications caused by necrotizing granulomatous lesions of small vessels [1, 2, 11, 12, 17]. CNS involvement depends on the presence of vasculitis, contiguous extension, or remote granulomatous spread. Granulomas cause basilar meningitis, temporal lobe dysfunction, and venous sinus occlusion [19]. Of 324))patients with WG described by Nishino and colleagues in 1993, 90 (28%) had cranial neuropathy in 6%, external ophthalmoplegia in 5%, cerebrovascular events in 4%, seizures in 3%, cerebritis in 2%, and miscellaneous events in 8%. Of note, necrotizing vasculitis ,of the coronary vessels can result in myocardial infarction or sudden death.

A rationale for B-cell-targeted therapy has emerged from the presence of B cells at sites of inflammation. Thus, cyclophosphamide, as B-cell-specific immunosuppressant agent, could be an effective option. Given their ability for B-cell depletion, rituximab and infliximab are effective in refractory disease [17, 20]. Thirty-three patients with active disease were enrolled in an open prospective trial that reviewed adding infliximab to standard therapy, aiming to achieve remission within a mean follow-up period of 12 months [21]. No benefit was demonstrated with the use of antitumor necrosis factor alpha agents. Current treatment strategies have substantial short-term and long-term adverse effects, and relapses are frequent; thus, less-toxic and more-effective approaches are needed.

9.1.4   Variable Vessel Vasculitis

9.1.4.1   Behçet Syndrome

This multisystem disorder of unknown, etiology predominantly affects men with oral and genital ulceration and uveitis, based on the International Criteria for Behçet Disease [22]. The histology reveals vasculitis of small vessels and perivascular deposition of inflammatory cells in the meninges of nervous system.

However, immunopathogenesis ,still remains enigmatic. There is robust evidence of infectious agents in predisposed genetical people, but no concrete proof of how these factors initiate the immunological response. IL-12 and IL-18 are produced by APCs toward an immune response Th1. Additionally, enhanced production of IFN-c, TNF-a, IL-8, IL-17, and IL-18 either by APCs or hypersensitivity of T cells might lead to neutrophil hyperactivity. Neutrophils secrete other cytokines which contribute further to Th1 polarization [23].

CNS involvement, so-called neuro-Behçet syndrome (NB), includes parenchymal forms, acute meningoencephalitis and nonparenchymal (dural sinus thrombosis or vena cava syndrome with intracranial hypertension), venous (papilledema, headache, focal neurological defects, seizures, nerve palsies, and altered consciousness), and artery thrombosis (intracerebral or infarcts) [24]. By contrast, chronic progressive NB is characterized by intractable slowly progressive dementia, ataxia, and dysarthria, with persistent elevation of cerebrospinal fluid (CSF) interleukin 6 (IL-6) activity (more than 20 pg/mL). CSF IL-1, IL-6, IL-8, TNF-α, and IFN-γ may reflect a nonspecific inflammatory pattern. Furthermore, the target for IL-33 in NBD is another key, unanswered question that requires histological studies, as both microglia and astrocytes express IL-33 receptors. Cerebellar symptoms at the onset of the disease, a rapidly progressive course, and the presence of elevated protein levels and pleocytosis in the CSF were negative prognostic factors, whereas initial presentation with headache was associated with favorable outcome [24].

Chronic progressive NB is resistant to conventional treatment with steroids, cyclophosphamide, or azathioprine. Recent studies have reported on the efficacy of low-dose methotrexate in chronic progressive NB [25]. Nevertheless, symptomatic management is limited to intravenous high-dose methylprednisolone, followed by a prolonged oral taper. On the other hand, preventive treatment includes azathioprine, cyclophosphamide, INF-alpha, and anti-TNF-a agents for long term, although there is no evidence in multicenter studies ,about their efficacy [26, 27]. Both TNF-a inhibitors and tocilizumab (humanized anti-IL-6R monoclonal antibody) were effective in patients with active NB who fail glucocorticoids alone.

9.1.5   Single-Organ Vasculitis

9.1.5.1   Primary Angiitis of the Central Nervous System

Primary angiitis of the CNS (PACNS) is a rare inflammatory disorder that may involve both small- and medium-sized arteries and veins such as leptomeningeal, cortical, and subcortical [28]. The pathogenesis of PACNS is unknown. Similar to other autoimmune diseases, certain viruses (Epstein-Barr virus, varicella-zoster virus, human immunodeficiency virus) have been reported as triggers for vasculitic lesions.

Th1 cytokines contribute to granulomatous vascular lesions in humans. Intracerebral injections of interferon-gamma have been shown to trigger inflammatory lesions and vasculitis in rats. TNF and IL-6 proinflammatory functions may also play a role in vascular inflammation in PACNS. TNF/TNF receptor p75 transgenic mice develop multifocal CNS ischemic injury secondary to vasculitis [29].

Diagnostic criteria include newly acquired neurological deficits, unexplained by another CNS)or systemic process, in the presence of a highly suggestive angiogram and/or biopsy. The histological findings of PACNS comprise granulomatous inflammation, fibrinoid necrosis of vessel walls, or exclusively lymphocytic cell infiltrates. CNS nonspecific symptoms include migraine seizures, ataxia, and cognitive dysfunction [28]. Reversible cerebral vasoconstriction syndrome is a main condition that mimics PACNS, with recurrent thunderclap headache, with or without neurological deficit, and normal CSF analysis findings. Magnetic resonance angiography shows reversible diffuse segmental vasospasm of intracranial vessels [28].

Since our understanding of the pathophysiology of PACNS is poor, little progress has been made in management of affected patients. In the largest reported series (Mayo Clinic cohort), combination of steroids and pulse cyclophosphamide has a favorable effect than steroids alone (frequent relapses) [30]. In the French cohort study, 32 of 52 (61.5%) patients responded to treatment with improved modified Rankin scale scores for disability [31]. Azathioprine was the most frequently used maintenance therapy; the higher mortality observed in the Mayo Clinic cohort seems less likely related to the type of therapy used and more likely because of case selection. A better outcome in patients with lymphocytic vasculitis that represented the prevalent histopathologic pattern in the French cohort may also partially explain this difference.)

9.1.6   Vasculitides Secondary to Connective Tissue Diseases

9.1.6.1   Rheumatoid Arthritis (RA)

RA is a chronic autoimmune inflammatory disorder with multisystemic complications. Antigen-presenting cells, including dendritic cells, macrophages, and activated B cells, present arthritis-associated antigens to T cells. CD4+ T cells secrete proinflammatory (IL)-1β or TNF, which are able to excite or lower thresholds of afferent nociceptive and afferent vagal nerve fibers. In this way, these cytokines seems to play a role in communication from immune system to central nervous system. Release of TNF-a, IL-6, and IL-1 from synovial tissue alters the function of distant tissues, including adipose tissue, skeletal muscle, and the vascular endothelium [32]. Elevated IL-6 plasma concentrations are associated with potentially detrimental cardiovascular consequences.

CNS involvement is uncommon in RA and presents vasculitis-like symptoms, such as stroke, seizures, and meningitis (probably due to vasculitis and damage resulting from the pressure applied by rheumatoid nodules) [1, 3, 33, 34]. Cervical spinal instability results in ligament laxity and bone erosion due to synovitis. Since neurological deficits are observed in only 7–34% of cases, many patients with pain and radiographic criteria for instability do not develop neurological sequelae. However, 10% of patients die due to brainstem compression [35].

The concept of a TNF-dependent proinflammatory cytokine cascade resolved the dilemma of which cytokine was a potential therapeutic target [32]. However, TNF antagonists are accompanied with a risk of severe adverse effects (lymphoma, heart failure, multiple sclerosis) [36]. Other therapies including IL-1 and IL-6, in addition to T- and B-cell inhibitors or in combination with MTX, have been effective in patients with RA. Nevertheless, it is unclear the mechanism by which inflammation is actually reduced. On the other hand, morbidity and mortality rates remain high, despite aggressive treatment with cyclophosphamide or biologic agents.

9.1.6.2 Systemic Lupus Erythematosus (SLE)

SLE is a heterogeneous autoimmune disease characterized by multisystemic microvasculopathy that follows a remitting—relapsing course [37]. Neuropsychiatric SLE (NPSLE) compromises a wide range of clinical manifestations affecting the CNS (from 33 to 75%) such as psychoses, seizures, headaches, cognitive dysfunction, chorea, and stroke [38, 39]. So far, the pathogenic mechanisms underlying these CNS symptoms are not well defined. Serum or CSF titers of aPL antibodies, particularly lupus anticoagulant, anticardiolipin, and anti-β2GP1 antibodies, are by far the most widely investigated autoantibodies in NPSLE. However, a meta-analysis showed that their diagnostic value is not enough for differentiating various disease phenotypes (such as psychosis, mood disorder, and other diffuse or focal manifestations).

The hallmark of pathogenesis of SLE includes loss of immune tolerance and production of autoantibodies and immune complexes leading to systemic inflammation and atherosclerosis. The pathogenic responses in NPSLE and cardiovascular disease (CVD) share some characteristics, such as impaired clearance of apoptotic cells, skewed T- and B-cell activation, and LDL oxidation. Vascular occlusion, tissue, and neuronal damage mediated by autoantibodies and proinflammatory cytokines (IL-1, IL-6, IL-8, IL-17, tumor necrosis factor [TNF], colony-stimulating and macrophage-stimulating factors), as well as direct neuronal cell death, are implicated in both SLE and related CVD. One other common feature among patients with SLE and CVD is a continuous activation of the type I interferon (IFN) system, which manifests as increased serum levels of IFN-α and/or an increased expression of type I IFN-induced genes has been defined as type I IFN signature. This type I IFNs can be involved in the accelerated CVD observed in SLE, as these IFNs enhance macrophage migration and foam cell formation [40].

Many studies have examined autoantibodies against phospholipids, ribosomal P peptides, glial fibrillary acidic protein (GFAP), the NMDA receptor, microtubule-associated protein 2 (MAP-2), and matrix metalloproteinase 9 (MMP-9) as potential biomarkers of endothelial dysfunction, thrombosis, and vascular damage [41]. Larger studies should further elucidate the pathogenic mechanisms underlying NPSLE and correlate these mechanisms with specific NPSLE phenotypes.

To date, new drugs have not been studied in patients with severe active NPSLE involving the CNS. Limited data for NPSLE include antibody therapies targeting BAFF or other B-cell markers, such as CD22 (epratuzumab) and CD20 (rituximab); IL-6, IFN-α, IFN-α receptor, and TWEAK; mediators of lymphocyte activation (abatacept, a CTLA-4-Ig fusion protein that binds to CD80 and CD86); and non-antibody agents, such as the T-cell-modulator peptide P140. There is also very low-quality evidence that cyclophosphamide is more effective in reducing symptoms of neuropsychiatric involvement in SLE compared with methylprednisolone [41].

9.1.6.3   Systemic Sclerosis (SSc)

SSc is characterized by widespread microvasculopathy and diffuse tissue fibrosis affecting the skin and other systemic organs, particularly the heart, CNS, lungs, and gastrointestinal tract.

The exact immunological mechanisms are still unexplained. Most data support a role for pathogenic T cells from tissues undergoing fibrosis in SSc by outlining the preferential production of IL-4, a Th2 cytokine [42]. Accordingly, increased levels of the Th2-cell-derived cytokines IL-4, IL-10, IL-13, and IL-17 were observed in SSc. IL-4 and TGF- are crucial fibrogenic cytokines in SSc. IL-4 increases collagen production in fibroblasts in patients with SSc and induces the production of TGF-. TGF- stimulates the synthesis of various collagens, proteoglycans, and fibronectin and inhibits extracellular matrix degradation by decreasing the synthesis of matrix metalloproteinases (MMP) and by increasing the synthesis of the tissue inhibitor of MMP. IL-17, a T-cell cytokine that can be produced by both Th1 and Th2 cells, and B cells are activated in SSc, as indicated by hypergammaglobulinemia, the presence of autoantibodies, the overexpression of the B-cell transduction molecule CD19 in peripheral blood, expanded naive B cells, and activated, but diminished, memory B cells [42]. Furthermore, in animal models of fibrosis, deficiency of CD19 suggests that B cells may also contribute to fibrosis. In particular, myocardial involvement has been associated with repeated focal ischemia leading to myocardial fibrosis with irreversible lesions [43]. Activated B cells are known to produce IL-6 and

IL-10, and both these may promote a predominant Th2 immune response that induces collagen synthesis. The production of IL-6, as well as TGF- by activated B cells, may also induce directly tissue fibrosis in SSc.

Previously considered a rare event, neurological complications in systemic sclerosis have been increasingly recognized [1, 43]. In a recent review of 180 studies, CNS involvement in systemic sclerosis was characterized by headache (23.73%), seizures (13.56%), and cognitive impairment (8.47%). Depression and anxiety were frequently observed (73.15 and 23.95%, respectively) [44].

As immunological activity in SSc is considered to be a key stimulus to vascular abnormalities and fibrosis, novel therapies (i.e. autologous stem cell transplantation, tolerance to type I collagen) may be promising agents. Corticosteroids and cyclophosphamide may be effective [44].

9.1.6.4 Sjögren's Syndrome

SS is a chronic inflammatory disorder characterized by both organ-specific and multisystem organ involvement. An environmental trigger (e.g., coxsackieviruses) leads to disturbed antigen clearance and/or neoantigen presentation based upon a genetic background (HLA A1, B8, DR3, DQ2 haplotype). SS is characterized by T-cell (CD4+) infiltration and destruction of salivary and lacrimal glands leading to loss of tears (keratoconjunctivitis sicca) and saliva (xerostomia). Multiple proinflammatory cytokines, such as TNF-a, IL-1b, and IL-6, have been implicated. B-cell-activating factor (BAF) is another trigger of B-cell hyperactivation and (auto) antibody production. Activation or apoptosis of glandular epithelial cells in genetically predisposed individuals drives to activation of T-cell-dependent autoimmune response [45].

Neurological manifestations may precede the sicca symptoms in 40–93% of the cases. CNS complications observed in 15% of patients include trigeminal neuralgia, stroke, hemorrhage, seizures, aseptic meningoencephalitis, and transverse myelitis; [46] however, the spectrum of neurological complication is not well defined. The vascular injury may be related to the presence of antineuronal antibodies and anti-Ro antibodies [2]. Additionally, SS with CNS disease may mimic MS, suggesting other mechanisms rather than vasculopathy [1, 2]. It was recently observed that antibodies against the type III muscarinic receptor may eventually explain part of the broader autonomic dysfunction found in patients with SS [47].

Clinical improvement has seen with intravenous immunoglobulin therapy and anti- TNF alpha. Anti-CD20 treatment with rituximab exhibited benefit in both pSS and its malignant complication, mucosa-associated lymphoid tissue type lymphoma, although two pSS patients developed severe serum sickness [45]. Because BAFF/BlyS is significantly elevated, treatment with anti-BLyS monoclonal antibody could be a plausible strategy in pSS. Another choice such as organ-targeted gene transfer is in progress.

References

1. Riggs JE. Neurological consequences of systemic disease. In: Bradley W, Daroff R, Fenichel G, Marsden D, editors. Neurology in clinical practice. Boston: Butterworth-Heinemann; 1991. p. 841–60.
2. Jennette JC, Falk RJ, Bacon PA, Basu N, Cid MC, Ferrario F, et al. 2012 revised International Chapel Hill Consensus conference nomenclature of vasculitides. Arthritis Rheum. 2013;65:1–11.
3. Salvarani C, Cantini F, Boiardi L, Hunder GG. Polymyalgia rheumatica and giant-cell arteritis. N Engl J Med. 2002;347:261–71.
4. Weyand C, Joyce Liao Y, Goronzy JJ. The immunopathology of giant cell arteritis: diagnostic and therapeutic implications. J Neuroophthalmol. 2012;32(3):259–65.
5. Nesher G. Neurologic manifestations of giant cell arteritis. Clin Exp Rheumatol. 2000;4(Suppl 20):S24–6.
6. Hoffman GS, Cid MC, Rendt-Zagar KE, Merkel PA, Weyand CM, Stone JH, et al. Infliximab-GCA study group. Infliximab for maintenance of glucocorticosteroid-induced remission of giant cell arteritis: a randomized trial. Ann Intern Med. 2007;146(9):621–30.
7. Pfadenhauer K, Roesler A, Golling A. The involvement of the peripheral nervous system in biopsy proven active giant cell arteritis. J Neurol. 2007;254(6):751–5.
8. Vishwanath S, Relan M, Shen L, Ambrus JL Jr. Update on the use of biologics in vasculitides. Curr Pharm Biotechnol. 2014;15(6):558–62.
9. Seko Y, Takahashi N, Tada Y, Yaqida H, Okumura K, Naqai R. Restricted usage of T-cell receptor Vγ-Vδ genes and expression of co-stimulatory molecules in Takayasu's arteritis. Int J Cardiol. 2000;75:S77–83.
10. Forbess L, Bannykh S. Polyarteritis nodosa. Rheum Dis Clin N Am. 2015;41(1):33–46.
11. Chalk C, Dyck J, Conn D. Vasculitic neuropathy. In: Thomas PK, Dyck PJ, editors. Peripheral neuropathy. Philadelphia: Saunders; 1993. p. 1424–143.
12. Midroni G, Bilbao J. Vasculitic neuropathy. In: Midroni G, Bilbao J, editors. Biopsy diagnosis of peripheral neuropathy, vol. 1995. Boston: Butterworth-Heinemann; 1995. p. 241–62.
13. Younger DS. Vasculitis of the nervous system. Curr Opin Neurol. 2004;17(3):317–36.
14. Masi AT, Hunder GG, Lie JT, Michel BA, Bloch DA, Arend WP, et al. The American College of Rheumatology 1990 criteria for the classification of Churg-Strauss syndrome (allergic granulomatosis and angiitis). Arthritis Rheum. 1990;33(8):1094–100.
15. Greco A, Rizzo MI, De Virgilio A, Gallo A, Fusconi M, Ruoppolo G, et al. Churg- Strauss syndrome. Autoimmun Rev. 2015;14(4):341–8.
16. Wolf J, Bergner R, Mutallib S, Buggle F, Grau AJ. Neurologic complications of Churg-Strauss syndrome--a prospective monocentric study. Eur J Neurol. 2010;17(4):582–8.
17. McKinney EF, Willcocks LC, Broecker V, Smith KGC. The immunopatology of ANCA- associated vasculitis. Semin Immunopathol. 2014;36(4):461–78.
18. Leavitt RY, Fauci AS, Bloch DA, Michel BA, Hunder GG, Arend WP, et al. The American College of Rheumatology 1990 criteria for the classification of Wegener's granulomatosis. Arthritis Rheum. 1990;33(8):1101–7.
19. Nishino H, Rubino FA, Parisi JE. The spectrum of neurologic involvement in Wegener's granulomatosis. Neurology. 1993;43(7):1334.
20. de Menthon M, Cohen P, Pagnoux C, Buchler M, Sibilia J, Détrée F, et al. Infliximab or rituximab for refractory Wegener's granulomatosis: long-term follow-up. A prospective randomised multicentre study on 17 patients. Clin Exp Rheumatol. 2011;29(1Suppl 64):S63–71.
21. Morgan MD, Drayson MT, Savage CO, Harper L. Addition of infliximab to standard therapy for ANCA-associated vasculitis. Nephron Clin Pract. 2011;117(2):c89–97.
22. International Team for the Revision of the International Criteria for Behcet's Disease. Revision of the International criteria for Behcet's disease (ICBD). Clin Exp Rheumatol. 2006;42:S14–5.
23. Dinc A, Erdem H, Simsek I, Pay S. Immunopathogenesis of Behcet's disease with special emphasize on the possible role of antigen presenting cells. Rheumatol Int. 2007;27:417–24.
24. Kidd D. Neurological complications of Behçet's syndrome. Curr Neurol Neurosci Rep. 2012;12(6):675–9.

25. Kikuchi H, Aramaki K, Hirohata S. Low dose MTX for progressive neuro-Behçet's disease. A follow-up study for 4 years. Adv Exp Med Biol. 2003;528:575–8.
26. Saip S, Akman-Demir G, Siva A. Neuro-Behçet syndrome. Handb Clin Neurol. 2014;121:1703–23.
27. Kararizou E, Davaki P, Karandreas N, Davou R, Vassilopoulos D. Nonsystemic vasculitic neuropathy: a clinicopathological study of 22 cases. J Rheumatol. 2005;32(5):853–8.
28. Hammad TA, Hajj-Ali RA. Primary angiitis of the central nervous system and reversible cerebral vasoconstriction syndrome. Curr Atheroscler Rep. 2013;15(8):346.
29. Alba MA, Espígol-Frigolé G, Prieto-González S, Tavera-Bahillo I, Martínez AG, Butjosa M, et al. Central nervous system vasculitis: still more questions than answers. Curr Neuropharmacol. 2011;9:437–48.
30. Salvarani C, Brown RD Jr, Christianson TJ, et al. Adult primary central nervous system vasculitis treatment and course: analysis of one hundred sixty-three patients. Arthritis Rheumatol. 2015;67:1637–45.
31. De Boysson H, Zuber M, Naggara O, et al. French Vasculitis Study Group and the French NeuroVascular Society. Primary angiitis of the central nervous system: description of the first fifty-two adults enrolled in the French cohort of patients with primary vasculitis of the central nervous system. Arthritis Rheumatol. 2014;66:1315–26.
32. Choy E. Understanding the dynamics: pathways involved in the pathogenesis of rheumatoid arthritis. Rheumatology. 2012;51(suppl 5):v3–v11.
33. Rosenbaum R. Neuromuscular complications of connective tissue diseases. Muscle Nerve. 2001;24(2):154–69.
34. Caballol Pons N, Montalà N, Valverde J, Brell M, Ferrer I, Martínez-Yélamos S. Isolated cerebral vasculitis associated with rheumatoid arthritis. Joint Bone Spine. 2010;77(4):361–3.
35. da Côrte FC, Neves N. Cervical spine instability in rheumatoid arthritis. Eur J Orthop Surg Traumatol. 2014;24(Suppl 1):S83–91.
36. Matsumoto T, Nakamura I, Miura A, Momoyama G, Ito K. New-onset multiple sclerosis associated with adalimumab treatment in rheumatoid arthritis: a case report and literature review. Clin Rheumatol. 2013;32(2):271–5.
37. Hochberg MC. Updating the American College of Rheumatology revised criteria for the classification of systemic lupus erythematosus. Arthritis Rheum. 1997;40(9):1725.
38. Greenberg BM. The neurologic manifestations of systemic lupus erythematosus. Neurologist. 2009;15(3):115–21.
39. Streifler JY, Molad Y. Connective tissue disorders: systemic lupus erythematosus, Sjögren's syndrome, and scleroderma. Handb Clin Neurol. 2014;119:463–73.
40. Wigren M, Nilsson J, Kaplan MJ. Pathogenic immunity in systemic lupus erythematosus and atherosclerosis: common mechanisms and possible targets for intervention. J Intern Med. 2015;278:494–506.
41. Jeltsch-David H, Muller S. Neuropsychiatric systemic lupus erythematosus: pathogenesis and biomarkers. Nat Rev Neurol. 2014;10(10):579–96.
42. Zuber JP, Spertini F. Immunological basis of systemic sclerosis. Rheumatology. 2006;45(suppl 3):iii23–5.
43. Allanore Y, Kahan A. Primary myocardial involvement in systemic sclerosis. Rheumatology. 2006;45:iv14–7.
44. Amaral TN, Peres FA, Lapa AT, Marques-Neto JF, Appenzeller S. Neurologic involvement in scleroderma: a systematic review. Semin Arthritis Rheum. 2013;43(3):335–47.
45. Agarwal P. Immunopathogenesis of Sjögren's syndrome. J Indian Rheumatol Assoc. 2003;11:71–5.
46. Gono T, Kawaguchi Y, Katsumata Y, Takagi K, Tochimoto A, Baba S, et al. Clinical manifestations of neurological involvement in primary Sjögren's syndrome. Clin Rheumatol. 2011;30(4):485–90.
47. Park K, Haberberger RV, Gordon TP, Jackson MW. Antibodies interfering with the type 3 muscarinic receptor pathway inhibit gastrointestinal motility and cholinergic neurotransmission in Sjögren's syndrome. Arthritis Rheum. 2011;63(5):1426–34.

Chapter 10
Cardiac Autoimmunity: Myocarditis

William Bracamonte-Baran and Daniela Čiháková

10.1 Myocarditis

Development of autoimmune diseases is a consequence of lack of self-tolerance, which can arise due to defective function of any of the features contributing to the unresponsive status of the immune system toward self-antigens, i.e., anergy, regulation, and clonal deletion [1, 2]. Autoimmunity requires a self-specific response, despite the fact that innate response might be involved. That is the main difference with the rare autoinflammatory diseases, in which an uncontrolled but unspecific response occurs, with minimal involvement of the adaptive response [3].

Myocarditis can be defined as the inflammatory process affecting the muscular tissues of the heart (myocardium). Myocarditis is considered an important cause of sudden death as has been shown by autopsy-based studies in the general population [4–7]. Regardless of its etiology, the acute inflammation may progress to subacute and chronic stages and finally to tissue remodeling, fibrosis, and loss of myocardium architecture and contractile function [4, 6, 8]. The latter chronic damage corresponds to development of dilated cardiomyopathy (DCM). Its overall incidence among myocarditis cases is not accurately known, but retrospective studies report that 9–16% of unexplained nonischemic DCM cases have histological evidence of myocarditis, thus suggesting a persistent/self-sustained autoimmune inflammatory progression as a requirement [4, 7, 9, 10]. Other studies

W. Bracamonte-Baran
Department of Pathology, Division of Immunology, Johns Hopkins University School of Medicine, 720 Rutland Ave., Baltimore, MD 21205, USA

D. Čiháková (✉)
Division of Immunology, Department of Pathology, Johns Hopkins University School of Medicine, 720 Rutland Ave., Baltimore, MD 21205, USA

W. Harry Feinstone Department of Molecular Microbiology and Immunology, Johns Hopkins University Bloomberg School of Public Health, Baltimore, MD 21205, USA
e-mail: dcihako1@jhmi.edu

© Springer International Publishing AG 2017
S. Sattler, T. Kennedy-Lydon (eds.), *The Immunology of Cardiovascular Homeostasis and Pathology*, Advances in Experimental Medicine and Biology 1003, DOI 10.1007/978-3-319-57613-8_10

estimate a wider range of 10–50% of DCM cases having evidence of myocarditis as could be determined by endomyocardial biopsy [11].

Thus, DCM is the most severe complication of myocarditis. DCM implies the dilatation of heart chambers leading to impairment of systolic function [5, 12]. The consequence of such systolic dysfunction is heart failure, for which the only definitive treatment is transplantation, since the fiber damage and fibrosis are, so far, irreversible processes [4, 5, 9]. Other complications might occur as consequence of tissue damage, like valve insufficiency due to rupture of papillary muscles, arrhythmias due to damage of conduction system, reentry phenomenon associated with myocardial fibrosis, and adrenergic stimulation by autoantibodies [4, 5].

10.1.1 Epidemiology

Myocarditis is a disease with an extreme wide range of clinical presentations, from asymptomatic to life-threatening, importantly including sudden death. This fact, in conjunction to the lack of noninvasive highly specific diagnostic methods and its overlapping symptoms with other more prevalent/incident cardiovascular diseases, makes it an underdiagnosed entity [8]. Myocarditis is the cause of sudden death in around 10% of cases [7, 13]. Important efforts had been made to develop noninvasive imaging diagnostic methods. Cardiac magnetic resonance (CMR) has been proposed as a reliable approach based on magnetic relaxation times suggesting regional myocardial edema and fluid leak. Lake Louise criteria seem to be an accurate diagnostic method based on evidence of myocardial edema on T2-weighted images plus capillary leak in T1 [4, 14–16].

Consequence of such diagnostic conundrum, retrospective studies based on autopsies have reported an extremely wide range of association of myocarditis with sudden death, from 2 to 42% [17, 18]. Importantly all of them are relatively small studies with lack of multicentric approach, thus probably biased by environmental and genetic factors.

On the other hand, prospective studies analyzing progression of myocarditis diagnosed by gold-standard biopsy parameters, an ideal clinical-epidemiologic design, report a consistent progression of myocarditis to DCM of about 30% [5, 19–21]. Post-myocarditis DCM patients have a poor prognosis, and when American Heart Association (AHA) heart failure functional classes III–IV are reached, only heart transplantation provides a definitive resolution [5].

Viral myocarditis is thought to be the most frequent type, mostly affecting children and young adults. Studies report that 60% of children diagnosed with acute myocarditis have a transplant-free survival of 10 years [21]. Also, 25–40% of DCM patients have viral genome detected in the endomyocardial biopsy [22].

10.1.2 Clinical Presentation

The presentation of acute myocarditis is extremely variable and frequently subclinical. Acute myocarditis can either lead to acute complications or progress relatively asymptomatically to chronic heart failure, then debuting clinically with chronic late-stage complications like heart failure due to DCM. As a consequence, a high level of suspicion is required by the clinician for deciding to rule out myocarditis with specific tests. The gold standard for myocarditis diagnosis is still a positive endomyocardial biopsy, an invasive procedure which requires a high clinical pretest likelihood and low risk/benefit ratio to be performed [10]. The main clinical presentation features of myocarditis are:

10.1.2.1 Acute Coronary Syndrome-Like Symptoms

Considering the overwhelmingly higher incidence of "real" acute coronary syndrome (ACS, consequence of coronary artery disease or vasculopathy) as compared with myocarditis, this is probably the presentation needing higher clinical suspicion index. In that regard, consideration of classic risk factors for ACS like age, sex, family history, and metabolic disturbances is of extreme importance in clinical care. Angiographic studies lacking evidence of coronary atherosclerosis or vasculopathy, the latter typical of transplant chronic allorejection, strongly suggest myocarditis rather than ACS [10, 23]. Functional cardiac tests (echocardiography and cardiac magnetic resonance (CMR)) or indexes of myocardial damage (like cardiac troponin T or I, cTnT or cTnI) may show results equivalent to ACS, as unspecifically reflect cardiac tissue injury. Even more important is the fact that electrocardiogram (EKG), the first-line diagnostic test for ACS in clinical practice, may show similar findings in myocarditis as compared with ACS, mainly ST segment elevation/depression and T-wave inversion. Inflammation-associated coronary vasospasm had been identified as one of the main mechanisms leading to ACS-like symptoms in myocarditis, thus also involving transient ischemia [24].

10.1.2.2 New Onset or Worsening of Heart Failure Symptoms in the Absence of Coronary Artery Disease (CAD) or Other Typical Causes

In this regard, it must be considered that CAD, long-term high blood pressure and metabolic disturbances (like Diabetes Mellitus, which turns out to be pathophysiologically related to CAD and high blood pressure) are epidemiologically the main factor predisposing to heart failure. Acute decompensation of heart failure functional status without paralleling changes in underlying disease or, even more, the unexplained new onset of heart failure signs must lead to rule out myocarditis of any etiology [4–6].

10.1.2.3 Chronic and Persistent Symptoms Compatible with Heart Failure, but Not Implying Acute Worsening nor Typical Risk Factors

Patients with stable symptoms of heart failure as the ones enounced above, but lacking typical risk factors, must be considered potential myocarditis patients, despite the absence of acute signs of worsening or previous history/symptoms of acute myocarditis [4].

10.1.2.4 Acute Life-Threatening Cardiac Conditions

This category includes arrhythmias, aborted sudden death, and cardiogenic shock [6]. Evidently, in these cases, the priority is the resolution of the acute event, but afterward proper studies are needed to rule out myocarditis.

10.1.3 Histopathology

Myocarditis can be classified based on several parameters, mainly histopathology, time progression, and etiology. It is important to consider that once the acute inflammatory phase is surpassed, the long-term fibrosis and loss of myocardial architecture features are usually similar regardless of original type of myocarditis. The Dallas classification was defined in order to standardize the pathology reports and account for the technical issues associated with endomyocardial biopsy sampling process. It is based on conventional staining procedures (hematoxylin-eosin) and not immunohistochemistry. It categorizes myocarditis in (a) myocarditis with/without fibrosis, (b) borderline myocarditis, and (c) no myocarditis (subsequent biopsies should be classified in persistent, healing, or healed myocarditis) [25, 26]. Nevertheless, it is not particularly useful in pathophysiologic and immunologic grounds, and its usefulness has decayed over time [25]. Based on the immunopathology findings, myocarditis is classified in:

10.1.3.1 Acute Lymphocytic Myocarditis

Acute lymphocytic myocarditis is characterized by a predominant myocardial patchy infiltration of T lymphocytes, typically identified in immunohistochemistry [IHC] by CD3 expression, with minimal fibrosis. As expected, areas of lymphocyte infiltration co-localize with CD68+ macrophages. This is the most common pathologic type of myocarditis and is most frequently of viral etiology, mainly Coxsackievirus B and adenoviruses [5, 8].

10.1.3.2 Chronic Lymphocytic Myocarditis (CLM)

CLM is thought to be a chronic stage of acute lymphocytic myocarditis; this entity is pathologically characterized by existence of myocardial fibrosis but still accompanied by leukocyte infiltration. The timing for such progression from acute to chronic inflammation is variable and currently unpredictable. In this case, the areas of fibrosis are consequence of the persistent evolution of the inflammatory processes [4].

10.1.3.3   Giant Cell Myocarditis

Giant cell myocarditis is characterized by unique histological features and particular aggressiveness and capacity to progress to chronic and subacute life-threatening complications like DCM. The prevalence of progression to DCM is considered to be up to 80% [8]. In fact, despite immunosuppressive therapy, two studies have shown that only around 10% of giant cell myocarditis patients survive 4 years without transplantation, compared with 44% of lymphocytic myocarditis [10, 27]. Although other studies reported improved transplant-free survival between 40 and over 70%, some of these studies might have not included the most severe cases with early complications and mortality [28, 29]. Giant cell myocarditis is thought to be a consequence of autoimmunity. That autoimmune origin is also supported by association of giant cell myocarditis with numerous autoimmune diseases and post-transplantation appearance of giant cells in heart grafts [30–35]. Histologically, giant cell myocarditis is characterized also by a prominent leukocyte infiltration. In this case, the inflammatory areas are more extensive, but with myeloid cell (mainly CD68+ macrophages) predominance as compared with T cell infiltration. Interestingly, eosinophils are also often present in the cardiac infiltrate; however, eosinophils are not an independent predictor of mortality [9]. It is important to notice that the murine model of autoimmune myocarditis, experimental autoimmune myocarditis (EAM), resembles the features of this pathologic subtype [8].

10.1.3.4   Sarcoidosis

This is a systemic "idiopathic" disease in the frontier between autoimmunity and autoinflammatory disease, characterized by an antigen presenting cells (APC) dysfunction, generating chronic tissue inflammation and granulomatous lesions in organs like the lung, kidney, and heart. Sarcoidotic myocarditis display extensive infiltration by activated macrophages, leading to chronic inflammation and tissue damage [4, 23].

10.1.3.5   Eosinophilic Myocarditis

This form of myocarditis is observed in entities associated with peripheral eosinophilia (like primary idiopathic hypereosinophilia or chronic eosinophilia due to infectious causes). Eosinophilic myocarditis may also appear as a primary disease, most likely of autoimmune origin. Its landmark is the presence of eosinophils in significant proportions in myocardial infiltrates. This entity, like the giant cell myocarditis, shows also a poor long-term prognosis despite broad immunosuppressive treatment [4, 8, 10]. A murine model of this human type of myocarditis has been developed by our laboratory and will be described later in this chapter [36].

Different etiologic agents might lead to similar histological characteristics. Toxic (drug-induced), viral, radiation-associated, and autoimmune myocarditis might generate acute lymphocytic myocarditis with similar pathologic findings. Similarly, most cases of myocarditis associated with systemic autoimmune diseases (Sjögren's disease, systemic lupus erythematous, vasculitis) also have lymphocytic or giant cells as features [37, 38].

10.1.4 Etiology

Myocarditis is a very broad pathologic definition, as it does not account for the trigger or specific immunologic features involved in the disease. As a consequence, myocarditis can also be classified based on its etiology. Several factors might lead to development of myocarditis, including viral (believed to have the higher incidence and prevalence, being Coxsackievirus B and adenovirus the main causes), physical noxa (radiation), pharmacologic (like anthracyclines, 5-fluorouracil, alcohol, tricyclic antidepressants), hematologic (essentially the eosinophilic myocarditis, either associated with hypereosinophilic conditions or as primary Th2-skewed autoimmune response), and autoimmune, existing mechanistic overlap between those categories as will be described below. Other significantly less frequent infectious causes have been identified: *Mycobacterium* species, *Mycoplasma pneumoniae*, *Cryptococcus* species, and *Trypanosoma cruzi* [6]. It is controversial if HIV itself can trigger the myocardial inflammation or if the myocarditis occurs secondarily to AIDS-related complications like autoimmunity and/or opportunistic infections [39, 40]. Interestingly, the Smallpox Vaccination Program of the Department of Defense (targeting adults) was stopped for significant increase of myocarditis cases close to the vaccination time [41].

Autoimmune myocarditis may occur as an isolated entity, in which the primary (and usually only) targeted organ is the heart. Typically, that is the case of giant cell myocarditis and certain cases of eosinophilic myocarditis not associated with peripheral hypereosinophilia. Also, several systemic autoimmune diseases may affect heart tissues, generating myocarditis in the context of a broader autoimmune phenomenon. The disease most strongly associated with development of myocarditis is systemic lupus erythematosus (SLE), but it might also occur in association with Sjögren's syndrome (SS), vasculitis, and polymyositis [8, 37, 38].

In the enounced cases, autoimmune diseases lead mainly to lymphocytic acute/chronic myocarditis, strongly suggesting a T cell-mediated process. Accessory diagnostic tests are needed to determine the actual etiology/trigger of myocarditis and differentiate viral vs primary autoimmune causes. As myocarditis-associated viruses are epidemiologically common, a positive serology (IgG or IgM) should not be considered enough evidence to establish a viral etiology. Simultaneous evidence of active infection in myocardial tissues along with endomyocardial biopsy proof of myocarditis is the most accurate etiologic diagnosis [5, 6].

It is important to notice that the progression rate of myocarditis to irreversible tissue damage varies depending on the etiology. On the other hand, despite the causes, triggers, and initial immunologic driving forces may be different, the clinical and histological characteristics of DCM stage are similar for all the types and causes of myocarditis [42]. In that regard, it is possible that at certain point of the progression of the myocarditis, several etiologic types confluence in a common autoimmune pathogenic process leading to chronic inflammation, tissue remodeling, fibrosis, muscle fiber damage, systolic dysfunction, and finally DCM [43].

10.2   Murine Models of Myocarditis

Significant efforts have been made to study mechanistically the immunologic features associated with the trigger/initiation, acute phase, and progression of myocarditis to DCM. As with other several pathologies, animal models are extremely important to carry out those types of studies.

10.2.1   EAM and Eosinophilic EAM Models

Experimental autoimmune myocarditis (EAM) murine model was developed allowing to address the immunobiology of acute and chronic myocarditis. EAM has immunologic features paralleling and resembling the human entity, making it suitable to pursue pathophysiologic insights on myocarditis. Importantly, EAM mimics the most severe clinical course of giant cell myocarditis, allowing to study the entire temporal spectrum and progression of the disease to DCM. Another important feature of EAM models is a gender bias resembling the atypical pattern of human autoimmune myocarditis, in such a way that male mice are more susceptible to the induction of heart-specific autoimmunity [44].

EAM can be induced by immunization with cardiac myosin or with a myocarditogenic peptide derived from the α-cardiac myosin heavy chain emulsified in complete Freund's adjuvant (CFA) injected twice in the first 8 days to susceptible mice strains [45, 46]. The mice strain susceptibility to EAM seems to be partially related to MHC haplotypes. The main susceptible strains are cogenic A/J background (A/J H2^a, A.BY H2^b, A.CA H2^f, and A.SW H2^s) and Balb/c (H2^d). Susceptibility of certain C57BL/10 J background strain had also been described (B10.A H2^a, B10.S H2^s, and B10.PL H2^u) [47]. In the section dedicated to viral etiology and influence of HLA haplotypes, further discussion will be made regarding the influence of MHC and non-MHC genes.

In susceptible strains, the self-peptide presentation is mainly IA restricted, altogether pointing out the importance of that specific class II chain, equivalent to human HLA-DQ. Furthermore, as will be described below, transgenic nonobese diabetic mice expressing human HLA-DQ8 instead of IA^b spontaneously develop autoimmune myocarditis.

As might be expected according to the MHC molecular biology, the H2-restricted self-peptides associated with optimal autoimmunization are strain and haplotype-specific, also demonstrating a MHC bias with potential translational implication.

Thus, Balb/c mice are susceptible to immunization with α-myosin heavy chain peptide MyHCα$_{614-629}$, SWXJ to MyHCα$_{406-425}$, and MyHCα$_{1631-1650}$, whereas A/Js are susceptible to MyHCα$_{334-352}$ as well as cTnI$_{105-122}$ [48].

The rationale of the induction process is to elicit a cellular immune response simultaneously with an antigenic challenge with a cardiac-specific self-peptide in order to generate an adaptive self- and myocardium-specific immune response capable to overcome the regulatory mechanisms, thought to be suppressed in human autoimmune diseases. Myocardium-specific inflammatory process occurs peaking at day 21 after first immunization and progressing to late-stage DCM between day 40 and 60 [44, 48]. Cardiac inflammation at the peak of EAM on day 21 is characterized by a significant leukocyte infiltration in the myocardium, including innate cells like neutrophils, eosinophils, monocytes/macrophages, as well as lymphocytes, representing adaptive cellularity. The adaptive T cell-mediated response is the driving force in the development of this inflammatory process [48].

EAM models also employ the use of adjuvants and Toll-like receptor ligands. In the case of the widely studied Balb/c EAM, the protocol includes subcutaneous injection of MyHCα peptide emulsified in complete Freund's adjuvant (CFA) and supplemented with heat-inactivated *Mycobacterium tuberculosis* strain H37Ra to 5 mg/mL on day 0 and 7 of the induction protocol, plus 500 ng of intraperitoneal Pertussis toxin on day 0 [44]. The requirement of coadjuvants underlines the importance of innate immunity activation, presumably via TLRs, in the generation of a robust adaptive autoimmune response [49].

We have developed recently a murine model of eosinophilic experimental autoimmune myocarditis (EoEAM) using mice deficient in IL-17A and IFnγ and IL17A−/−IFNγ−/− double knockout (DKO) mice, immunized similarly to the general EAM model [36]. EAM in IL17A−/−IFNγ−/− DKO results in a condition in which the immune response is preferentially Th2, leading to a lethal eosinophilic myocarditis.

10.2.2 Other Murine Models of Autoimmune Myocarditis

In addition to EAM, troponin-induced myocarditis was developed, in which also susceptible mice are immunized in a similar manner than described above, but using a troponin-derived peptide instead of myosin peptides. It is unclear how closely this model resembles the real pathogenic events occurring in humans. It seems that in human myocarditis the main target of autoimmunity is the myosin heavy chain. Nevertheless, the rationale of the troponin-induced model is to have the possibility to use troponin levels and anti-troponin antibodies as an alternative readout [50].

Nonobese diabetic (NOD) mice which lack expression of the murine MHC-II molecule IA (IA^b−/−) but express the human class II haplotype HLA-DQ8 develop spontaneous myocarditis. It is important to clarify that those mice are not a humanized murine model but rather a transgenic strain expressing one human HLA haplotype in substitution of the murine one [51]. Despite the xenogenic differences, the mouse antigen-presenting cells can effectively present peptides in an HLA-restricted manner to mouse T cells, then allowing certain mechanistic studies regarding HLA-biased presentation during autoimmunity. Those studies are potentially translatable to human physiology, mainly in the case of presentation of peptides derived from phylogenetically preserved self-antigens.

Murine models have also focused on the involvement of deficient PD-1 signal on T cells in the development of myocarditis [52, 53]. PD-1 is a member of the CD28 family. Its ligation with PDL1/PDL2 expressed on antigen-presenting cells during the formation of the immune synapse generates a downregulation of effector T cell activation, via anergy, apoptosis, and/or induction of regulatory properties [54]. PD-1-deficient mice (Pd1−/−) develop more severe EAM [52]. That enhanced susceptibility is associated with increased CD4 and CD8 myocardial infiltration. Similar findings were observed using the MRL-Fas$^{lpr/lpr}$, a murine model of autoimmunity with lupus-like features as consequence of a loss-of-function mutation in the Fas gene. If a PD-1 KO condition is introduced in the MLR-Fas$^{lpr/lpr}$ strain, then a severe lethal myocarditis occurs spontaneously at 4–8 weeks after birth. The incidence of myocarditis was up to 96% in this murine model. The features were an increased T cell infiltration, characteristically with a Th1 bias. The latter has been proposed as a useful murine model of PD-1 influence in myocarditis development/progression [53]. This is of clinical relevance since cases of acute myocarditis have been reported in human patients as side effect of anti-PD-1 checkpoint treatment for cancer (melanoma and non-small cell carcinoma) [55–57].

10.2.3   Experimental Viral Myocarditis

The most widely used viral models imply the infection of the mouse strain with Coxsackievirus B3 (CVB3), an enterovirus of the *Picornaviridae* family which is one of the primary pathogens associated with human viral myocarditis [43, 58–60]. Two main models of CVB3-induced myocarditis have been described. First one induces severe acute myocarditis with significant tissue damage and sudden death occurring within the first week of direct intraperitoneal infection [59, 60]. In the second CVB3 myocarditis model, heart-passaged CVB3 viruses are used to induce milder acute myocarditis, which progresses to chronicity and DCM [43]. In this CVB3 model, myocarditis is induced by intraperitoneal injection of heart-passaged Coxsackievirus B3 in a susceptible mice strain. Inflammatory phase is developed 7–14 days postinfection, and progression to DCM occurs 28–56 postinfection [43]. Thus, the model using heart-passaged CVB3 viruses allows to study the whole spectrum of immune processes involved in the progression to DCM, including the post-viral autoimmune phenomena [43]. A similar gender bias than EAM and human viral myocarditis exists in this model, with greater male susceptibility [61]. The fact that CVB is also the main myocarditis-associated virus in human disease, as well as the immunopathogenic similarities between the model and the patients, makes it a powerful research tool.

It has been shown that mice with an A/J background and C57BL/10 J background can develop the inflammatory phase of CVB3-induced myocarditis but only A/J mice progress to a chronic stage and DCM [43, 62]. These facts strongly suggest that progression to sustained inflammation and chronic complications of viral myocarditis might follow a common immunopathogenic pathway with autoimmune myocarditis [8, 61, 63]. Cardiac-tropic viruses might act as initial triggers and "natural adjuvants" of autoimmune processes [61].

10.3 Specific Factors Triggering/Predisposing Myocarditis Development

As most of the autoimmune diseases, myocarditis is considered a multifactorial entity, in which several immunologic mechanisms are involved on its development and progression. Regarding the trigger and initiation of its pathogenesis, so far, no unique sufficient factor has been identified but rather multiple endogenous and environmental confluent factors, in such a way that the myocardium-specific autoimmune process is triggered and sustained (Fig. 10.1). The balance and relative influence of those factors is still unclear but seems to be variable and host-dependent.

10.3.1 Gender

In the case of myocarditis, the gender bias is unusual as myocarditis is more likely to occur in males, as compared with females, a feature which is mirrored in the murine models [4, 5, 8, 44, 64]. The reason for that bias is still a conundrum, but certain factors have been found as a possible explanation, importantly differences in TLR4 activation susceptibilities between sexes [4, 5, 8, 64, 65].

Using the CVB3 myocarditis murine model, it was found that myocarditis severity is significantly stronger in males, as well as the likelihood of progression to DCM [43, 66]. This occurs despite a similar viral load and replication rate among genders, suggesting the existence of sex-specific immunologic features not related to virus clearance. Males produce higher amounts of pro-inflammatory cytokines IL1β, IL18, and IFNγ during myocarditis. TLR4, an important inducer of IL1β and IL18 by monocytes/macrophages and mast cells upon ligation, is more strongly expressed in male APCs than in female hosts, in a IFNγ-independent manner. Furthermore, Tim-3, a key peripheral inducer of T regulatory cells (Tregs), is cross regulated in an inverse manner by TLR4 with estrogens as cofactor [49]. Finally, Treg development, which is proportional to Tim-3 expression/functionality, is stronger in females, even during viral myocarditis, in an estrogen-dependent manner. This fact provides not only a plausible explanation for the myocarditis gender bias but also a link between innate and adaptive immunity and the requirement for coadjuvants in EAMs, which typically involves TLR ligands [49].

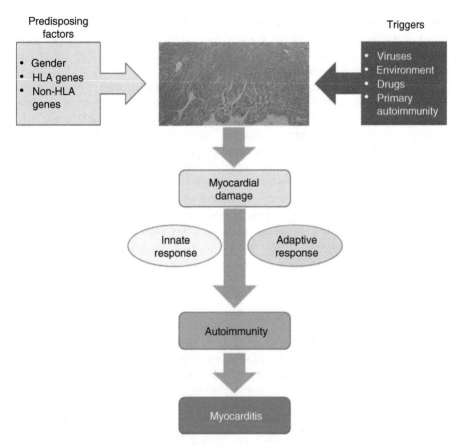

Fig. 10.1 Proposed model for myocarditis development. Coexistence of predisposing factors along with specific triggers of myocardium damage leads to exposure of cryptic self-antigens and a consequent inflammatory process. At this point, both the innate and the myocardium-specific adaptive response generate a self-sustained autoimmune phenomenon independent of the original trigger factor. That autoimmune process is responsible for development of myocarditis and progression to DCM

10.3.2 Environment

An important factor that observationally and mechanistically has been associated with development of human autoimmunity, with some successful animal model correlates, is the environmental influence [67].

Drugs such as digoxin, cephalosporins, diuretics (like furosemide), and tricyclic antidepressants are relatively weakly associated with myocarditis, as the incidence among patient taking those drugs is low. On the other hand, anthracyclines (like doxorubicin) are strongly associated with myocardial inflammation, even in a dose-dependent manner [64, 68, 69]. The mechanisms of drug-induced myocarditis are considered consequence of pleiotropic pharmacologic properties [64, 69]. There are also case reports of myocarditis associated with drug-induced eosinophilia. Despite the fact that no extensive mechanistic studies had been performed in those cases and most of the data is based on clinical reports, it is believed that in the latter cases myocardial inflammation is a consequence of eosinophilic infiltration rather than direct drug-induced damage [70].

Physical factors like radiation are also strongly associated with myocarditis in a dose-dependent manner. The risk of actinic myocarditis increases exponentially above 2Gy [71]. Radiation induces an acute immune response mediated by TNFα and IL1β, which seems to be the initiation mechanism if radiation noxa affects heart tissues [71].

The current concept is that pleiotropic properties of those pharmacologic and physical agents induce a direct myocardial damage. Nevertheless, this direct effect is not the only cause of myocarditis but rather its trigger. After that initial damage, an innate immune response occurs associated with exposure of intracellular self-antigens and eventually modification of those proteins in the inflammatory milieu generating neo-epitopes, altogether priming a myocardial-specific autoimmune adaptive response [64, 68].

10.3.3 Viruses

Viral myocarditis is considered sometimes an independent entity. Nevertheless, it seems that once the trigger infectious noxa exerts its effect, the final effector mechanisms are similar to the ones leading to autoimmune myocarditis progression and chronic complications. Myocardium-tropic viral infection acts as a trigger and "coadjuvant" generating a sustained myocardium-specific autoimmune response. The main viruses associated with myocarditis are the CVB3, adenovirus, influenza (A, B), parvovirus B19, cytomegalovirus, and Epstein-Barr virus. All these viruses cause myocarditis with similar inflammatory features, and all could lead to DCM. The real prevalence of progression to DCM for each specific virus is not known [6, 64, 72].

The current consensus is that both immune-mediated and viral cytotoxic mechanisms play an important role. *In vitro* experiments have demonstrated that low-level/low-rate enterovirus replication in myocytes generates viral proteins able to produce filament disruption of myocyte structure changes resembling the features observed *in vivo*. This filament disruption is induced by enteroviral protease [73–75]. Thus, beyond virus cytotoxicity, a low-level viral replication can induce cardiac cell damage even in the absence of production of fully mature and infectious viral particles.

During acute infection, one of the first infiltrating leukocytes to the myocardium are Natural Killer (NK) cells, which seem to play a short-term protective role by limiting the viral infection [76]. In support of that, NK-deficient mice develop a more severe inflammatory viral myocarditis (CVB3 model) [77]. Similar to CVB3 myocarditis, NK cells are protective in EAM model since NK cell depletion led to exacerbated inflammation, fibrosis, and loss of cardiac function [78]. We have shown that the mechanism of NK cell protection is mediated by antagonizing eosinophils trafficking to the heart [78]. Eosinophils, classically considered to exert an innate response, play a final effector role in myocarditis even in parallel to a robust adaptive T cell-mediated response [36].

A "second wave" of infiltrating leukocytes during viral myocarditis is mainly comprised of T cells, peaking 7–14 days after viral infection in murine models. T cells play an important role in the clearance of viruses. Specific T cell clones have the capacity to destroy and lysate infected cardiomyocytes, according to *in vitro* data [72, 76]. Overall, this antiviral response has a dual effect: (a) it controls viral infection and limits its cytotoxic effects, and (b) the tissue damage associated with the T cell response leads to exposure of cryptic antigens like myosin-derived peptides, which could eventually generate an autoimmune cardiac-specific response [79].

Several facts support the involvement of autoimmunity in the progression of viral myocarditis to a chronic stage. Mice develop cardiac-specific autoantibodies in both CVB3 myocarditis and in EAM. Furthermore, the mice susceptible or resistant to chronic CVB3 myocarditis are also susceptible or resistant to EAM, respectively (see above). C57BL/10 J mice expressing H2^b haplotype can develop acute inflammatory viral myocarditis, equivalent to A/J background strains, but are protected from chronic disease and progression to DCM [62]. A similar phenomenon has been described in mice sharing MHC haplotypes but no other non-MHC antigens (A/J B10.A H2^a vs. B10.A H2^a, resistant and susceptible to virus-associated DCM, respectively) [47]. Thus, both MHC and non-MHC genes are involved in the susceptibility to autoimmune myocarditis.

10.3.4 Mimicry

Recognition of antigens by T cell receptors (TCR), B cell receptors (BCR), and antibodies relies on the existence of specific complementarity of molecular regions of proteins, called epitopes, and the antigen-binding regions of the enounced receptors and antibodies (in a MHC-restricted manner in the case of TCR). Mimicry implies molecular similarity between non-self (microbial or alloepitopes) and self-epitopes, and the consequent cross-reactivity with T cell clones and/or antibodies (BCR are antibody-like surface receptors) [80, 81]. A paradigmatic example is the association of infections of *Campylobacter jejuni* with the development of Guillain-Barré syndrome [82].

It is still unclear if the molecular mimicry phenomenon is critical in the pathogenic process of myocarditis, but some studies suggest at least a partial contribution. The main proposed target of autoimmune response in myocarditis is the heavy chain of the myosin, specifically the isoform expressed in myocytes αMyHC [83, 84]. Multiple myosin isotypes had been identified, but myosin sequence is relatively phylogenetically preserved [85]. Using an A/J background murine model (H2^k haplotype), it was found that autoreactive T cell clones recognizing αMyHC peptides (specifically 334–352) in an IA^k-restricted manner have cross-reactivity with microbial epitopes derived from *Bacillus* spp., *Magnetospirillum gryphiswaldense*, *Zea mays*, and, even more important for its human clinical implications, *Cryptococcus neoformans* [84]. The latter fungi had shown a breakout within the last decades in association with the AIDS pandemic. That might have implication on the pathogenesis of myocarditis, mostly in patients susceptible to *C. neoformans* infections under chemotherapy or carrying clinical HIV infection.

Another particular kind of molecular mimicry was described in the context of myocarditis as similarity between self-antigens, myosin epitopes, and β-adrenergic receptors. Therefore, the autoantibodies generated during myocarditis against myosin peptides may cross-react with adrenergic receptors and exert an activating adrenergic effect upon ligation, thus potentially contributing to chronic sympathetic-mediated cardiac damage [86].

10.3.5 Exposure of Encrypted Self-Antigens

Another concept demonstrated to play a role in the development of autoimmunity is the exposure of self-antigens which are encrypted and unavailable to the immune system under physiologic conditions [87, 88]. Cardiac myosin (specifically αMyHC) is one of the most important self-targets in myocarditis. Importantly, myosin, which belongs to the contractile apparatus of the myocytes, is not significantly exported to the extracellular matrix.

Myh6, the gene encoding αMyHC, has been shown to not be expressed in medullary thymic epithelial cells (mTECs), which are the main responsible for T cell thymic negative selection, via promiscuous self-antigen presentation. αMyHC is not expressed neither in peripheral lymphoid stromal cells. As consequence, in physiologic conditions, specific self-reactive anti-αMyHC T cell clones escape from negative selection, reaching periphery as autoreactive cardiac-specific clones. That is an important feature predisposing development of myocarditis in mice and humans as long as other events or risk factors take place leading to release of αMyHC, a cryptic self-antigen. In fact, it was shown that transgenic mice, expressing *Myh6* in mTECs, are protected from EAM induction in association with clonal deletion of those autoreactive clones [89].

Either myocardial infection, toxins, ischemia or other insults can lead to myocardial damage and subsequent exposure of intracellular proteins (cryptic epitopes). That exposure, in the context of a proper pro-inflammatory microenvironment, triggers the adaptive immune response leading to myocarditis in genetically susceptible individuals [6, 72, 76]. Thus, different triggers could lead to myocarditis and eventually chronic autoimmune myocarditis.

10.3.6 MHC and Non-MHC Bias

Human Leukocyte Antigen (HLA) genes (human form of Major Histocompatibility Complex, MHC) are one of the most polymorphic genes in humans, as well as the coresponding MHC genes are in most mammals. This genetic variability has functional consequences in terms of the affinity of MHC molecules for specific peptides. Despite MHC molecules being promiscuous in terms of peptide presentation, certain biases exist as consequence of the avidity and affinity of MHC molecules for specific peptides [2].

The association of certain autoimmune diseases with specific HLA haplotypes is considered to be consequence of a higher affinity of certain haplotypes for preserved protein self-products.

HLA haplotypes are not sufficient, and may not be main determinants, in myocarditis initiation and progression. Nevertheless, certain associations between DCM of any cause and HLA haplotypes had been found. Specifically, HLA-DR4 is statistically associated with DCM based on retrospective studies [90–92]. Other DCM-HLA-positive associations had been reported, mainly HLA-DR12, DR15, and DRB*0601, as well as negative associations (HLA-DR11, DQB1*0301) [93–95].

Experimental facts observed in murine models of EAM and CVB3 myocarditis also support the influence of MHC haplotypes in the development of myocarditis and its progression to DCM. Mice with b haplotypes in A/J background are less susceptible than other non-H2^b A/J strains to EAM and CVB3 myocarditis including the acute inflammatory phase and DCM [96]. Furthermore, that b-associated protection on A/J background parallels development of lower titers of cardiac-specific autoantibodies [62, 96].

Similarly, transgenic nonobese diabetic mouse strain expressing human HLA-DQ8 instead of IA^b develops spontaneous myocarditis which progresses to DCM even with electrophysiologic disturbances like heart block (see Sect. 10.2) [51, 97]. Nevertheless, it is of notice that HLA-DQ8 is not within the haplotypes associated with DCM in human studies, which might limit the translational findings of this murine model and/or underscore the importance of other non-MHC genes.

There is a lack of myocarditis-specific association of MHC haplotypes in certain murine models of myocarditis as was shown by using specific strains sharing MHC haplotypes (MHC-full matched), but differing in non-MHC background-associated genes has been performed. A.SW (A/J background) and B10.S (B10 background), both H2^s, have differences in myosin-induced EAM susceptibility, being B10.S protected as compared with susceptible A.SW [98]. Similarly, mice with b haplotypes differ in susceptibility to EAM. C57BL/10 J are resistant, while A/J are very susceptible to EAM. That strongly suggests the influence of other non-MHC features in the development of myocardial-specific autoimmunity. Using simple sequence length polymorphism (SSLP) markers in the murine genome, two non-MHC loci were found to be associated with the development of EAM in H2^s equivalent strains. Those genes, named in mice *Eam1* and *Eam2* (located in proximal chromosome 1 and distal chromosome 6, respectively), are linked to myocarditis development. Interestingly, those loci and their human equivalents had been associated with SLE and diabetes, as well as autoimmune experimental encephalitis and orchitis in mouse [98]. Other studies using the CVB3 murine model and also SSLP tracking system found other non-MHC loci associated with viral myocarditis: *Vms1* (chromosome 1), *Vms2* (chromosome 4), and *Vms3* (chromosome 3) [99].

Finally, a specific 14 bp deletion in a region of the HLA-G gene (a human nonclassical MHC I molecule) was reported to be associated with DCM. Nevertheless, as linkage disequilibrium exists between HLA-G and HLA-DR and DQ and considering that the reported HLA-G 14 bp deletion occurs in the 3′-untranslated region of the gene, it remains unclear if the HLA-G bias corresponds to a real mechanistic association, or just a correlation whose mechanism relies on class II-linked haplotypes [100, 101].

Other polymorphisms have been identified in association with autoimmunity, mainly on the CTLA-4, PD-1, and ICOS genes. All these genes encode for functional proteins involved in the regulation of T cell activation mainly via induction of apoptosis and/or anergy. Specifically, mutations in PD-1 and ICOS are associated with the development of myocarditis in murine models but in the context of broader systemic autoimmune features [52, 53, 102, 103]. The case of PD-1 deserves particular attention considering the outbreak of the checkpoint blockade in cancer therapy. PD-1 blockade has been shown to provide benefit in certain cancers like non-small cell lung carcinoma and melanoma [55, 56]. Myocarditis has been found to be an infrequent side effect of PD-1 blockade. The histological features were that of acute lymphocytic myocarditis [57]. This validates the importance of the disruption of the PD1/PDL1 axis in the development of myocarditis observed in mice.

10.3.7   Autoimmune Regulator (AIRE)

Autoimmune regulator (AIRE) allows a promiscuous expression of self-antigens by medullary thymic epithelial cells (mTECs) [104, 105]. AIRE is involved in central deletion of effector T cells (Teff) and thymic Treg (tTreg) induction but also in peripheral Teff anergization and pTreg differentiation [104–106].

The absence of AIRE expression in murine models (AIRE−/− mice) leads to an increase of autoreactive effector T cells in the periphery [107]. AIRE also influence self-tolerance by directing autoreactive bone marrow-derived T cell clones into regulatory functions [107].

Taking these concepts to the field of myocardial autoimmunity, some experimental data have demonstrated that defective central (thymicdependent) tolerance and increase of autoreactive Teff (specific for myosin-derived epitopes) as well as decreased thymic Tregs (tTregs, formerly nTregs) with the same specificity are involved in the inflammatory phase of EAM [106, 108]. HLA-DQ8+ IA^b−/− NOD mice develop spontaneous myocarditis with cellular and humoral autoimmune responses directed toward epitopes of the α isoform of myosin heavy chain (αMyHC). The same model showed that EAM is dependent on the T cell-mediated anti-MyHC response [109]. Anti-myosin-specific T cells represent the majority of the myocardium-infiltrating Teff [89]. The development of myocarditis mediated by MyHC-specific Teff was associated with lack of expression of αMyHC by mTECs. With more complex genetic manipulations of that murine strain, it was shown that susceptibility to EAM was abrogated by expression of MyHC by mTECs, paralleling a decrease in that specific Teff autoreactive clones in the periphery. Further studies about the functional impact of AIRE in the expression of myosin by human mTECs as a factor determining development of autoimmune myocarditis are needed [89].

10.3.8   Fefz2

It was discovered recently that nuclear factor Fezf2, similarly to AIRE, directs tissue-restricted antigen expression in thymic medulla stromal cells. [110]. Fefz2-deficient mice (Fefz2−/−) develop systemic disease distinct from AIRE−/− mice [110]. Discovery of the importance of Fezf2 in the development of central tolerance is relatively recent. So far, no evidence exists associating autoimmune myocarditis with functional or genetic modifications of Fezf2. Nevertheless, it is a topic that probably will be under scrutiny in the near future.

10.4   Immunopathogenesis of Myocarditis

Studies performed in murine models and observational data from humans have demonstrated that CD4 T cell response is the main driving force of autoimmune myocarditis.

Autoimmunity is characterized by a highly antigen-specific immune response, yet the activation of innate response is required to prime the adaptive response [1]. Its importance in the context of autoimmune myocarditis has been demonstrated by the fact that EAM murine models require the use of coadjuvants (like complete Freund's adjuvant (CFA)) and unspecific stimulation by pathogen-associated molecular patterns (PAMPs) provided by *Mycobacterium* antigens. Importantly, the coadjuvant challenge must be provided simultaneously to the exposure of cardiac self-antigens in order to generate the cardiac-specific sustained autoimmunity. If timing is not properly set, then the self-specific immune response is not mounted, even if the innate response is successfully stimulated by the adjuvants [8]. Innate cellular response is required not only for initiation of autoimmunity but also for the maintenance of the adaptive T cell-mediated response and progression to chronicity. Myocardial infection by specific microbes, beyond a direct virus-dependent cytolytic effect, seems to play the role of "coadjuvant" to the autoimmune adaptive response (Fig. 10.1) [61, 81]. In this section, the specific features of this complex cross talk will be described.

10.4.1   Adaptive Cellular Response

The adaptive cellular immune response is characterized by its antigen specificity and high inflammatory efficiency. Its major mediators are the T cells, which specificity relies in the molecular structure of clonal TCRs, able to "recognize" characteristic peptide/MHC complexes.

The classic dichotomist Th1/Th2 model does not provide an accurate representation of the normal immune response [111, 112]. That became evident in the last decades after discovery of other important pro-inflammatory Teff subsets, like Th17 (but also including Th9 and Th22), as well as anti-inflammatory subpopulations, mainly Tregs and Tr1. Furthermore, a high plasticity of T cell subsets has been described, involving not only central (thymic) but also peripheral T cell fate induction [112]. Dysfunction of Th17 and Treg has been widely found to be a key factor in autoimmunity, including myocarditis. Importantly Treg and Th17 activation/differentiation shares certain cytokine requirements, remarkably TGFβ, needed for both subsets but in a concentration-dependent manner. In the presence of TGFβ, IL6/IL-1β *vs* IL10 balance is responsible for the Th17 *vs* Treg differentiation [112].

10.4.1.1 Th1 Response

As in other autoimmune diseases, the overall activity of self-specific Th1 response is one of the main mediators of the inflammatory phase of myocarditis [111]. Supporting the importance of Th1 response in myocarditis, several studies had focused on IL12 as primary mediator. It was shown that mice lacking IL12Rβ1 and STAT4 signal (thus unresponsive to IL12) are resistant to myocarditis, whereas exogenous IL12 exacerbates EAM [113]. Notwithstanding, the same study demonstrated that blockade of IFNγ worsen the disease, starting to draw the picture of a counterbalance of IFNγ-IL12 axis and a potential dual role of IFNγ [113].

IL12 family main members and its subunits are IL12 (p35 p40), IL23 (p19 p40), IL27(p28 EBI3), and IL35 (p35 EBI3) [114]. The existence of shared subunits between the cytokines makes difficult the determination of the specific role of each member. Furthermore, IL12Rβ is a receptor chain shared by IL12 and IL23 [114]. Several attempts have been made to elucidate the differential role of IL12 family cytokines. The first studies analyzed the differential EAM phenotype between IL12p40 −/− and IL12p35−/− [115]. It was found that IL23 and IL-12 dual-deficient mice (IL12p40 −/−) were protected from EAM in contrast to IL12-deficient mice (IL12p35−/−), suggesting predominant pathogenic role of IL23 over IL12 [115]. Importantly, IL23 is key in the development and stabilization of the Th17 response [112]. Also, it must be considered that IL12p35 is a subunit shared with the recently discovered IL35, a potent anti-inflammatory cytokine [116]. Furthermore, that study was not able to induce specific knockout of IL23, and the conclusions are rather inferred from the differences between IL12p40 −/− and IL12p35−/−.

In later studies, our laboratory was able to determine the specific role of IL23 in myocarditis using an IL12p19−/− strain (IL23 KO), which is deficient only in IL23, because as far as is known, IL12p19 subunit is not shared with other members of the family [117]. We found that IL23 is transiently required during the early stages to induce CD4 T cell pathogenicity. That process was dependent on GM-CFS. IL23 was required in the early stages but dispensable once the GM-CSF-dependent T cell-mediated autoimmunity is established; thus, IL23 is a required "switch" for the initiation process of EAM [117].

In congruence with the complex regulatory network of the immune system, results observed in IFNγ-deficient models showed paradoxical effects as compared with IL12 family-deficient studies. IFNγ KO (*Ifng−/−*), IFNγ receptor KO (*Ifngr−/−*), and mice receiving anti-IFNγ antibody treatment developed more severe inflammatory myocarditis than WT strains [113, 118, 119]. In addition, mice deficient in Tbet (*Tbx21−/−*), nuclear factor required for Th1 T cell differentiation/development, develop more severe EAM than WT [120]. Similar findings regarding the effect of depletion of IFNγ were observed in CVB3 myocarditis model [121]. The severe CVB3 myocarditis in the absence of IFNγ was not associated with lack of antiviral response but with an enhanced IL1β, IL4, and TGFβ production [121].

An important feature observed in DCM on IFNγ-deficient mice is the severity of the fibrosis and even the development of constrictive hemodynamic complications [122]. The latter might be associated with the regulatory influence of IFNγ on the mediators of tissue remodeling and fibrosis, including monocytes and fibroblasts. IFNγ has multiple potential sources in the context of myocarditis, including T cells, monocytes, macrophages, dendritic cells, and innate lymphoid cells.

As final consequence, Th1 response occurs during the development of myocarditis, with IL12 and TNFα playing essentially a pro-inflammatory role but with IFNγ being dual, thus modulating and homeostatically dampening the immune response and limiting sustained inflammation and fibrosis.

10.4.1.2 Th2 Response

In the murine model of Th2-mediated eosinophilic myocarditis, EoEAM, a massive and severe inflammatory eosinophilic myocarditis progressing to DCM, is observed in a transgenic strain lacking the main Th1 and Th17 final effector cytokines, i.e., IL17A−/−IFNγ−/−, after EAM induction. The lack of Th1 and Th17 responses generates a Th2-biased inflammation leading to eosinophilic myocarditis, resembling the features and severity of the eosinophilic human disease. The main final effectors of the myocardial damage are eosinophils, despite the T cell requirement [36].

Pointing out the complexity of the regulatory process, IL4 and IL13, both classic pro-inflammatory Th2 cytokines, seem to have an opposite effect in the development of EAM- and CVB3-induced myocarditis. Those Th2 cytokines are under the same promoter and are typically dependent on the activation of the nuclear factor GATA3 in T cells [48]. Mice lacking IL4 expression (*Il4−/−*) develop a milder inflammatory myocarditis and a less severe systolic dysfunction and progression to chronic stages when EAM is induced in an A/J background. However, Balb/c IL4 KO mice develop a disease similar to WTs [123, 124]. This unveils strain-specific immunologic differences but, on the other hand, shows that IL4 pro-inflammatory capacity is variable during EAM but certainly is not a protective mediator. Oppositely, we described that IL13−/− mice on Balb/c background develop more severe EAM- and CVB3-induced myocarditis and progress to severe DCM and the associated heart failure [123].

The latter observation in IL13−/− mice takes us back to the cross talk between adaptive T cell response and the innate cellular response. In fact, IL13 exert a protective role in the development and progression of myocarditis by regulating the macrophage differentiation. Aggressive acute inflammatory features and the important chronic impairment in systolic function during DCM phase were associated with a typical upregulation of a macrophage-derived cytokine cluster: IL1β, IL18, IFNγ, and TGFβ [123]. Aside from an increase in macrophage-derived cytokines, a specific upregulation of CD204+ CD206+ pro-inflammatory/activated macrophages was observed in IL13 KO mice, strongly suggesting a suppressive effect of IL13 in the macrophage side of the innate-adaptive cross talk.

10.4.1.3 Th17 Response

IL17A, the main pro-inflammatory Th17-derived mediator, unexpectedly is not necessary for development of acute inflammatory stages of myocarditis in EAM model [125]. On the other hand, we have found that IL-17A is strictly required for progression to DCM, cardiac fibrosis, and loss of cardiac function. In other words, the acute inflammation can take place in the absence of IL17A; however without IL17A, myocarditis does not progress to DCM [125].

Importantly, the Th17 response required for progression from myocarditis to DCM is not only dependent on leukocytes. We demonstrated that beyond inflammatory Ly6C^{high} monocytes, also cardiac fibroblasts play an important role in the inflammatory process. IL17A−/− mice, protected from DCM but not acute EAM, have a diminished myocardial infiltration of neutrophils and Ly6C^{high} inflammatory monocytes [126]. Interestingly, a conversion of Ly6C^{high} monocytes to Ly6C^{lo} monocytes protects WT host from DCM, strongly suggesting that Ly6C^{high} monocytes are associated with the pro-fibrotic IL17A effect. We have found that granulocyte-monocyte colony-stimulating factor (GM-CSF) is required, in conjunction with IL17A, for Ly6C^{high} monocyte infiltration in myocardium during EAM. We showed that IL-17A is able to induce high amount of GM-CSF and other myeloid cytokines and chemokines from cardiac fibroblasts. Thus, we have discovered an active Th17-fibroblast-monocyte cross talk in the pathogenesis of myocarditis. To summarize, T cell-derived IL17A plus fibroblast-derived GM-CSF contributes to Ly6C^{high} monocyte chemotaxis/activation, which plays an active role in fibrosis and sustains inflammatory process (Fig. 10.2) [126].

As described above, a very specific milieu of cytokines is needed for Th17 cell differentiation and establishment of the so-called Th17 environment. That milieu includes IL6, IL23, and TGFβ. Importantly, IL23 is needed for Th17 terminal differentiation and Th17 "stabilization" [111, 112]. We demonstrated the requirement of IL23 (p19) during EAM development [117]. Specifically, CD4 T cell stimulation by IL23 is required during the acute phase of autoimmunity for an effective myocarditis (EAM) and consequent DCM development. The key effect of such IL23

Fig. 10.2 Schematic immunopathogenesis of post-myocarditis DCM development. CD4 T cell autoimmune response induces a Th17-dependent pro-inflammatory process associated with DCM development. T cell-derived IL17A induces cardiac fibroblasts to produce GM-CSF, which in turns activates monocytes toward a highly inflammatory function. Those activated monocytes are required final effectors in the progression to chronic tissue damage and DCM

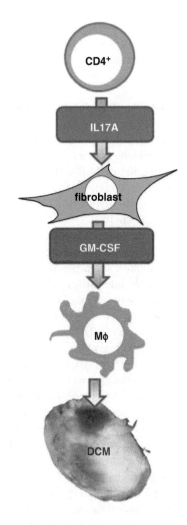

stimulation was proven to be the GM-CSF production by T cells. Furthermore, IL23 effect is only transiently required during the acute phase (early after EAM induction), as later influence cannot restore the EAM development [117].

An important translational study supporting the latter concepts was published recently [127]. That study supports the influence of Th17 in human myocarditis and its progression to DCM. Th17 CD4 T cells were found to be associated with myocarditis, influencing inflammation via IL6, TGFβ, and IL23. Also, an association exists with GM-CSF producing monocytes (CD14+). This interaction was related with TLR2 expression on those inflammatory monocytes, an interestingly finding unveiling the role of this particular TLR type in human myocarditis. Consistently, a decreased classic Treg population (Foxp3+) was observed in association with the enounced features [127].

Those seminal studies made evident potential Th17 response-focused therapeutic targets, not only to treat acute inflammatory myocarditis but also its late-stage complications.

10.4.1.4 T Regulatory Cells

Treg deficiency is associated with autoimmune severity, including in myocarditis models. A mechanism, already described above, is associated with the cross regulation of TLR4-Tim3, which is preferentially associated with Treg development in females. It is a mechanism explaining the constitutive protection of females to myocarditis, both autoimmune and viral associated, as compared with male hosts [49].

In the same way, a possible explanation for the preferential susceptibility of A.SW H2^s to EAM as compared with B10.S H2^s, despite an identical H2 genotype, is a constitutive strain-specific lower frequency of classic Tregs (CD4 + CD25 + Foxp3+) in A.SW. Interestingly, this Treg profile seems to be really constitutive and not associated with specific myosin-targeted responses, as demonstrated by ovalbumin immunization. Importantly, Tregs showed an opposite trend in terms of frequency with respect to Th17 cells in those strains in the context of EAM [128].

Interestingly, Tregs also provide protection to viral myocarditis, as demonstrated in the CVB3 myocarditis model. Importantly, Tregs not only diminished tissue damage but also were associated with improved viral clearance. Those phenomena were associated with secretion of TGFβ, again demonstrating the multiple roles of that cytokine-like factor [129].

Recently, the severity of EAM was found to be attenuated by cannabidiol (a non-psychoactive constituent of marijuana), in relation with a decrease of CD4 T cells. The mechanism was not entirely elucidated, but the possibility of a change in the Treg/Teff balance is a plausible hypothesis [130]. Overall, the current concept is that a defective Treg function is associated with development of autoimmune diseases, including autoimmune myocarditis, providing a potential therapeutic target, which so far had been elusive.

10.4.2 Adaptive Humoral Response

Despite the existence of clearly humoral-mediated autoimmune diseases (like post-streptococcal glomerulonephritis, Berger disease, and Goodpasture disease), the influence of those autoantibodies on the pathogenesis of most autoimmune diseases is still controversial, at least on its initiation phase. Myocarditis is a cellular-mediated process, and several myocarditis-associated autoantibodies are specific to encrypted antigens that are not available to antibody ligation without tissue damage and cell disruption [87]. As consequence, the generation of autoantibodies by clonal selection of self-reactive B cell clones is secondary to T cell activation, T-B cross talk, and release of intracellular or matrix-encrypted proteins after tissue damage [131, 132].

In myocarditis, this lack of pivotal role during initiation is supported by the fact that up to two-thirds of acute myocarditis patients have no detectable cardiac-specific antibodies at the moment of diagnosis or clinical onset [83, 132]. On the other hand, its correlation with disease progression and detection in symptom-free relatives of DCM patients suggest that they occasionally may be early markers paralleling myocardial damage after its initiation, with minimal to null causative influence in the initial phase [132].

Eighty percent of patients with DCM-related myocarditis develop cardiac-specific antibodies, but also up to 60% of patients with heart failure of any cause have circulating antibodies targeting heart-specific epitopes. The latter supports the idea of the necessity of tissue damage of any cause for development of humoral autoimmunity, as well as the paucity of its inflammatory influence [83, 132–134].

A plethora of autoantibodies has been described in myocarditis, including anti-αMyHC, troponin I and T, and β1-adrenergic receptor. Also, non-cardiac-specific autoantibodies are frequently found in myocarditis patients, including anti-actin, tropomyosin, laminin, and anti-muscarinic receptor [4]. Of those, the ones receiving most attention are the anti-αMyHC and the anti-adrenergic receptor. Anti-αMyHC antibodies have been described to correlate with disease progression (including diminished titers after adequate clinical response) and are also found in murine models [132]. Anti-adrenergic receptor antibodies are also correlated with disease progression, and interestingly a significant proportion of the clones are activating antibodies, so those antibodies might contribute to hemodynamic alterations via autonomic modulation [4, 83, 132, 133, 135, 137].

Antibodies targeting specific receptors might induce persistent activation of such receptors, i.e., induce a sustained positive intracellular signaling, similar to the one generated by physiologic ligands, but abnormally sustained over time. This is not the case of all receptor-specific antibodies but seems to be the case of several clones involved in myocarditis targeting adrenergic receptors [133]. The case of cross-reaction of anti-myosin antibodies with adrenergic receptors was already described above in the section dedicated to mimicry [84].

In the case of activating β1-adrenergic antibodies (with a prevalence of 70–80% among patients with dilated cardiomyopathy of any cause and 60% on patients with myocarditis), they seem to exert their persistent adrenergic effect by stabilizing an activated molecular conformation of the receptor upon ligation. Also, the cross-link of two receptors, generating a stable dimerization, contributes to that effect [132, 133].

A pathogenic sustained β-adrenergic activation has been demonstrated to be able to induce cardiomyocyte apoptosis [137, 138]. Furthermore, once systolic dysfunction begins, the increased adrenergic tone (sympathetic) has deleterious hemodynamic effects [139, 140]. It is believed that beneficial effect of β blocker drugs in patients with heart failure of any cause is related both with the improvement of hemodynamic status and the decrease of the proapoptotic effect. Nevertheless, theoretically, such drugs cannot reverse *per se* the stabilization of the receptors induced by the activating autoantibodies. In that regard, the turnover rate and upregulation of those receptors must be considered [140].

Therapeutic approaches are focused on the depletion or neutralization of anti-adrenergic activating autoantibodies. Plasmapheresis and immunoadsorption of those antibodies were tested in case-control clinical studies in patients with dilated cardiomyopathy [141]. Interestingly, also benefit from the removal of cardio-depressant autoantibodies by immunoadsorption was also found [142]. Patients receiving immunoadsorption have improved cardiac function. After a 12-month follow-up, anti-β-adrenergic receptor autoantibodies did not return to the original titers [143].

Another treatment strategy with a similar goal is the neutralization of those antibodies using aptamers in the apheresis technology. As aptamers are synthetic oligonucleotide ligands with high specificity to targets like the Fab region of antibodies, its use is proposed as a mean to optimize the removal of autoantibodies by apheresis and decrease toxic and immunogenic complications described for immunoadsorption [144, 145]. The overall utility of this approach has not been fully elucidated.

10.4.3   Innate Immune Response

Innate leukocytes are those ones defined for lacking an antigen-specific receptors, thus responding in an unspecific manner via cytokine chemoattraction and/or non-specific receptors such as Toll-like receptors (TLRs) and responding with phagocytosis and nonspecific cytotoxic chemical species. The main innate immune cells involved in myocarditis are natural killers (NKs), neutrophils, eosinophils, and monocyte/macrophages [8]. It is important to notice that innate lymphoid cells (ILCs), a specific subset of leukocytes having lymphoid properties but lacking antigen-specific receptor, were described recently. ILCs are involved in mucosae patrol and in several immune responses, including antihelminthic responses and immune-mediated diseases like Crohn disease, psoriasis, dermatitis, and airway hyperreactivity [146]. Little is known about its biology in the heart. Nevertheless, NK cells, a particular TCR-lacking subset of lymphocytes with cytolytic capacity, are currently considered ILCs type 1 [147]. Regarding NK cells, its role in the immune response during autoimmune myocarditis (EAM model) and viral myocarditis (CVB3 models) has been described above.

Eosinophils are not only involved in the development of the severely Th2-skewed EoEAM but also in the classic EAM [36]. Eosinophils behave as final effectors and infiltrate and produce myocardial inflammation even once the adaptive T cell response is established.

Neutrophils also infiltrate myocardium during EAM, exerting an inflammatory role, with long-term impact even in the impairment of the cardiac function [48]. Neutrophil activation and recruitment are dependent on the Th17 response via IL17A and GM-CSF [125]. Also, in an OVA-TCR transgenic system of heart inflammation, it was found that neutrophil cross talk with heart-infiltrating CD8 T cells sustains its T cytotoxic response [148].

Finally, one of the most important heart-infiltrating innate cells during myocarditis are the macrophages [48, 149]. Some of its interactions with specific cytokines and T cell responses were described above.

Several attempts have been made to classify macrophages. For instance, depending on its pattern of activation and inflammatory capacities, they are divided into M1 and M2. M1 macrophages (or "classic") are activated by IFNγ in association with the Th1 response and have strong antigen-presenting and pro-inflammatory capacities. On the other hand, M2 "alternative" differentiation occurs in anti-inflammatory environments and is induced by IL10 and TGFβ. It is proposed that M2 macrophages have a significantly weaker antigen presentation capacity [149]. However, M1-M2 dichotomy is difficult to reproduce and detect *in vivo*. Also, based on its monocyte precursors and final inflammatory capacities, mouse macrophages are classified *in vivo* as Ly6C^{high} inflammatory and Ly6C^{low} regulatory subsets. Human CD14^{high} monocyte/macrophages correspond to mouse Ly6C^{high}, whereas CD14^{int} are equivalent to Ly6C^{low}. M1/M2 and Ly6C$^{high/low}$ classifications do not completely overlap. A significant plasticity exists in the monocyte/macrophage populations [149]. As consequence, it is considered that such a rigid categorization does not correspond to the real immunobiology of these cells.

Specifically in EAM, monocytes and macrophages are early myocardial-infiltrating cells. Not all myocardial macrophages are strictly "infiltrating cells" but rather derived from resident monocyte differentiation [149]. Even before that massive infiltration, the TLR ligation (mainly 2 and 4) in monocytes/macrophages is crucial in the initiation process of myocarditis and also the targets of coadjuvants in the EAM model [8, 61, 149].

The pro-inflammatory molecule called high-mobility group box 1 (HMGB1) has been found to be important during the initiation process of EAM in studies performed with TnT-EAM model [150]. This is a ligand of a macrophage receptor called receptor for advanced glycation end products (RAGE). This interaction induces a M1-like phenotype/functionality of macrophages, boosting its inflammatory impact on myocarditis. Importantly, TLRs are redundant receptors of HMGB1, which activation is independent of RAGE [150, 151].

It has been found that once in an inflammatory Ly6C^{high} status, macrophages express IL17 receptor. Heart-infiltrating macrophages during EAM have these characteristics. In that way, macrophages, along with neutrophils, belong to the innate cells associated with Th17 responses during myocarditis. After IL17A stimulation, Ly6C^{high} macrophages produce a particular cluster of cytokines, GM-CSF, already described as an important mediator of EAM, IL3, IL9, CCL4, and CCL5 [152].

Overall, macrophages are potent inflammatory cells during myocarditis and potentially the most abundant in endomyocardial biopsies. These cells are critical in the initiation process. Nevertheless, they are also responsible for the progression of the disease. Macrophages are orchestrated with the T cell response, in such a way that several compensatory and regulatory mechanisms which dampen the severity of EAM (like IFNγ) can target macrophages, as described above.

10.5   Therapeutics

Unfortunately, this is one of the less developed areas in the myocarditis field. To begin with, some clinical studies lack a clear diagnostic and etiologic definition, and several times, the term "virus-positive" or "virus-negative" myocarditis is based only on peripheral blood serology [153, 154].

That generates a huge conundrum on how to analyze the results of the therapeutic trials. The trigger is unclear in most of the cases of the "virus-negative" patients. Even more important is the fact that it is unknown at which point of the temporal evolution of the autoimmune process is the patients when enrolled in the therapeutic trials. That makes us hypothesize that case and control groups had been heterogeneous in immunopathogenic terms, in such a way that it is hard to analyze the data from a strict evidence-based medicine perspective.

Notwithstanding, it is understandable that the potential severity and the relatively low incidence of myocarditis, along with the immunologic and diagnostic complexities/limitations enounced above, make almost impossible to carry out optimally designed clinical trials as the ones performed for other high prevalent /incident entities as high blood pressure and diabetes.

Fortunately, there is a growing body of therapeutic knowledge which, despite frequently based on case reports and uncontrolled trials, suggests that immune modulation/suppression is a useful approach in myocarditis, even in viral-triggered cases if it is used together with proper antiviral treatment [72, 153].

10.5.1   Immunosuppression

The rationale of this therapeutic approach is to target the pro-inflammatory mediators of the disease. Immunosuppression is used in treatment of myocarditis types considered to be autoimmune such as giant cell myocarditis. So far, broad immunosuppressive drugs rather than targeted treatments have been used. The main drugs tested for myocarditis are steroids (prednisone, prednisolone), cyclosporine, and azathioprine [9, 30]. These drugs are mostly used in combination; however, the benefits for individual subtypes of myocarditis need to be evaluated in proper clinical comparative studies. Some studies showed significant or at least some improvement in terms of ejection fraction [155], but another study reported no benefit on ejection fraction or survival as compared with placebo [156]. Notwithstanding, differences in the study design exist, and importantly the study reporting benefit was made on nonviral myocarditis cases, whereas in the one reporting no benefit no viral status discrimination was made.

Another interesting study analyzed the effect of muromonab-CD3 (a monoclonal antibody targeting CD3) plus cyclosporine and steroids in a prospective cohort of 12 patients. This study included specifically patients with giant cell myocarditis. Despite there was no control group (which is understandable due to the high severity and lethality of this type of myocarditis), an improved survival was reported [28–30, 157].

10.5.2 Immunomodulation

As described in the section of humoral response, plasmapheresis/immunoadsorption has been studied by several groups. A consistent benefit was observed in hemodynamic terms, mainly improvement of ejection fraction. Those protocols include the coadministration of immunoglobulin. Interestingly, those studies enrolled patients with DCM, which supports the hemodynamic deleterious effect of cardiac autoantibodies. Importantly, DCM patients of any cause were included, which expands the usefulness of this approach to non-myocarditis cases [141, 159–161].

High doses of immunoglobulin exert a beneficial effect (improved survival and ejection fraction) in acute myocarditis patients. Several data come from small case studies [153], but a randomized controlled study on acute myocarditis patients supports the observation [161]. It is of notice that one controlled study reports conflicting data by not finding improvements of the ejection fraction [162]. Also, in those studies, no clear etiologic definition was made.

10.5.3 Antiviral

The main antiviral drugs studied in myocarditis have been acyclovir, peramivir, ganciclovir, ribavirin, and artesunate, in well-defined viral myocarditis patients (etiology was specifically determined: parvovirus B19, influenza, cytomegalovirus, parainfluenza, herpesvirus, respectively) [6, 72, 153]. All of them have been either small studies or case reports, but overall the benefit of antiviral treatment seems to be consistent in terms of ejection fraction, survival, and decreased viral load. All protocols had included immunosuppressive and/or immunomodulatory treatment, as steroids and/or immunoglobulin [153]. The latter is consistent with the described importance of the immune-mediated damage in conjunction with viral cytotoxic effects in the development of viral myocarditis.

Also, interferon α and β were analyzed in viral myocarditis. Interferon α was found beneficial in enterovirus-confirmed DCM, based on hemodynamic parameters and viral clearance. Interferon β significantly improved ejection fraction and viral load in a cohort of acute viral myocarditis [163], whereas no benefit was observed in a cohort of patients treated at DCM stage [164].

10.5.4 Future Therapeutic Challenges

In general, the future directions should focus on a proper diagnostic, not only on the etiologic aspect but also on the specific stage of evolution of the immune/inflammatory process. That would allow to determine specific treatments depending on the underlying cause and also on the predominant immune process taking place in the patient at the moment of the intervention. Targeted treatments should be generated in the near future, addressing the specific immunopathogenic process predominating in the patient, i.e., more effective antiviral treatments, induction of self-tolerance, boost of Treg response, dampening Teff response, and blockade of innate response-associated receptors, among others, including modulation of the immunologic role of stromal cells like fibroblast and endothelial cells. The positive side of the story is the exponentially growing knowledge about the immunopathogenesis of myocarditis, which certainly will end up in development of effective diagnostic, prognostic, and therapeutic strategies.

10.6 Concluding Remarks

Myocarditis is an extremely complex immune-mediated process. Several risk factors and biologic issues predisposing its trigger and progression have been identified. Those include gender-associated immunologic properties, HLA and non-HLA genetic characteristics, exposure of cryptic antigens, mimicry, systemic autoimmune diseases, drugs, and viral infections. Also, the current concept is that once the initial myocardial inflammation is established, then a T cell-dependent autoimmune process takes place despite differences in the specific etiologic factor (Fig. 10.1). That autoimmune process is responsible for the self-sustained inflammation and progression to tissue damage leading to DCM. In general, it has been found that IFNγ play a paradoxical protective role, in opposition to other Th1 cytokines like IL12. Similar counterbalancing system exists between Th2 cytokines like IL4 and IL13. Notwithstanding, the Th17 response, and importantly its timing, is key in the progression of the acute disease to chronic damage and DCM, clinically the most severe complication of myocarditis. IL17A is not required during the acute phase, but IL23 is required to induce a pathogenic priming of self-reactive T cell clones in a GM-CSF-dependent manner. Importantly, the Th17 system is strictly required for the progression to DCM (Fig. 10.2). Despite the growing body of knowledge about the immunopathogenesis of myocarditis, the specific triggers and factors leading to progression in patients are still a conundrum. Also, since no risk or etiologic factor seems to be sufficient for the initiation and progression processes, post-myocarditis progression to DCM is still unpredictable in clinical practice. Advances exist in therapeutics, but still relying in global immunosuppression and unspecific immunomodulation, with is still suboptimal results. The expectation is that future basic and translational studies might provide even deeper insights in the pathogenesis of myocarditis. That would lead to development of better diagnostic tools allowing characterization and stratification of stages of myocarditis progression in each patient. Finally, that translational knowledge would make possible the development of individualized targeted treatments.

References

1. Mackay IR, Leskovsek NV, Rose NR. Cell damage and autoimmunity: a critical appraisal. J Autoimmun. 2008;30(1–2):5–11.
2. Bracamonte-Baran W, Burlingham W. Non-inherited maternal antigens, pregnancy, and allotolerance. Biom J. 2015;38(1):39–51.

3. Ozen S, Bilginer Y. A clinical guide to autoinflammatory diseases: familial Mediterranean fever and next-of-kin. Nat Rev Rheumatol. 2014;10(3):135–47.
4. Caforio AL, et al. Current state of knowledge on aetiology, diagnosis, management, and therapy of myocarditis: a position statement of the European Society of Cardiology Working Group on Myocardial and Pericardial Diseases. Eur Heart J. 2013;34(33):2636–48, 2648a–2648d.
5. Kindermann I, et al. Update on myocarditis. J Am Coll Cardiol. 2012;59(9):779–92.
6. Pollack A, et al. Viral myocarditis-diagnosis, treatment options, and current controversies. Nat Rev Cardiol. 2015;12(11):670–80.
7. Fabre A, Sheppard MN. Sudden adult death syndrome and other non-ischaemic causes of sudden cardiac death. Heart. 2006;92(3):316–20.
8. Cihakova D, Rose NR. Pathogenesis of myocarditis and dilated cardiomyopathy. Adv Immunol. 2008;99:95–114.
9. Ekstrom K, et al. Long-term outcome and its predictors in giant cell myocarditis. Eur J Heart Fail. 2016;18(12):1452–8.
10. Cooper LT, et al. The role of endomyocardial biopsy in the management of cardiovascular disease: a scientific statement from the American Heart Association, the American College of Cardiology, and the European Society of Cardiology. Endorsed by the Heart Failure Society of America and the Heart Failure Association of the European Society of Cardiology. J Am Coll Cardiol. 2007;50(19):1914–31.
11. Kindermann I, et al. Predictors of outcome in patients with suspected myocarditis. Circulation. 2008;118(6):639–48.
12. Daubeney PE, et al. Clinical features and outcomes of childhood dilated cardiomyopathy: results from a national population-based study. Circulation. 2006;114(24):2671–8.
13. Doolan A, Langlois N, Semsarian C. Causes of sudden cardiac death in young Australians. Med J Aust. 2004;180(3):110–2.
14. Baccouche H, et al. Diagnostic synergy of non-invasive cardiovascular magnetic resonance and invasive endomyocardial biopsy in troponin-positive patients without coronary artery disease. Eur Heart J. 2009;30(23):2869–79.
15. Abdel-Aty H, et al. Diagnostic performance of cardiovascular magnetic resonance in patients with suspected acute myocarditis: comparison of different approaches. J Am Coll Cardiol. 2005;45(11):1815–22.
16. Aletras AH, et al. ACUT2E TSE-SSFP: a hybrid method for T2-weighted imaging of edema in the heart. Magn Reson Med. 2008;59(2):229–35.
17. Basso C, et al. Postmortem diagnosis in sudden cardiac death victims: macroscopic, microscopic and molecular findings. Cardiovasc Res. 2001;50(2):290–300.
18. Gore I, Saphir O. Myocarditis; a classification of 1402 cases. Am Heart J. 1947;34(6): 827–30.
19. Richardson P, et al. Report of the 1995 World Health Organization/International Society and Federation of Cardiology Task Force on the Definition and Classification of cardiomyopathies. Circulation. 1996;93(5):841–2.
20. Felker GM, et al. The spectrum of dilated cardiomyopathy. The Johns Hopkins experience with 1,278 patients. Medicine (Baltimore). 1999;78(4):270–83.
21. Towbin JA, et al. Incidence, causes, and outcomes of dilated cardiomyopathy in children. JAMA. 2006;296(15):1867–76.
22. Cooper LT. Molecular biologic detection of virus infection in myocarditis and dilated cardiomyopathy. In: Cooper LT, editor. Myocarditis: from bench to bedside. Totowa: Humana Press; 2002. P. 295–324.
23. Leone O, et al. 2011 consensus statement on endomyocardial biopsy from the Association for European Cardiovascular Pathology and the Society for Cardiovascular Pathology. Cardiovasc Pathol. 2012;21(4):245–74.
24. Yilmaz A, et al. Coronary vasospasm as the underlying cause for chest pain in patients with PVB19 myocarditis. Heart. 2008;94(11):1456–63.
25. Baughman KL. Diagnosis of myocarditis: death of Dallas criteria. Circulation. 2006;113(4):593–5.

26. Aretz HT. Myocarditis: the Dallas criteria. Hum Pathol. 1987;18(6):619–24.
27. Okura Y, et al. A clinical and histopathologic comparison of cardiac sarcoidosis and idiopathic giant cell myocarditis. J Am Coll Cardiol. 2003;41(2):322–9.
28. Cooper LT Jr, et al. Usefulness of immunosuppression for giant cell myocarditis. Am J Cardiol. 2008;102(11):1535–9.
29. Maleszewski JJ, et al. Long-term risk of recurrence, morbidity and mortality in giant cell myocarditis. Am J Cardiol. 2015;115(12):1733–8.
30. Cooper LT Jr, Berry GJ, Shabetai R. Idiopathic giant-cell myocarditis – natural history and treatment. Multicenter Giant Cell Myocarditis Study Group Investigators. N Engl J Med. 1997;336(26):1860–6.
31. Cooper LT Jr, et al. Giant cell myocarditis. J Heart Lung Transplant. 1995;14(2):394–401.
32. Kong G, et al. Response of recurrent giant cell myocarditis in a transplanted heart to intensive immunosuppression. Eur Heart J. 1991;12(4):554–7.
33. Gries W, et al. Giant cell myocarditis: first report of disease recurrence in the transplanted heart. J Heart Lung Transplant. 1992;11(2 Pt 1):370–4.
34. Grant SC. Giant cell myocarditis in a transplanted heart. Eur Heart J. 1993;14(10):1437.
35. Grant SC. Recurrent giant cell myocarditis after transplantation. J Heart Lung Transplant. 1993;12(1 Pt 1):155–6.
36. Barin JG, et al. Fatal eosinophilic myocarditis develops in the absence of IFN-gamma and IL-17A. J Immunol. 2013;191(8):4038–47.
37. Busteed S, et al. Myocarditis as a prognostic indicator in systemic lupus erythematosus. Postgrad Med J. 2004;80(944):366–7.
38. Levin MD, Zoet-Nugteren SK, Markusse HM. Myocarditis and primary Sjogren's syndrome. Lancet. 1999;354(9173):128–9.
39. Barbaro G. Cardiovascular manifestations of HIV infection. Circulation. 2002;106(11):1420–5.
40. Frustaci A, et al. Biopsy-proven autoimmune myocarditis in HIV-associated dilated cardiomyopathy. BMC Infect Dis. 2014;14:729.
41. Halsell JS, et al. Myopericarditis following smallpox vaccination among vaccinia-naive US military personnel. JAMA. 2003;289(24):3283–9.
42. Root-Bernstein R, Fairweather D. Unresolved issues in theories of autoimmune disease using myocarditis as a framework. J Theor Biol. 2015;375:101–23.
43. Fairweather D, Rose NR. Coxsackievirus-induced myocarditis in mice: a model of autoimmune disease for studying immunotoxicity. Methods. 2007;41(1):118–22.
44. Cihakova D, et al. Animal models for autoimmune myocarditis and autoimmune thyroiditis. Methods Mol Med. 2004;102:175–93.
45. Donermeyer DL, et al. Myocarditis-inducing epitope of myosin binds constitutively and stably to I-Ak on antigen-presenting cells in the heart. J Exp Med. 1995;182(5):1291–300.
46. Pummerer CL, et al. Identification of cardiac myosin peptides capable of inducing autoimmune myocarditis in BALB/c mice. J Clin Invest. 1996;97(9):2057–62.
47. Li HS, Ligons DL, Rose NR. Genetic complexity of autoimmune myocarditis. Autoimmun Rev. 2008;7(3):168–73.
48. Barin JG, Cihakova D. Control of inflammatory heart disease by CD4+ T cells. Ann N Y Acad Sci. 2013;1285:80–96.
49. Frisancho-Kiss S, et al. Cutting edge: cross-regulation by TLR4 and T cell Ig mucin-3 determines sex differences in inflammatory heart disease. J Immunol. 2007;178(11):6710–4.
50. Goser S, et al. Cardiac troponin I but not cardiac troponin T induces severe autoimmune inflammation in the myocardium. Circulation. 2006;114(16):1693–702.
51. Elliott JF, et al. Autoimmune cardiomyopathy and heart block develop spontaneously in HLA-DQ8 transgenic IAbeta knockout NOD mice. Proc Natl Acad Sci U S A. 2003;100(23):13447–52.
52. Tarrio ML, et al. PD-1 protects against inflammation and myocyte damage in T cell-mediated myocarditis. J Immunol. 2012;188(10):4876–84.

53. Wang J, et al. PD-1 deficiency results in the development of fatal myocarditis in MRL mice. Int Immunol. 2010;22(6):443–52.
54. Keir ME, et al. PD-1 and its ligands in tolerance and immunity. Annu Rev Immunol. 2008;26:677–704.
55. Naidoo J, Page DB, Wolchok JD. Immune modulation for cancer therapy. Br J Cancer. 2014;111(12):2214–9.
56. Page DB, et al. Immune modulation in cancer with antibodies. Annu Rev Med. 2014;65:185–202.
57. Laubli H, et al. Acute heart failure due to autoimmune myocarditis under pembrolizumab treatment for metastatic melanoma. J Immunother Cancer. 2015;3:11.
58. Henke A, et al. The role of CD8+ T lymphocytes in coxsackievirus B3-induced myocarditis. J Virol. 1995;69(11):6720–8.
59. Huber SA, Gauntt CJ, Sakkinen P. Enteroviruses and myocarditis: viral pathogenesis through replication, cytokine induction, and immunopathogenicity. Adv Virus Res. 1998;51:35–80.
60. Fuse K, et al. Myeloid differentiation factor-88 plays a crucial role in the pathogenesis of Coxsackievirus B3-induced myocarditis and influences type I interferon production. Circulation. 2005;112(15):2276–85.
61. Fairweather D, Frisancho-Kiss S, Rose NR. Viruses as adjuvants for autoimmunity: evidence from Coxsackievirus-induced myocarditis. Rev Med Virol. 2005;15(1):17–27.
62. Wolfgram LJ, et al. Variations in the susceptibility to Coxsackievirus B3-induced myocarditis among different strains of mice. J Immunol. 1986;136(5):1846–52.
63. Fairweather D, et al. IL-12 protects against coxsackievirus B3-induced myocarditis by increasing IFN-gamma and macrophage and neutrophil populations in the heart. J Immunol. 2005;174(1):261–9.
64. Feldman AM, McNamara D. Myocarditis. N Engl J Med. 2000;343(19):1388–98.
65. Mahfoud F, et al. Blood pressure and heart rate predict outcome in patients acutely admitted with suspected myocarditis without previous heart failure. J Hypertens. 2012;30(6):1217–24.
66. Fairweather D, Frisancho-Kiss S, Rose NR. Sex differences in autoimmune disease from a pathological perspective. Am J Pathol. 2008;173(3):600–9.
67. Parks CG, et al. Expert panel workshop consensus statement on the role of the environment in the development of autoimmune disease. Int J Mol Sci. 2014;15(8):14269–97.
68. Ansari A, Maron BJ, Berntson DG. Drug-induced toxic myocarditis. Tex Heart Inst J. 2003;30(1):76–9.
69. Feenstra J, et al. Drug-induced heart failure. J Am Coll Cardiol. 1999;33(5):1152–62.
70. Lo MH, et al. Drug reaction with eosinophilia and systemic symptoms syndrome associated myocarditis: a survival experience after extracorporeal membrane oxygenation support. J Clin Pharm Ther. 2013;38(2):172–4.
71. Madan R, et al. Radiation induced heart disease: pathogenesis, management and review literature. J Egypt Natl Canc Inst. 2015;27(4):187–93.
72. Rose NR. Viral myocarditis. Curr Opin Rheumatol. 2016;28(4):383–9.
73. Wessely R, et al. Transgenic expression of replication-restricted enteroviral genomes in heart muscle induces defective excitation-contraction coupling and dilated cardiomyopathy. J Clin Invest. 1998;102(7):1444–53.
74. Wessely R, et al. Low-level expression of a mutant coxsackieviral cDNA induces a myocytopathic effect in culture: an approach to the study of enteroviral persistence in cardiac myocytes. Circulation. 1998;98(5):450–7.
75. Badorff C, et al. Enteroviral protease 2A cleaves dystrophin: evidence of cytoskeletal disruption in an acquired cardiomyopathy. Nat Med. 1999;5(3):320–6.
76. Kearney MT, et al. Viral myocarditis and dilated cardiomyopathy: mechanisms, manifestations, and management. Postgrad Med J. 2001;77(903):4–10.
77. Lodge PA, et al. Coxsackievirus B-3 myocarditis. Acute and chronic forms of the disease caused by different immunopathogenic mechanisms. Am J Pathol. 1987;128(3):455–63.

78. Ong S, et al. Natural killer cells limit cardiac inflammation and fibrosis by halting eosinophil infiltration. Am J Pathol. 2015;185(3):847–61.
79. Yao HL, et al. Gene expression analysis during recovery process indicates the mechanism for innate immune injury and repair from Coxsackievirus B3-induced myocarditis. Virus Res. 2016;213:314–21.
80. Benvenga S, Guarneri F. Molecular mimicry and autoimmune thyroid disease. Rev Endocr Metab Disord. 2016;17(4):485–98.
81. Fairweather D, et al. From infection to autoimmunity. J Autoimmun. 2001;16(3):175–86.
82. Phongsisay V. The immunobiology of Campylobacter jejuni: innate immunity and autoimmune diseases. Immunobiology. 2016;221(4):535–43.
83. Caforio AL, Mahon NJ, McKenna WJ. Cardiac autoantibodies to myosin and other heart-specific autoantigens in myocarditis and dilated cardiomyopathy. Autoimmunity. 2001;34(3):199–204.
84. Massilamany C, et al. Identification of novel mimicry epitopes for cardiac myosin heavy chain-alpha that induce autoimmune myocarditis in A/J mice. Cell Immunol. 2011;271(2):438–49.
85. Tzolovsky G, et al. Identification and phylogenetic analysis of *Drosophila melanogaster* myosins. Mol Biol Evol. 2002;19(7):1041–52.
86. Li Y, et al. Mimicry and antibody-mediated cell signaling in autoimmune myocarditis. J Immunol. 2006;177(11):8234–40.
87. Moudgil KD, Sercarz EE. Crypticity of self antigenic determinants is the cornerstone of a theory of autoimmunity. Discov Med. 2005;5(28):378–82.
88. Park AC, et al. Mucosal administration of collagen V ameliorates the atherosclerotic plaque burden by inducing interleukin 35-dependent tolerance. J Biol Chem. 2016;291(7):3359–70.
89. Lv H, et al. Impaired thymic tolerance to alpha-myosin directs autoimmunity to the heart in mice and humans. J Clin Invest. 2011;121(4):1561–73.
90. Carlquist JF, et al. HLA class II (DR and DQ) antigen associations in idiopathic dilated cardiomyopathy. Validation study and meta-analysis of published HLA association studies. Circulation. 1991;83(2):515–22.
91. Limas CJ, Limas C. HLA antigens in idiopathic dilated cardiomyopathy. Br Heart J. 1989;62(5):379–83.
92. Martinetti M, et al. HLA and immunoglobulin polymorphisms in idiopathic dilated cardiomyopathy. Hum Immunol. 1992;35(3):193–9.
93. Liu W, et al. Association of HLA class II DRB1, DPA1 and DPB1 polymorphism with genetic susceptibility to idiopathic dilated cardiomyopathy in Chinese Han nationality. Autoimmunity. 2006;39(6):461–7.
94. Rodriguez-Perez JM, et al. MHC class II genes in Mexican patients with idiopathic dilated cardiomyopathy. Exp Mol Pathol. 2007;82(1):49–52.
95. Lozano MD, et al. Human leukocyte antigen class II associations in patients with idiopathic dilated cardiomyopathy. Myocarditis Treatment Trial Investigators. J Card Fail. 1997;3(2):97–103.
96. Neu N, et al. Cardiac myosin induces myocarditis in genetically predisposed mice. J Immunol. 1987;139(11):3630–6.
97. Taneja V, et al. Spontaneous myocarditis mimicking human disease occurs in the presence of an appropriate MHC and non-MHC background in transgenic mice. J Mol Cell Cardiol. 2007;42(6):1054–64.
98. Guler ML, et al. Two autoimmune diabetes loci influencing T cell apoptosis control susceptibility to experimental autoimmune myocarditis. J Immunol. 2005;174(4):2167–73.
99. Aly M, et al. Complex genetic control of host susceptibility to coxsackievirus B3-induced myocarditis. Genes Immun. 2007;8(3):193–204.
100. Lin A, et al. 14 bp deletion polymorphism in the HLA-G gene is a risk factor for idiopathic dilated cardiomyopathy in a Chinese Han population. Tissue Antigens. 2007;70(5):427–31.

101. Hviid TV, Christiansen OB. Linkage disequilibrium between human leukocyte antigen (HLA) class II and HLA-G – possible implications for human reproduction and autoimmune disease. Hum Immunol. 2005;66(6):688–99.
102. Seko Y, et al. Roles of programmed death-1 (PD-1)/PD-1 ligands pathway in the development of murine acute myocarditis caused by coxsackievirus B3. Cardiovasc Res. 2007;75(1):158–67.
103. Futamatsu H, et al. Attenuation of experimental autoimmune myocarditis by blocking activated T cells through inducible costimulatory molecule pathway. Cardiovasc Res. 2003;59(1):95–104.
104. Abramson J, Goldfarb Y. AIRE: From promiscuous molecular partnerships to promiscuous gene expression. Eur J Immunol. 2016;46(1):22–33.
105. Abramson J, Husebye ES. Autoimmune regulator and self-tolerance – molecular and clinical aspects. Immunol Rev. 2016;271(1):127–40.
106. Metzger TC, Anderson MS. Control of central and peripheral tolerance by Aire. Immunol Rev. 2011;241(1):89–103.
107. Malchow S, et al. Aire enforces immune tolerance by directing autoreactive T cells into the regulatory T cell lineage. Immunity. 2016;44(5):1102–13.
108. Metzger TC, Anderson MS. Myocarditis: a defect in central immune tolerance? J Clin Invest. 2011;121(4):1251–3.
109. Smith SC, Allen PM. Myosin-induced acute myocarditis is a T cell-mediated disease. J Immunol. 1991;147(7):2141–7.
110. Takaba H, et al. Fezf2 orchestrates a thymic program of self-antigen expression for immune tolerance. Cell. 2015;163(4):975–87.
111. Damsker JM, Hansen AM, Caspi RR. Th1 and Th17 cells: adversaries and collaborators. Ann N Y Acad Sci. 2010;1183:211–21.
112. Kleinewietfeld M, Hafler DA. The plasticity of human Treg and Th17 cells and its role in autoimmunity. Semin Immunol. 2013;25(4):305–12.
113. Afanasyeva M, et al. Interleukin-12 receptor/STAT4 signaling is required for the development of autoimmune myocarditis in mice by an interferon-gamma-independent pathway. Circulation. 2001;104(25):3145–51.
114. Pope RM, Shahrara S. Possible roles of IL-12-family cytokines in rheumatoid arthritis. Nat Rev Rheumatol. 2013;9(4):252–6.
115. Sonderegger I, et al. Neutralization of IL-17 by active vaccination inhibits IL-23-dependent autoimmune myocarditis. Eur J Immunol. 2006;36(11):2849–56.
116. Olson BM, Sullivan JA, Burlingham WJ. Interleukin 35: a key mediator of suppression and the propagation of infectious tolerance. Front Immunol. 2013;4:315.
117. Wu L, et al. Pathogenic IL-23 signaling is required to initiate GM-CSF-driven autoimmune myocarditis in mice. Eur J Immunol. 2016;46(3):582–92.
118. Eriksson U, et al. Dual role of the IL-12/IFN-gamma axis in the development of autoimmune myocarditis: induction by IL-12 and protection by IFN-gamma. J Immunol. 2001;167(9):5464–9.
119. Eriksson U, et al. Lethal autoimmune myocarditis in interferon-gamma receptor-deficient mice: enhanced disease severity by impaired inducible nitric oxide synthase induction. Circulation. 2001;103(1):18–21.
120. Rangachari M, et al. T-bet negatively regulates autoimmune myocarditis by suppressing local production of interleukin 17. J Exp Med. 2006;203(8):2009–19.
121. Fairweather D, et al. Interferon-gamma protects against chronic viral myocarditis by reducing mast cell degranulation, fibrosis, and the profibrotic cytokines transforming growth factor-beta 1, interleukin-1 beta, and interleukin-4 in the heart. Am J Pathol. 2004;165(6):1883–94.
122. Fairweather D, et al. Complement receptor 1 and 2 deficiency increases coxsackievirus B3-induced myocarditis, dilated cardiomyopathy, and heart failure by increasing macrophages, IL-1beta, and immune complex deposition in the heart. J Immunol. 2006;176(6):3516–24.

123. Cihakova D, et al. Interleukin-13 protects against experimental autoimmune myocarditis by regulating macrophage differentiation. Am J Pathol. 2008;172(5):1195–208.
124. Afanasyeva M, et al. Experimental autoimmune myocarditis in A/J mice is an interleukin-4-dependent disease with a Th2 phenotype. Am J Pathol. 2001;159(1):193–203.
125. Baldeviano GC, et al. Interleukin-17A is dispensable for myocarditis but essential for the progression to dilated cardiomyopathy. Circ Res. 2010;106(10):1646–55.
126. Wu L, et al. Cardiac fibroblasts mediate IL-17A-driven inflammatory dilated cardiomyopathy. J Exp Med. 2014;211(7):1449–64.
127. Myers JM, et al. Cardiac myosin-Th17 responses promote heart failure in human myocarditis. JCI Insight. 2016;1(9).
128. Chen P, et al. Susceptibility to autoimmune myocarditis is associated with intrinsic differences in CD4(+) T cells. Clin Exp Immunol. 2012;169(2):79–88.
129. Shi Y, et al. Regulatory T cells protect mice against coxsackievirus-induced myocarditis through the transforming growth factor beta-coxsackie-adenovirus receptor pathway. Circulation. 2010;121(24):2624–34.
130. Brusko TM, Putnam AL, Bluestone JA. Human regulatory T cells: role in autoimmune disease and therapeutic opportunities. Immunol Rev. 2008;223:371–90.
131. Cheng HM, Chamley L. Cryptic natural autoantibodies and co-potentiators. Autoimmun Rev. 2008;7(6):431–4.
132. Caforio AL, et al. Circulating cardiac autoantibodies in dilated cardiomyopathy and myocarditis: pathogenetic and clinical significance. Eur J Heart Fail. 2002;4(4):411–7.
133. Wallukat G, Schimke I. Agonistic autoantibodies directed against G-protein-coupled receptors and their relationship to cardiovascular diseases. Semin Immunopathol. 2014;36(3):351–63.
134. Neumann DA, et al. Circulating heart-reactive antibodies in patients with myocarditis or cardiomyopathy. J Am Coll Cardiol. 1990;16(6):839–46.
135. Caforio AL, et al. Identification of alpha- and beta-cardiac myosin heavy chain isoforms as major autoantigens in dilated cardiomyopathy. Circulation. 1992;85(5):1734–42.
136. Caforio AL, et al. Idiopathic dilated cardiomyopathy: lack of association between circulating organ-specific cardiac antibodies and HLA-DR antigens. Tissue Antigens. 1992;39(5):236–40.
137. Gu C, et al. Apoptotic signaling through the beta-adrenergic receptor. A new Gs effector pathway. J Biol Chem. 2000;275(27):20726–33.
138. Staudt Y, et al. Beta1-adrenoceptor antibodies induce apoptosis in adult isolated cardiomyocytes. Eur J Pharmacol. 2003;466(1–2):1–6.
139. Christ T, et al. Autoantibodies against the beta1 adrenoceptor from patients with dilated cardiomyopathy prolong action potential duration and enhance contractility in isolated cardiomyocytes. J Mol Cell Cardiol. 2001;33(8):1515–25.
140. Lymperopoulos A, Rengo G, Koch WJ. Adrenergic nervous system in heart failure: pathophysiology and therapy. Circ Res. 2013;113(6):739–53.
141. Herda LR, et al. Effects of immunoadsorption and subsequent immunoglobulin G substitution on cardiopulmonary exercise capacity in patients with dilated cardiomyopathy. Am Heart J. 2010;159(5):809–16.
142. Trimpert C, et al. Immunoadsorption in dilated cardiomyopathy: long-term reduction of cardiodepressant antibodies. Eur J Clin Investig. 2010;40(8):685–91.
143. Muller J, et al. Immunoglobulin adsorption in patients with idiopathic dilated cardiomyopathy. Circulation. 2000;101(4):385–91.
144. Haberland A, et al. Aptamer neutralization of beta1-adrenoceptor autoantibodies isolated from patients with cardiomyopathies. Circ Res. 2011;109(9):986–92.
145. Marquis JK, Grindel JM. Toxicological evaluation of oligonucleotide therapeutics. Curr Opin Mol Ther. 2000;2(3):258–63.
146. Artis D, Spits H. The biology of innate lymphoid cells. Nature. 2015;517(7534):293–301.
147. Eberl G, Di Santo JP, Vivier E. The brave new world of innate lymphoid cells. Nat Immunol. 2015;16(1):1–5.

148. Grabie N, et al. Neutrophils sustain pathogenic CD8+ T cell responses in the heart. Am J Pathol. 2003;163(6):2413–20.
149. Barin JG, Rose NR, Cihakova D. Macrophage diversity in cardiac inflammation: a review. Immunobiology. 2012;217(5):468–75.
150. Bangert A, et al. Critical role of RAGE and HMGB1 in inflammatory heart disease. Proc Natl Acad Sci U S A. 2016;113(2):E155–64.
151. Su Z, et al. HMGB1 facilitated macrophage reprogramming towards a proinflammatory M1-like phenotype in experimental autoimmune myocarditis development. Sci Rep. 2016;6:21884.
152. Barin JG, et al. Macrophages participate in IL-17-mediated inflammation. Eur J Immunol. 2012;42(3):726–36.
153. Jensen LD, Marchant DJ. Emerging pharmacologic targets and treatments for myocarditis. Pharmacol Ther. 2016;161:40–51.
154. Escher F, et al. Long-term outcome of patients with virus-negative chronic myocarditis or inflammatory cardiomyopathy after immunosuppressive therapy. Clin Res Cardiol. 2016;105(12):1011–20.
155. Frustaci A, Russo MA, Chimenti C. Randomized study on the efficacy of immunosuppressive therapy in patients with virus-negative inflammatory cardiomyopathy: the TIMIC study. Eur Heart J. 2009;30(16):1995–2002.
156. Mason JW, et al. A clinical trial of immunosuppressive therapy for myocarditis. The Myocarditis Treatment Trial Investigators. N Engl J Med. 1995;333(5):269–75.
157. Menghini VV, et al. Combined immunosuppression for the treatment of idiopathic giant cell myocarditis. Mayo Clin Proc. 1999;74(12):1221–6.
158. Felix SB, et al. Hemodynamic effects of immunoadsorption and subsequent immunoglobulin substitution in dilated cardiomyopathy: three-month results from a randomized study. J Am Coll Cardiol. 2000;35(6):1590–8.
159. Knebel F, et al. Reduction of morbidity by immunoadsorption therapy in patients with dilated cardiomyopathy. Int J Cardiol. 2004;97(3):517–20.
160. Staudt A, et al. Effects of immunoadsorption on the nt-BNP and nt-ANP plasma levels of patients suffering from dilated cardiomyopathy. Ther Apher Dial. 2006;10(1):42–8.
161. Kishimoto C, et al. Therapy with immunoglobulin in patients with acute myocarditis and cardiomyopathy: analysis of leukocyte balance. Heart Vessel. 2014;29(3):336–42.
162. McNamara DM, et al. Controlled trial of intravenous immune globulin in recent-onset dilated cardiomyopathy. Circulation. 2001;103(18):2254–9.
163. Kuhl U, et al. Interferon-beta treatment eliminates cardiotropic viruses and improves left ventricular function in patients with myocardial persistence of viral genomes and left ventricular dysfunction. Circulation. 2003;107(22):2793–8.
164. Zimmermann O, et al. Interferon beta-1b therapy in chronic viral dilated cardiomyopathy – is there a role for specific therapy? J Card Fail. 2010;16(4):348–56.

Part IV
The Immune System in Repair and Regeneration After Myocardial Infarct

Chapter 11
Lymphocytes at the Heart of Wound Healing

Vânia Nunes-Silva, Stefan Frantz, and Gustavo Campos Ramos

11.1   Introduction

It has always been a crucial challenge to understand and foster wound healing - from the injuries suffered by our hunter-gather ancestors to the rise of modern pathology under the lenses of Virchow's microscope [1]. And if nowadays bows and arrows are no longer a relevant cause of wounds in modern society, it could be argued that the shifts in our ways of living over the past few millennia have also brought us unprecedented sources of tissue injury.

Emerging concepts in cardiology now suggest that the infarcted myocardium could be also perceived as a "wounded" tissue under frank repair process [2]. Thus, besides the classical concerns with the haemodynamic conditions, now the immune-inflammatory phenomena underlying myocardial healing process have started receiving attention. Such repair-oriented perspective of MI has expanded our concerns beyond the borders of cardiology and has raised new interesting possibilities to cope with infarcted patients. In the present chapter, we picture the infarcted heart from a "wound healing" perspective and focus on how lymphocyte-mediated phenomena contribute to myocardial repair.

V. Nunes-Silva
Instituto Gulbenkian de Ciência, PT-2781-901 Oeiras, Portugal

S. Frantz
Department of Internal Medicine III, University Clinic Halle, 06120 Halle, Germany

G.C. Ramos (✉)
Department of Internal Medicine III, University Clinic Halle, 06120 Halle, Germany

Martin-Luther-Universität Halle-Wittenberg Universitätsklinik und Poliklinik für Innere Medizin III, Ernst-Grube-Str. 40, 06120 Halle, Germany
e-mail: gustavo.ramos@uk-halle.de

© Springer International Publishing AG 2017   225
S. Sattler, T. Kennedy-Lydon (eds.), *The Immunology of Cardiovascular Homeostasis and Pathology*, Advances in Experimental Medicine and Biology 1003, DOI 10.1007/978-3-319-57613-8_11

11.1.1 Myocardial Injury and Repair

Myocardial infarction (MI) is defined as myocardial cell death triggered by pro-longed ischemia. Cardiomyocytes cannot endure persistent anoxic conditions, as their metabolism heavily relies on oxygen supply. Thus, obstructions in the coro-nary circulation (e.g. the rupture of an atherosclerotic plaque in human patients) normally cause myocardial necrosis and inflammation and impose a life-threatening acute functional impairment [3]. The prevalence of MI is extremely high in Western countries, being the single most frequent cause of death worldwide. It is estimated that every sixth man and every seventh woman in Europe will die from MI [3]. Although recent advances in medical attention have helped reducing the MI-induced mortality rates, the surviving patients often develop long-term complications such as adverse remodelling and heart failure [4]. This occurs because the adult mam-malian myocardium normally repairs injuries via replacing the contractile cells by a fibrotic scar, as cardiomyocytes exhibit negligible mitotic activity [5, 6]. Thus, in order to improve post-MI conditions, we need to understand in details the immuno-logical mechanisms underlying myocardial healing.

A schematic representation depicting the major events following a MI is pre-sented in Fig. 11.1. In brief, neutrophils and pro-inflammatory monocytes readily accumulate into the injured tissue, promoting the clearance of cell debris, digestion of extracellular matrix (ECM), and eventually causing secondary cardiomyocyte

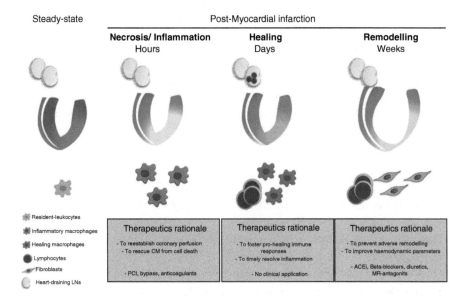

Fig. 11.1 Healing after myocardial infarction is studied in three major overlapping phases termed inflammatory, healing and remodelling (see text for details). Therapeutic approaches aimed at reducing infarct size (in acute term) or at holding the progression to HF (at late term) are widely available. However, until now, no approach aiming at improving the myocardial repair conditions is available for clinical applications

cell death [7]. Excessive myocardial inflammation can promote collateral damage and contribute to infarct expansion. However, it should be stressed that *in situ* inflammation is not necessarily harmful, as it is a necessary step towards tissue repair. It has been reported that insufficient removal of necrotic cell debris can also lead to thrombi formation and increased mortality rates [8].

Within a few days post-MI, T-cells are primed against cardiac antigens and expand at the heart-draining lymph nodes [9]. At the end of the first week, the early inflammatory reaction gives way to a healing phase in which a new ECM and new blood vessels are rebuild. The infiltration of T- and B-cells peaks at this stage [10]. Dying neutrophils are cleared by local macrophages that switch their phenotypic polarization to support healing rather than inflammation [11]. This switch occurs, at least in part, in a mechanism dependent on $Foxp3^+CD4^+$ T-cells/macrophage signalling cross talk [12]. Because cardiomyocytes cannot be generated at reasonable amount in the mammalian adult myocardium, the tissue repair follows a fibrotic path. The effective construction of a fibrous scar tissue in the heart is important to avoid cardiac rupture. However, excessive fibrosis and remodelling may result in gross alterations in the cardiac geometry and impact the overall contractile function, often leading to HF [6]. Despite the preponderant role played by the immune system in mediating myocardial repair, all the therapeutic approaches currently available to treat MI patients have been designed to modulate cardiovascular rather than immunological mechanisms. In acute term, the therapeutic rationale is primarily designed to preserve the myocardium at risk and minimise the damage (e.g. anticoagulants, reperfusion). In later (chronic) stages, the therapeutic strategies focus in controlling the haemodynamic conditions that contribute to the HF progression (e.g. beta-blockers, diuretics, Angiotensin-II Receptor antagonists). To address this therapeutical gap and provide new tools to foster myocardial repair is therefore a major task of the raising field of immunocardiology (Fig. 11.1).

The contribution of monocytes, macrophages, neutrophils and other innate mechanisms to the post-MI inflammation and repair has been a subject of intensive research over the last decades [7, 8, 13]. In sharp contrast, the role played by lymphocytes in these conditions has only recently started to be uncovered [14]. From a lymphocyte perspective, MI is an odd situation. It is a sterile injury coupled to massive necrosis of a unique tissue. It is not rare to observe human patients showing MI area comprising >30% of the left ventricle, and in the murine LAD ligation model, the injured area can easily surpass 50%. Thus, upon MI, there is an enormous amount of tissue-restricted cytosolic proteins (e.g. cardiac myosin heavy chain and troponin-I) that are abruptly released in the circulation and lymph and that become available to interact with lymphocytes in an inflamed context. Furthermore, it has been demonstrated that the cardiac-specific myosin heavy chain isoform is not expressed in the thymus of mice and humans, indicating that immunological central tolerance to this heart-restricted protein might be impaired, as compared to other auto-antigens [15].

Beyond causing the release of a considerable amount of heart-specific antigens, the MI situation also imposes a unique context for lymphocyte activation. Because the cardiac function is so central to body maintenance, the acute post-infarction cardiac impairment triggers important autonomic reflexes (e.g. sympathetic overdrive) that can also impact lymphocytes' physiology in nonclassical fashion.

Thus, on the one hand, the MI situation pushes the limits of cardiology, by bringing the "inflammation/repair" problem into the centre of a cardiovascular-oriented field. On the other hand, by framing lymphocyte activity in an unusual cardiovascular context, the MI condition also expands the borders of immunology towards a more physiological perspective.

11.2   B-Cells and Autoantibodies in Myocardial Injury and Repair

Back in 1890, von Behring and Kitasato created the term antikörper (antibodies) to describe antitoxins present in the serum of immunized animals. It took nearly 50 years until serum gamma globulins could be identified as structural counterpart of antibodies and another 15 years until the plasma cells were discovered as antibody-producing cells. It was not before 1965 that the lymphocyte division of labour was considered, so that B (from *b*ursa of Fabricius/*b*one marrow)- and T (*t*hymus)-cells were described as distinct lymphocyte subsets. This means that our knowledge on antibodies is about 75 years older than on B-cells [16, 17], a historical fact that still echoes in our current knowledge. It is therefore not surprising to observe that the literature on heart-specific autoantibodies highly outnumbers the few studies addressing the cellular aspects of post-MI B-lymphocyte activity [18–21].

11.2.1   *Autoantibodies*

Antibodies reactive to cardiac antigens have been found in the sera of rodents and patients in several conditions such as ischemia/reperfusion injury [22, 23], myocardial infarction [21], chronic heart failure [20], Chagas disease [24] and autoimmune myocarditis [25]. The immunoglobulin reactivity profile described in all those different pathological conditions exhibits a high degree of similarity, and most specificities fall into three major categories: (1) antibodies recognizing contractile elements, including myosins, actins and troponins [19, 21]; (2) anti-receptor antibodies, often exhibiting agonistic effects [26]; and (3) natural autoantibodies recognizing conserved epitopes presented on the surface of altered/dying cells [23]. Yet, it remains under dispute whether autoantibodies targeting cardiac antigens should be perceived as disease-modifying agents or simply as biomarkers for cardiac injury.

Besides specificity, other factors such as immunoglobulin *isotype* and *timing* might also be considered, as they can critically influence the outcome of immune responses. For instance, whereas IgM and the murine IgG3 can activate the complement system and start a local inflammatory reaction, other IgG isotypes and IgAs primarily act via signalling through Fc-receptors [27, 28].

The timing of antibody response to the injured myocardium is also of major importance, although it is often a neglected issue. For the sake of clarification, we herein

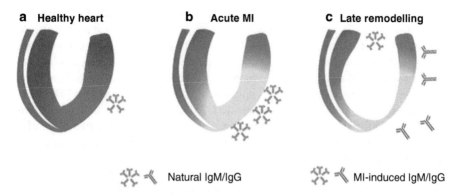

Fig. 11.2 The role of autoantibodies at different stages of myocardial ischemic injury and repair. Natural autoantibodies reactive to ischemia-related antigens and to apoptotic cells can be detected in the sera of healthy subjects, under physiological conditions (**a**). Thus, with the onset of myocardial infarction, such pre-existing natural autoantibodies can readily accumulate at the ischemic heart and trigger in situ inflammation by means of activating the complement system (**b**). In addition, the massive myocardial necrosis results in a leakage of several heart-associated proteins into the lymph and circulation, bringing about neoreactivities against heart components at later stages (**c**). Thus, whereas the pre-existing natural IgMs may engage in early inflammatory/healing processes, the MI-induced IgGs have been implicated in the long-term heart failure progression

approach this subject in two different topics: (1) the role of natural (i.e. pre-existing) autoantibodies in the early onset of myocardial ischemic diseases and (2) the role of injury-triggered neoreactivities in modulating the late cardiac remodelling (Fig. 11.2).

11.2.1.1 Natural Autoantibodies in Acute Myocardial Injury

Most of the literature on antibody production has focused on ill patients or on animals challenged with specific antigens. In such situations, immunoglobulin production peaks within a few days upon injury/challenge, as it relies on the activation, expansion and differentiation of antigen-specific B-cells. In the context of MI, this would indicate that neoreactivities directed to heart antigens released by dying cells are most likely to influence the late post-MI remodelling, but not the early in situ inflammatory and healing processes. Indeed, the vast majority of the literature on autoantibodies and MI has focused on late remodelling/HF events. However, it should be stressed that healthy subjects (and mice which haven't been through the hands of immunologists) contain an enormous and diverse pool of circulating immunoglobulins (circa 5–10 mg/ml) that can potentially recognize antigens exposed in the ischemic myocardium [22, 23, 29–33]. Such antibodies that spontaneously arise under physiological conditions and in the absence of overt specific antigenic stimulation are referred to as "natural antibodies" [29]. Of particular relevance to the myocardial infarction context (which is a sterile injury), it should be stressed that the vast majority of natural antibodies primarily recognize self-antigens [29, 30, 33–36]. In fact, the production of natural IgMs is largely independent on external antigenic contacts, as germ-free mice produce a normal IgM repertoire [31]. This reinforces the idea that natural autoantibodies are not mere side products of previous immunizations and might rather have physiological roles.

In the context of tissue injury and repair, it has been shown that natural immunoglobulins can readily accumulate (within 6–24 h) in the wounded skin [37], ischemic intestine [38], muscle [39] and heart [22, 23]. Some of these immunoglobulins have been reported to recognize antigens presented on altered/damaged cells, triggering subsequent local inflammatory reaction [23] and facilitating the clearance of apoptotic corpses in injured tissue [40].

Experimental evidences raised back at the 1990s first indicated that some natural IgMs can recognize ischemia-associated antigens and subsequently elicit complement-mediated local inflammatory responses [39, 41]. In this context, Zhang et al. [38] isolated an IgM-producing B-cell clone (CM22) that recognizes a specific neoantigen expressed on the surface of ischemic cells [38]. Of note, this B-cell clone was isolated from resident peritoneal cells harvested from healthy (non-immunized) mice, i.e. it was by definition a natural autoantibody-producing B-cell clone. Further analysis identified the cognate antigen as being the non-muscle myosin heavy chain type II (NMHC-II) [42]. This myosin isoform shares 40% homology with the cardiac myosin heavy chain and can be constitutively found in the cytoplasm of most cell types where it modulates cytokinesis, cell motility and shape. According to these authors, the non-motor myosin isoform is translocated to the outer cytoplasmic membrane under hypoxic conditions, getting therefore accessible to natural IgMs. A schematic representation of the major epitopes described in different myosin molecules is presented in Fig. 11.3.

Carroll's group have convincingly demonstrated that the "NMHC-II - natural IgM - complement system" axis work in tandem to start inflammation in different tissues submitted to ischemia/reperfusion injury, including the myocardium [23, 42, 44]. Furthermore, these authors reported that blocking such anti-NMHC-II natural autoantibodies using a mimicking peptide resulted in attenuated ischemia-induced myocardial injury [23]. Additional evidences coming from other independent groups give further support to the idea that natural IgMs can contribute to the myocardial ischemia-reperfusion injury [22, 45].

Taken together, the above-mentioned studies indicate that natural IgMs can fuel the inflammatory response that occurs in the early stages of ischemia/reperfusion injury and therefore contribute to tissue damage. Still, one might be careful not to assume that myocardial inflammation is only detrimental. Although destructive, inflammation paves the way for tissue repair [46]. Thus, it should be pondered that natural autoantibodies could also mediate salutary events. This has been proven to be the case in the context of atherosclerosis [47] and cutaneous wound healing [37], situations in which natural IgMs facilitated the clearance of necrotic cell debris and accelerated the tissue repair process.

It is therefore plausible to consider that, beyond driving myocardial inflammation, natural IgMs could also influence other myocardial healing processes, such as angiogenesis, phenotypic polarization of infiltrating cells and extracellular matrix remodelling. These points should be further addressed in future investigations.

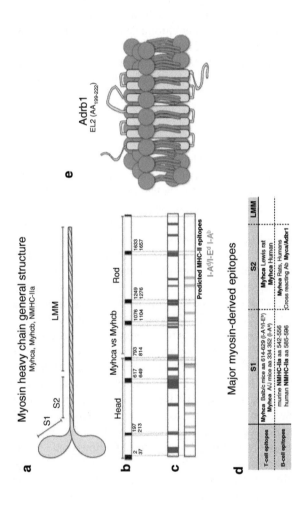

Fig. 11.3 Deciphering the major cardiac antigens. The cardiac myosin has been reported to be a major antigenic source for both B- and T-lymphocytes. (**a**) General structure of the myosin-II family members. Proteolysis protocols to dissect the myosin structure revealed two major myosin fragments, a larger N-terminal heavy meromyosin (HMM) and a C-terminal light meromyosin (LMM). The HMM is consisted of two globular heads (termed sub-fragment S1), connected to a hinge structure (S2), bridging HMM to a long dimeric coiled-coil rod (LMM). (**b**) Although myosin heavy chains alpha (myhca) and beta (myhcb) share 93% homology, the differences are enough to trigger nonoverlapping specific immune responses. The major regions of discrepancy between the myca and myhcb are presented as *black* bars in the protein linear structure. Important amino acid residues are described (Figure adapted from Pummerer et al. [43]). (**c**) In silico prediction of the capacity of myca-derived specific peptides to be presented at different murine MHC-II haplotypes is shown in *blue* (I-A^d) and in *green* (I-A^b) (according to the IEDB Analysis Resource tool, National institute of Allergy and Infectious Disease). (**d**) Most of myosin-reacting autoantibodies produced in mice, rats and humans recognize epitopes at the S2 regions, whereas most T-cell MHC-II-restricted antigens are distributed rather at the S1 region. (**e**) Antibodies targeting the second extracellular loop of the adrenergic receptor beta-1 often exhibit agonistic effects (see text)

11.2.1.2 Injury-Induced Autoantibodies and Heart Failure

Besides the natural autoantibodies that are readily available to react to the infarcted myocardium, heart-directed neoreactivities have also been reported in MI patients and rodents [21]. In this case, it is assumed that myocardial necrosis will cause a leakage of several cardiac proteins to the mediastinal lymph nodes and the circulation. These antigens can then be accessed by B- and T-cells in an inflammatory context, propitious to raise specific immune responses. The injury-induced autoantibodies (mainly IgGs) have been linked to rather chronic/late events such as post-MI myocardial remodelling and heart failure (Fig. 11.2) [20]. In the next few lines, we will review the major cardiac antigenic sources triggering autoantibody-mediated responses in the context of myocardial infarction and heart failure progression.

Cardiac Myosin

The myosin heavy chain alpha (myhca, a product of the *Myh6* gene) is the major isoform expressed in the cardiac muscle, in contrast to the isoform beta (myhcb) that is expressed in skeletal muscle cells and in embryonic cardiomyocytes. The two myosin isoforms share circa 93% similarity, but this apparently slight difference is enough to trigger specific immune responses that are able to discriminate between cardiac and skeletal muscle tissues [43]. The NMHC-II (above-discussed) is also a member of the same protein family. The cardiac isoform of the myosin heavy chain converges several unique features that make them a particularly relevant source of cardiac antigens in the MI context. It is a tissue-restricted protein, expressed at high levels in cardiomyocytes, and it is not expressed in the thymus, meaning that central tolerance to this protein is not operational [15]. Several independent studies have reported presence of anti-myosin, anti-actin and anti-troponin autoantibodies in the sera of patients with MI, ischemic HF and even under physiological conditions [21, 33, 48, 49]. Furthermore, in some clinical studies, it has been observed that the anti-myosin antibody titres correlate with poorer prognosis, indicating that anti-myosin antibodies could be of clinical relevance [50]. Still, the question whether such autoantibodies targeting contractile elements that are normally confined to the intracellular space could contribute to post-MI remodelling is a highly debatable issue.

On the one hand, a plausible interpretation of these clinical findings could be that elevated anti-myosin antibody titres are simply a readout for myocardial damage, with no direct implication to disease progression. Supporting this line of reasoning, Dangas et al. [48] observed that higher anti-myosin and anti-actin antibody titres correlated with higher circulating levels of troponin-I, which is a biomarker for cardiomyocyte necrosis.

On the other hand, experimental evidence suggesting an active role of anti-myosin antibodies in mediating post-MI remodelling and heart failure have also been reported. Warraich et al. [51] demonstrated that specific anti-myosin IgGs purified from patients with ischemic heart disease can directly impair the contractility of cardiomyocytes in culture. Furthermore, it has been demonstrated that the administration of myhca adsorbed in adjuvants can induce autoimmune myocarditis and the deposition of heart-reactive autoantibodies in some susceptible mouse strains [52]. In the same line of arguments, Caforio et al. [53] observed that affinity-purified IgGs isolated from myocarditis patients can induce heart failure when transferred into BALB/c recipient mice. Last but not least, experimental evidence coming from Cunningham's lab indicates that some anti-myosin autoantibodies produced in rats can cross-react to epitopes on beta-1-adrenergic receptors and stimulate downstream signalling pathway [54]. Taken together, these findings suggest that myosin-like antigenic determinants can be expressed on the surface of cardiomyocytes even under steady-state conditions and thus that myosin-specific antibodies could mediate disease progression.

Antibodies Targeting Adrenergic Receptors

During the past decades, independent groups have also reported the presence of autoantibodies targeting beta-1-adrenergic receptors (Adrb1) in patients with myocardial infarction and heart failure [26, 55–57]. Further analysis identified that autoantibodies targeting epitopes on the second extracellular loop of the Adrb1 (ECL2) can stimulate downstream signalling and directly influence cardiomyocytes' activity [55, 58–60]. A clinical study reported the presence of agonistic anti-Adrb1 antibodies in 26% and 13% of patients with dilated cardiomyopathy (DCM) and ischemic cardiomyopathy patients (ICM), respectively [61]. Furthermore, the presence of such adrenergic-stimulating autoantibodies correlated with increased mortality (49% versus 80% all-cause mortality in ICM patients negative or positive for anti-Adbr1, respectively) [61]. Supporting the notion that such autoantibodies can actively promote myocardial disease, Jahns et al. [62] demonstrated that rats immunized with a peptide derived from the adrenergic receptor's ECL2 develop progressive left ventricular dilation and dysfunction [55, 62]. In this context, a cyclic peptide (COR-1) able to neutralize the anti-Adrb1 pathogenic antibodies is currently being tested in a phase I clinical trial [63]. A schematic representation of the major epitopes described in different myosin molecules is presented in Fig. 11.3.

11.2.2 Beyond Autoantibodies: The Roles of B-Cells in Myocardial Diseases

B-cells are not mere precursors of antibody-secreting cells. They can influence tissue repair via several other mechanisms, including the production of cytokines, chemokines and growth factors, or via direct cell-cell contact. Furthermore, B-lymphocytes also express high levels of innate pattern recognition receptors (including TLR4) that can also trigger strong polyclonal B-cell activation that is independent of their specificity [64–67].

Previous studies revealed that B-cells are readily recruited to the murine infarcted heart, peaking at around 5–7 days post-MI [10, 68]. The infiltrating B-cells were characterized as being mainly mature cells expressing $CD19^+ IgD^+IgM^{low}$. A similar kinetics of B-cell infiltration has also been observed in experimental models for cutaneous wound healing [69]. Whether infiltrating B-cells receive antigenic stimulation (via BCRs) or simply respond to rather unspecific inflammatory signals (via TLRs) remains an open question.

Regarding to the role played by such acutely infiltrating B-cells in post-MI in situ inflammation, Zouggari et al. [68] found that the myocardial B-cells express Ccl7, a chemokine that mediates monocyte recruitment via the CCR2 receptor. Furthermore, after performing B-cell depletion with an anti-CD20 monoclonal antibody, authors observed reduced monocyte recruitment and infarct size.

In a different experimental setup, Goodchild et al. [70] reported that intramyocardial injection of bone marrow-derived B-lymphocytes into infarcted Sprague Dawley rats had rather beneficial effects, as it reduced in situ apoptosis and helped in preserving ejection fraction. An important difference between those studies is that Goodchild et al. [70] might have transferred immature bone marrow B-cells, which are believed to be resistant to CD20mAB-mediated B-cell depletion used by Zouggari et al. [68].

These conflicting results indicate that, although promising, the emerging field of immunocardiology has so far accumulated more questions than answers. Yet, targeting B-cells in the MI context might hold interesting therapeutical perspectives, for several reasons. B-cells can readily respond to unspecific inflammatory stimulation and accumulate in the injured myocardium where they can fine-tune the local molecular milieu [71]. In addition, B-cells can also mediate long-lasting effects via bridging innate and adaptive immune mechanisms, especially via interacting with T-cells [72]. Further experimental studies addressing those questions shall shed some light in this incipient field.

11.3   T-Cell Biology and Overall Role in Tissue Repair

T-cells can be distinguished from other cell lineages by the presence of a T-cell receptor (TCR) on their surface, which is constructed after somatic recombination of V (variable), D (diversity) and J (joining) gene segments, in addition to a constant (C) region [73]. The TCR is a heterodimer composed by two protein chains that are complexed on the membrane with different CD3 chains. The most frequent subset of T-cells rearranges the TCR alpha and beta chains (hence, termed as $\alpha\beta$-T-cells), while only a minority subset rearranges the TCR gamma and delta chains ($\gamma\delta$-T-cells) [73].

Different to B-cells that can directly interact with soluble antigens, $\alpha\beta$-T-cells can only recognize peptides presented by other cells on the major histocompatibility complex (MHC), a phenomenon termed as MHC restriction. In this context, $\alpha\beta$-T-cells can be subdivided into cytotoxic (CD8$^+$ T-cells) and helper (CD4$^+$ T-cells). CD8$^+$T-cells interact with peptides presented on MHC-I complexes, expressed on all nucleated cells, whereas CD4$^+$T-cells interact with antigens presented on MHC-II molecules, known to be most commonly expressed in antigen presenting cells (APC) such as macrophages, dendritic cells and B-cells. Peptides loaded on MHC-I molecules are typically composed of eight to nine amino acid residues, whereas antigens presented on MHC-II context can be longer, reaching 14–20 residues in length [74–76].

Besides TCR interaction with its cognate antigen via MHC interaction, other co-stimulatory and inhibitory molecules presented on the surface of APCs also influence the outcome of T-cell activation (e.g. via interacting with CD28 and PD-1 receptors on T-cells). It is generally assumed that these co-stimulatory signals received by T-cells during priming will shape their cytokine and chemokine expression profile upon activation, hence defining their function and migratory patterns [74–76]. For instance, it was recently proposed that T-cell priming in the presence of hepatocyte growth factor (HGF) confers cardiotropism to T-cells by inducing a specialized homing signature c-Met$^+$ CCR4$^+$ CXCR3$^+$. Of note, HGF is expressed by cardiomyocytes and can accumulate in the heart-draining lymph nodes [77].

T-cells are often classified into different functional categories, according to their phenotypic polarization. The first subdivision of CD4$^+$ T-cell subsets based on the cytokine expression profile was made in the 1980s, after comparing the response patterns of different mouse strains. Accordingly, it was observed that CD4$^+$ T-cells obtained from C57BL/6 mice typically responded to in vitro stimulation by producing IFNy, TNF and IL12, whereas CD4$^+$ T-cells obtained from Balb/C mice primarily produced IL4, IL-5 and IL-13. These observations lead to the creation of a dichotomy ceasing T-helper cells into two subsets: the Th1 and Th2 [78]. Most recently further subsets were identified expressing other unique cytokine profiles (e.g. Th3, Th17, Th9), considerably expanding the list of T-helper subsets. Nevertheless, it should be stressed that T-cell phenotypes not always fall into completely discrete categories (especially human T-cells) and that interchange between classical phenotypes can occur under some circumstances [79].

Additional CD4$^+$ and CD8$^+$ T-cell subsets have also been characterized based on their ability to counterbalance classical immune responses. In this context, the most well-characterized T-cell subset exhibiting "homeostatic" functions is the so-called "regulatory CD4$^+$ T-cells" (Tregs) expressing the transcription factor Forkhead box P3 (Foxp3) [80–83].

Tregs are important components maintaining immune system homeostasis and are mostly known for their ability to suppress pro-inflammatory and "classic" immune responses. However, apart from their classical role in suppressing immune responses, Tregs have also been implicated in other physiological contexts, such as the regulation of metabolic indices in visceral adipose tissue and in tissue repair. For instance, Mathis' group has recently described a novel-specific Treg population that readily accumulates in the injured skeletal muscle and promotes tissue regeneration by signalling to local stem cells [84]. These muscle Tregs presented a skewed TCR repertoire diversity (suggestive of clonal expansion) and express high levels of IL-10 and amphiregulin. Interleukin-10 is a potent anti-inflammatory mediator with clear anti-fibrotic effects, whereas amphiregulin is a growth factor that induces differentiation of the muscle-resident progenitor cells [84].

Foxp3+ and Foxp3− CD4+ T-cell subsets display different (though overlapping) TCR repertoires. Foxp3+ Tregs exhibit enriched reactivity to self-antigens and lower activation threshold, making them more likely than conventional T-cells to become rapidly activated in the presence of auto-antigens [85, 86]. These features might have relevant implications to sterile inflammatory conditions such as MI. Of note, Arpaia et al. [87] recently demonstrated that different Treg functions imply distinct activation clues. Using an influenza infection model, they propose that whereas TCR stimulation is required for Tregs to mediate immune suppression, the amphiregulin production (leading to tissue repair) was reported to rely on cytokine signalling, rather than on antigenic stimulation.

11.3.1   T-Cell Dynamics In Myocardial Injury

It takes days to mount specific T-cell responses, as it relies on antigen processing/presentation and subsequent proliferation of antigen-specific cells. This would indicate that T-cells would not be relevant in the early events following a MI. However, recent experimental evidences challenge this common sense as they indicate that T-lymphocytes can readily infiltrate the infarcted myocardium (Fig. 11.4) and influence local inflammation and healing processes.

Using an experimental model of ischemia/reperfusion (I/R), Yang et al. [88] reported a decrease in peripheral blood lymphocytes 60 min after reperfusion. In parallel, the number of CD3+ T-lymphocytes was significantly increased in the myocardium (most likely in the coronary circulation) within 2 min after the initiation of reperfusion. No further increase was observed during the first hour of reperfusion. In the permanent coronary occlusion model, infiltrating CD4+T-cells, CD8+T-cells and γδT-cells started to increase gradually and peak on day 7 after MI [10]. IFNγ-producing T-cells (Th1) as well as Foxp3+Tregs were the predominant subsets of CD4+T cells seen after MI, whereas other cytokine-producing T-cell responses were barely detected [9].

Beyond the recruitment of T-cells from the circulation to the infarcted myocardium, another possibility to be considered is the putative contribution of tissue-resident cells to post-MI inflammation and healing. Emerging evidences have

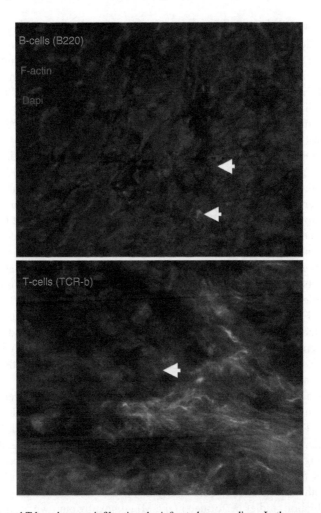

Fig. 11.4 B- and T-lymphocytes infiltrating the infarcted myocardium. In the *upper* micrograph, it is possible to distinguish the viable cardiomyocytes (*green*, Factin⁺) and the necrotic area, with a massive cellular infiltrate (nuclei stained with DAPI, *blue*). Sparse B-cells are seen in *red* (CD19⁺ cells) amongst other non-identified infiltrating cells. In the *lower* micrograph, it is possible to observe an infiltrating T-cell (TCRβ⁺) in a necrotic area, characterized by the presence of disarranged F-actin filaments (Own unpublished data)

reported the presence of tissue-resident T-cells in several organs at steady state [89, 90], including the heart [91]. In tissues other than the myocardium, such tissue-resident T-cells have been reported to exhibit a differentiated phenotype and to readily respond to tissue injury. It remains therefore to be established whether resident lymphocytes can contribute to reactions to MI.

The roles of T-cells in myocardial repair seem to vary according to the injury model studied (transient vs permanent coronary artery ligation) and also depending on time (acute vs chronic) [92]. CD4[+] T-cells seem to have detrimental effects in the early set of I/R injury (transient LAD ligation), as they can contribute to exacerbate inflammation and trigger further myocardial damage. However, the same T-cell compartment has been shown to later facilitate the resolution of inflammation and to foster the healing phase of myocardial repair in a model of permanent LAD ligation [92].

Early evidences indicating that T-cells can influence myocardial I/R injury came from Yang et al. [88]. By measuring the extent of myocardial injury 60 min after I/R, they showed that lymphocyte-deficient RAG1KO animals had smaller lesions after LAD ligation as compared to WT animals. By using antibody depletion prior to I/R injury in WT animals, they were able to show that CD4[+] T-cells, but not CD8[+], were involved in enhancing disease severity. Reconstitution of Rag1KO animals with WT CD4[+] T-cells was sufficient to revert the protective effect of lymphocyte deficiency. Although several reports show that Treg activation protects against experimental I/R injury in other organs, such as the liver and kidney, little is known about the role of this subset in myocardial I/R [93]. On the one hand, Fang et al. reported that Tregs contribute to the rosuvastatin-induced cardioprotection against myocardial I/R injury [94]. On the other hand, Mathes et al. recently reported that specific ablation of Foxp3[+] Tregs resulted in decreased infarct size, uncovering a potentially detrimental effect of Tregs in the myocardial I/R injury model [95].

The involvement of T-cells in MI was further dissected in a model with permanent LAD-ligation. Hofmann et al. [9] showed that at day 7 after MI, both conventional and Treg subsets became activated in the mediastinal heart-draining lymph node. An accumulation of CD4[+] T-cells in the injured myocardium was also reported. By inducing MI on CD4 KO, MHC class II KO and OT-II mice (bearing a transgenic TCR for an irrelevant antigen), it was shown that impairment of CD4 activation through TCR resulted in healing defects.

Treg ablation studies performed in the MI context by our own group [12] and by others [96–100] revealed that the Foxp3[+] CD4[+] cells critically mediate myocardial repair and foster the formation of a stable scar. Accordingly, Treg-depleted mice presented reduced survival rates, reduced fractional shortening and accentuated myocardial dilation upon MI [12, 97]. In addition, it has also been reported that increasing the frequency activity of Foxp3[+] CD4[+] cells, either by adoptive cell transfer or by with a CD28 superagonist antibody, positively impacts the post-MI healing outcome [96, 97, 99, 100].

Data from our group has shown that macrophages co-cultured with Tregs upregulated the expression level of genes associated with the healing process like Osteopontin, arginase-1 and CD206 [12]. Furthermore, the same genes were found to be upregulated in the scar of mice treated with the anti-CD28 superagonist, an antibody known to promote the preferencial expansion of Tregs over Tconvs [101]. Saxena et al. [99] observed that cardiac fibroblasts cultured in the presence of Tregs presented reduced alpha-SMA and MMP-3 mRNA expression, indicating that Tregs may attenuate the pro-remodelling activity of cardiac fibroblasts. In addition, Tang et al. [100] observed that Tregs can also exert direct effects on cardiomyocytes. By using a co-culture experimental setup, these authors observed that Tregs protected rat neonatal cardiomyocytes from the LPS-induced cell death. Taken together, these studies indicate that modulating the activity or frequency of Foxp3+CD4+ T-cells in the MI context could be of clinical value [102].

Because the MI situation sufficiently differs from other classical immunological diseases and models, it is plausible to assume that other unconventional lymphocyte subsets might also influence post-MI responses in unprecedented fashions. For instance, Curato et al. [103] described a subset of CD8+ T-cells expressing the angiotensin II receptor 2 (ATR2) that expanded in response to myocardial ischemic injury and produced IL-10 in response to angiotensin II stimulation. More recently, Skorska et al. [104] reported a similar anti-inflammatory ATR2+ CD4+ T-cell subset. These findings are particularly interesting and relevant because they frame T-cell activation in the cardiovascular context. A schematic presentation on the roles played by T-cells in post-MI inflammation and healing is presented in Fig. 11.5.

Last but not least, it is important to stress that even though pro-inflammatory factors are usually described as enhancers of tissue damage, evidences showing they can positively influence cardiac disease progression also exist. In experimental auto-immune myocarditis model (e.g. mice injected with myosin adsorbed in adjuvants),

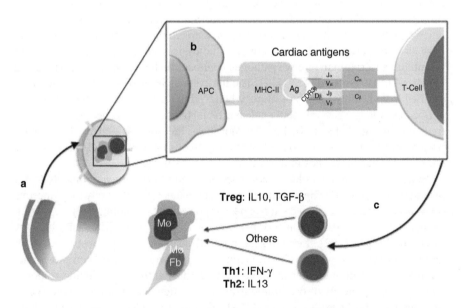

Fig. 11.5 Activation of T-cells following MI. Ischemia-induced cardiomyocyte necrosis promotes the release of several intracellular cardiac proteins that could eventually be presented to T-cells in an inflammatory context. In principle, other danger-associated molecular patterns and cytokines can also influence T-cells, which modulate the healing outcome by mainly interacting with macrophages and fibroblasts

INFγ was first shown to be a central player in promoting disease progression [105]. However, contrary to expected, injected IFNγ-deficient mice exhibit worsened myocarditis because this inflammatory arm of the immune system is also critical to trigger subsequent anti-inflammatory compensatory responses [106, 107]. Furthermore, in a model of spinal cord injury, it has been shown that autoreactive effector T-cells can foster tissue repair. Of note, these are the same autoreactive clones that, in other different context, can promote experimental autoimmune encephalomyelitis [108–110]. In conclusion, autoimmunity is not necessarily harmful and depending on the circumstances it can also benefit self-maintenance.

11.4 Therapeutic Approaches Targeting Lymphocytes and Autoantibodies in the MI and HF Context

Several approaches targeting either B-cells or autoantibodies have been tested in preclinical and clinical contexts. Yet, whether any of them will be proved effective remains an open question. Regarding to autoantibodies, different preclinical studies reported the successful use of specific peptides mimicking the cardiac epitopes as an efficient approach to block some specific autoantibodies [23, 55]. Despite the success of such approaches in rodent models of MI and HF, it is plausible to assume that blocking a single antibody reactivity may not be sufficient to counteract rather polyclonal B-cell responses. Thus, other nonspecific approaches designed to modulate the pathological effects of heart-reactive autoantibodies in myocardial diseases have also been proposed. In some clinical studies, it has been observed that the use of immunoadsorption to remove pathogenic autoantibodies from circulation may be beneficial to HF patients [111, 112]. The intravenous infusion of immunoglobulins purified from healthy donors (a strategy believed to neutralize the pathogenic autoantibodies amongst several other unclear effects) has been also tested, showing contradicting results [113, 114]. Last but not least, the anti-CD20mAb (Rituximab) used by Zouggari et al. [68] to deplete mature B-cells has been already approved by the FDA for human studies in other autoimmune contexts.

Emerging immunomodulatory approaches tested in experimental models of MI also suggest that interfering with the CD4+ T-cell phenotypic plasticity may improve myocardial repair. For instance, it has been reported that promoting Treg expansion using an anti-CD28 superagonist or performing Treg adoptive cell transfer benefits myocardial repair [102]. Targeting the post-MI adaptive immune responses in an antigen-specific fashion may also be an interesting approach. It has been shown that the induction of immunological tolerance to cardiac antigens (including troponin and myosin) by means of oral immunization can attenuate myocardial damage in different models of cardiac disease [115–119]. Similarly, Choo et al. recently demonstrated that adoptive transfer of tolerogenic dendritic cells loaded with cardiac antigens also improved myocardial healing and attenuated adverse remodelling

Box 11.1: Take-Home Messages
What Triggers T- and B-Cell Activation After MI?

The questions whether lymphocytes receive antigenic stimulation or simply respond to unspecific inflammatory signals (i.e., Toll-Like and cytokine Receptors) remain unsolved. Evidences suggesting that specific antigenic stimulation may occur have been reported. However, it is also plausible to assume that TCR- and BCR-independent activation mechanisms may co-exist.

What Fine-Tunes Post-MI Lymphocyte Responses?

The MI situation imposes a unique context for lymphocyte activation. Besides classical DAMPS that can be released by dying cardiomyocytes (e.g. HSPs), several other nonclassical mediators might also play a role. MI triggers sympathetic overdrive with prominent secretion of catecholamines, and changes in volumetric conditions trigger a renal reflex with consequent overproduction of angiotensin-II. In principle, both systems can modulate lymphocyte responses to cardiac antigens, as T- and B-cells express high levels of beta-2-adrenergic receptors and angiotensin receptors type 1.

What Brings Lymphocytes to the Injured Myocardium?

The infarcted myocardium expresses chemokines able to attract activated T-cells (CCL5) and B-cells (CXCL13). Furthermore, it has been recently reported that T-cells receiving antigenic stimulation at the heart-draining LNs develop cardiotropism in a mechanism dependent on HGF-c-met signalling.

How Do Lymphocytes Influence the Local Molecular Milieu?

Myocardial B-cells boost monocyte recruitment via secretion of CCL7. CD4+Foxp3+ T-cells shape the monocyte/macrophages' polarization towards a pro-healing phenotype. T-cells can also cross talk to fibroblasts at later stages.

The therapeutical gap.

Most of therapeutical strategies currently available to treat MI/HF patients focus in modulating cardiovascular rather than immuno-inflammatory mechanisms. Will novel immunotherapeutic strategies succeed in improving cardiac repair and help preventing the development of ischemic HF?

[120]. Yet, it should be pondered that this field is still in its infancy and such novel therapeutic approaches are still in a premature stage.

11.5   Conclusions

The capacity to maintain and restore the integrity of tissues is crucial for the survival of all organisms. Yet, the pathways leading to tissue repair can largely vary depending on the organism, tissue and developmental stage [121]. Salamanders, zebra fishes and newborn mice are capable of completely reconstructing a new functional myocardium, upon injury [122], whereas most other vertebrates normally replace the injured myocardium with a fibrous tissue [123]. Still, as Metchnikoff put forward more than a hundred years ago, it should be emphasized that inflammation is the common unifying mechanism underlying all those situations involving tissue injury and repair [121, 124].

Although potentially destructive, inflammation is a sine qua non condition towards tissue reconstruction, no matter whether it works as re-establishing the status quo ante or in promoting a fibrotic repair [46, 125–127]. It is widely accepted that MI patients receiving immunosuppressive therapies with corticosteroids exhibit a worse outcome due to impaired healing response [128]. Similarly, the myocardial regenerative capacity seen in zebra fishes and neonatal mice is lost when the inflammation is blocked [129–131]. This might implicate that novel therapeutic approaches aimed at improving myocardial repair should focus on fostering the pro-healing arms of the immune system rather than simply silencing it.

References

1. Majno G. The healing hand. Man and wound in the ancient world. 1st ed. Cambridge: Harvard University Press; 1975.
2. Ertl G, Frantz S. Wound model of myocardial infarction. Am J Physiol Heart Circ Physiol. 2005;288(3):H981–3. doi:10.1152/ajpheart.00977.2004.
3. Task Force on the management of STseamiotESoC, Steg PG, James SK, Atar D, Badano LP, Blomstrom-Lundqvist C, Borger MA, Di Mario C, Dickstein K, Ducrocq G, Fernandez-Aviles F, Gershlick AH, Giannuzzi P, Halvorsen S, Huber K, Juni P, Kastrati A, Knuuti J, Lenzen MJ, Mahaffey KW, Valgimigli M, van 't Hof A, Widimsky P, Zahger D. ESC Guidelines for the management of acute myocardial infarction in patients presenting with ST-segment elevation. Eur Heart J. 2012;33(20):2569–619. doi:10.1093/eurheartj/ehs215.
4. McMurray JJ, Adamopoulos S, Anker SD, Auricchio A, Bohm M, Dickstein K, Falk V, Filippatos G, Fonseca C, Gomez-Sanchez MA, Jaarsma T, Kober L, Lip GY, Maggioni AP, Parkhomenko A, Pieske BM, Popescu BA, Ronnevik PK, Rutten FH, Schwitter J, Seferovic P, Stepinska J, Trindade PT, Voors AA, Zannad F, Zeiher A, Guidelines ESCCfP. ESC Guidelines for the diagnosis and treatment of acute and chronic heart failure 2012: the task force for the diagnosis and treatment of acute and chronic heart failure 2012 of the European Society of Cardiology. Developed in collaboration with the Heart Failure Association (HFA) of the ESC. Eur Heart J. 2012;33(14):1787–847. doi:10.1093/eurheartj/ehs104.
5. Ertl G, Frantz S. Healing after myocardial infarction. Cardiovasc Res. 2005;66(1):22–32. doi:10.1016/j.cardiores.2005.01.011.

6. Frangogiannis NG. Inflammation in cardiac injury, repair and regeneration. Curr Opin Cardiol. 2015;30(3):240–5. doi:10.1097/HCO.0000000000000158.
7. Nahrendorf M, Pittet MJ, Swirski FK. Monocytes: protagonists of infarct inflammation and repair after myocardial infarction. Circulation. 2010;121(22):2437–45. doi:10.1161/CIRCULATIONAHA.109.916346.
8. Frantz S, Hofmann U, Fraccarollo D, Schafer A, Kranepuhl S, Hagedorn I, Nieswandt B, Nahrendorf M, Wagner H, Bayer B, Pachel C, Schon MP, Kneitz S, Bobinger T, Weidemann F, Ertl G, Bauersachs J. Monocytes/macrophages prevent healing defects and left ventricular thrombus formation after myocardial infarction. FASEB J. 2013;27(3):871–81. doi:10.1096/fj.12-214049.
9. Hofmann U, Beyersdorf N, Weirather J, Podolskaya A, Bauersachs J, Ertl G, Kerkau T, Frantz S. Activation of CD4+ T lymphocytes improves wound healing and survival after experimental myocardial infarction in mice. Circulation. 2012;125(13):1652–63. doi:10.1161/CIRCULATIONAHA.111.044164.
10. Yan X, Anzai A, Katsumata Y, Matsuhashi T, Ito K, Endo J, Yamamoto T, Takeshima A, Shinmura K, Shen W, Fukuda K, Sano M. Temporal dynamics of cardiac immune cell accumulation following acute myocardial infarction. J Mol Cell Cardiol. 2013;62:24–35. doi:10.1016/j.yjmcc.2013.04.023.
11. Harel-Adar T, Ben Mordechai T, Amsalem Y, Feinberg MS, Leor J, Cohen S. Modulation of cardiac macrophages by phosphatidylserine-presenting liposomes improves infarct repair. Proc Natl Acad Sci U S A. 2011;108(5):1827–32. doi:10.1073/pnas.1015623108.
12. Weirather J, Hofmann UD, Beyersdorf N, Ramos GC, Vogel B, Frey A, Ertl G, Kerkau T, Frantz S. Foxp3+ CD4+ T cells improve healing after myocardial infarction by modulating monocyte/macrophage differentiation. Circ Res. 2014;115(1):55–67. doi:10.1161/CIRCRESAHA.115.303895.
13. Frantz S, Nahrendorf M. Cardiac macrophages and their role in ischaemic heart disease. Cardiovasc Res. 2014;102(2):240–8. doi:10.1093/cvr/cvu025.
14. Hofmann U, Frantz S. Role of lymphocytes in myocardial injury, healing, and remodeling after myocardial infarction. Circ Res. 2015;116(2):354–67. doi:10.1161/CIRCRESAHA.116.304072.
15. Lv H, Havari E, Pinto S, Gottumukkala RV, Cornivelli L, Raddassi K, Matsui T, Rosenzweig A, Bronson RT, Smith R, Fletcher AL, Turley SJ, Wucherpfennig K, Kyewski B, Lipes MA. Impaired thymic tolerance to alpha-myosin directs autoimmunity to the heart in mice and humans. J Clin Invest. 2011;121(4):1561–73. doi:10.1172/JCI44583.
16. Cooper MD. The early history of B cells. Nat Rev Immunol. 2015;15(3):191–7. doi:10.1038/nri3801.
17. LeBien TW, Tedder TF. B lymphocytes: how they develop and function. Blood. 2008;112(5):1570–80. doi:10.1182/blood-2008-02-078071.
18. Bornholz B, Roggenbuck D, Jahns R, Boege F. Diagnostic and therapeutic aspects of beta1-adrenergic receptor autoantibodies in human heart disease. Autoimmun Rev. 2014;13(9):954–62. doi:10.1016/j.autrev.2014.08.021.
19. De Scheerder I, Vandekerckhove J, Robbrecht J, Algoed L, De Buyzere M, De Langhe J, De Schrijver G, Clement D. Post-cardiac injury syndrome and an increased humoral immune response against the major contractile proteins (actin and myosin). Am J Cardiol. 1985;56(10):631–3.
20. Kaya Z, Leib C, Katus HA. Autoantibodies in heart failure and cardiac dysfunction. Circ Res. 2012;110(1):145–58. doi:10.1161/CIRCRESAHA.111.243360.
21. O'Donohoe TJ, Schrale RG, Ketheesan N. The role of anti-myosin antibodies in perpetuating cardiac damage following myocardial infarction. Int J Cardiol. 2016;209:226–33. doi:10.1016/j.ijcard.2016.02.035.
22. Busche MN, Pavlov V, Takahashi K, Stahl GL. Myocardial ischemia and reperfusion injury is dependent on both IgM and mannose-binding lectin. Am J Physiol Heart Circ Physiol. 2009;297(5):H1853–9. doi:10.1152/ajpheart.00049.2009.

23. Haas MS, Alicot EM, Schuerpf F, Chiu I, Li J, Moore FD, Carroll MC. Blockade of self-reactive IgM significantly reduces injury in a murine model of acute myocardial infarction. Cardiovasc Res. 2010;87(4):618–27. doi:10.1093/cvr/cvq141.
24. Medei EH, Nascimento JH, Pedrosa RC, Carvalho AC. Role of autoantibodies in the physiopathology of Chagas' disease. Arq Bras Cardiol. 2008;91(4):257–62. 281-256
25. Rose NR. Myocarditis: infection versus autoimmunity. J Clin Immunol. 2009;29(6):730–7. doi:10.1007/s10875-009-9339-z.
26. Deubner N, Berliner D, Schlipp A, Gelbrich G, Caforio AL, Felix SB, Fu M, Katus H, Angermann CE, Lohse MJ, Ertl G, Stork S, Jahns R, Etiology, Titre-Course, and Survival-Study Group. Cardiac beta1-adrenoceptor autoantibodies in human heart disease: rationale and design of the Etiology, Titre-Course, and Survival (ETiCS) Study. Eur J Heart Fail. 2010;12(7):753–62. doi:10.1093/eurjhf/hfq072.
27. Sorman A, Zhang L, Ding Z, Heyman B. How antibodies use complement to regulate antibody responses. Mol Immunol. 2014;61(2):79–88. doi:10.1016/j.molimm.2014.06.010.
28. Mkaddem SB, Christou I, Rossato E, Berthelot L, Lehuen A, Monteiro RC. IgA, IgA receptors, and their anti-inflammatory properties. Curr Top Microbiol Immunol. 2014;382:221–35. doi:10.1007/978-3-319-07911-0_10.
29. Coutinho A, Kazatchkine MD, Avrameas S. Natural autoantibodies. Curr Opin Immunol. 1995;7(6):812–8.
30. Dighiero G, Lymberi P, Holmberg D, Lundquist I, Coutinho A, Avrameas S. High frequency of natural autoantibodies in normal newborn mice. J Immunol. 1985;134(2):765–71.
31. Haury M, Sundblad A, Grandien A, Barreau C, Coutinho A, Nobrega A. The repertoire of serum IgM in normal mice is largely independent of external antigenic contact. Eur J Immunol. 1997;27(6):1557–63. doi:10.1002/eji.1830270635.
32. Jerne NK. The Nobel Lectures in Immunology. The Nobel Prize for Physiology or Medicine, 1984. The generative grammar of the immune system. Scand J Immunol. 1993; 38(1):1–9.
33. Merbl Y, Zucker-Toledano M, Quintana FJ, Cohen IR. Newborn humans manifest autoantibodies to defined self molecules detected by antigen microarray informatics. J Clin Invest. 2007;117(3):712–8. doi:10.1172/JCI29943.
34. Lacroix-Desmazes S, Kaveri SV, Mouthon L, Ayouba A, Malanchere E, Coutinho A, Kazatchkine MD. Self-reactive antibodies (natural autoantibodies) in healthy individuals. J Immunol Methods. 1998;216(1–2):117–37.
35. Nobrega A, Haury M, Grandien A, Malanchere E, Sundblad A, Coutinho A. Global analysis of antibody repertoires. II. Evidence for specificity, self-selection and the immunological "homunculus" of antibodies in normal serum. Eur J Immunol. 1993;23(11):2851–9. doi:10.1002/eji.1830231119.
36. Quintana FJ, Cohen IR. The natural autoantibody repertoire and autoimmune disease. Biomed Pharmacother. 2004;58(5):276–81. doi:10.1016/j.biopha.2004.04.011.
37. Nishio N, Ito S, Suzuki H, Isobe K. Antibodies to wounded tissue enhance cutaneous wound healing. Immunology. 2009;128(3):369–80. doi:10.1111/j.1365-2567.2009.03119.x.
38. Zhang M, Austen WG Jr, Chiu I, Alicot EM, Hung R, Ma M, Verna N, Xu M, Hechtman HB, Moore FD Jr, Carroll MC. Identification of a specific self-reactive IgM antibody that initiates intestinal ischemia/reperfusion injury. Proc Natl Acad Sci U S A. 2004;101(11):3886–91. doi:10.1073/pnas.0400347101.
39. Weiser MR, Williams JP, Moore FD Jr, Kobzik L, Ma M, Hechtman HB, Carroll MC. Reperfusion injury of ischemic skeletal muscle is mediated by natural antibody and complement. J Exp Med. 1996;183(5):2343–8.
40. Silverman GJ. Protective natural autoantibodies to apoptotic cells: evidence of convergent selection of recurrent innate-like clones. Ann N Y Acad Sci. 2015;1362:164–75. doi:10.1111/nyas.12788.
41. Williams JP, Pechet TT, Weiser MR, Reid R, Kobzik L, Moore FD Jr, Carroll MC, Hechtman HB. Intestinal reperfusion injury is mediated by IgM and complement. J Appl Physiol (1985). 1999;86(3):938–42.

42. Zhang M, Alicot EM, Chiu I, Li J, Verna N, Vorup-Jensen T, Kessler B, Shimaoka M, Chan R, Friend D, Mahmood U, Weissleder R, Moore FD, Carroll MC. Identification of the target self-antigens in reperfusion injury. J Exp Med. 2006;203(1):141–52. doi:10.1084/jem.20050390.

43. Pummerer CL, Luze K, Grassl G, Bachmaier K, Offner F, Burrell SK, Lenz DM, Zamborelli TJ, Penninger JM, Neu N. Identification of cardiac myosin peptides capable of inducing autoimmune myocarditis in BALB/c mice. J Clin Invest. 1996;97(9):2057–62. doi:10.1172/JCI118642.

44. Sihag S, Haas MS, Kim KM, Guerrero JL, Beaudoin J, Alicot EM, Schuerpf F, Gottschall JD, Puro RJ, Madsen JC, Sachs DH, Newman W, Carroll MC, Allan JS. Natural IgM blockade limits infarct expansion and left ventricular dysfunction in a swine myocardial infarct model. Circ Cardiovasc Interv. 2016;9(1):e002547. doi:10.1161/CIRCINTERVENTIONS.115.002547.

45. Diepenhorst GM, Ciurana CL, Diaz Padilla N, Boekholdt SM, Krijnen PA, Lagrand WK, Niessen HW, Hack CE. IgM antibodies against apoptotic cells and phosphorylcholine in patients with acute myocardial infarction in relation to infarct size and inflammatory response. Adv Clin Exp Med. 2012;21(4):455–67.

46. Parnes O. From interception to incorporation: degeneracy and promiscuous recognition as precursors of a paradigm shift in immunology. Mol Immunol. 2004;40(14–15):985–91. doi:10.1016/j.molimm.2003.11.021.

47. Kyaw T, Tipping P, Bobik A, Toh BH. Protective role of natural IgM-producing B1a cells in atherosclerosis. Trends Cardiovasc Med. 2012;22(2):48–53. doi:10.1016/j.tcm.2012.06.011.

48. Dangas G, Konstadoulakis MM, Epstein SE, Stefanadis CI, Kymionis GD, Toutouza MG, Liakos C, Sadaniantz A, Cohen AM, Chesebro JH, Toutouzas PK. Prevalence of autoantibodies against contractile proteins in coronary artery disease and their clinical implications. Am J Cardiol. 2000;85(7):870–2. A876, A879

49. De Scheerder I, Vandekerckhove J, De Schrijver G, Hoste M, Clement D, Wieme R, Pannier R. Detection of anti-contractile antibodies after cardiac surgery using ELISA assay. Clin Exp Immunol. 1985;60(2):403–6.

50. Pang H, Liao Y, Wang Z, Dong J, Lu Q. Effect of anti-cardiac myosin antibody on prognosis of patients with acute myocardial infarction. J Tongji Med Univ. 2000;20(1):46–8.

51. Warraich RS, Griffiths E, Falconar A, Pabbathi V, Bell C, Angelini G, Suleiman MS, Yacoub MH. Human cardiac myosin autoantibodies impair myocyte contractility: a cause-and-effect relationship. FASEB J. 2006;20(6):651–60. doi:10.1096/fj.04-3001com.

52. Neumann DA, Lane JR, Wulff SM, Allen GS, LaFond-Walker A, Herskowitz A, Rose NR. In vivo deposition of myosin-specific autoantibodies in the hearts of mice with experimental autoimmune myocarditis. J Immunol. 1992;148(12):3806–13.

53. Caforio AL, Angelini A, Blank M, Shani A, Kivity S, Goddard G, Doria A, Schiavo A, Testolina M, Bottaro S, Marcolongo R, Thiene G, Iliceto S, Shoenfeld Y. Passive transfer of affinity-purified anti-heart autoantibodies (AHA) from sera of patients with myocarditis induces experimental myocarditis in mice. Int J Cardiol. 2015;179:166–77. doi:10.1016/j.ijcard.2014.10.165.

54. Li Y, Heuser JS, Cunningham LC, Kosanke SD, Cunningham MW. Mimicry and antibody-mediated cell signaling in autoimmune myocarditis. J Immunol. 2006;177(11):8234–40.

55. Boivin V, Beyersdorf N, Palm D, Nikolaev VO, Schlipp A, Muller J, Schmidt D, Kocoski V, Kerkau T, Hunig T, Ertl G, Lohse MJ, Jahns R. Novel receptor-derived cyclopeptides to treat heart failure caused by anti-beta1-adrenoceptor antibodies in a human-analogous rat model. PLoS One. 2015;10(2):e0117589. doi:10.1371/journal.pone.0117589.

56. Caforio AL, Tona F, Bottaro S, Vinci A, Dequal G, Daliento L, Thiene G, Iliceto S. Clinical implications of anti-heart autoantibodies in myocarditis and dilated cardiomyopathy. Autoimmunity. 2008;41(1):35–45. doi:10.1080/08916930701619235.

57. Wallukat G, Fu ML, Magnusson Y, Hjalmarson A, Hoebeke J, Wollenberger A. Agonistic effects of anti-peptide antibodies and autoantibodies directed against adrenergic and cholinergic receptors: absence of desensitization. Blood Press Suppl. 1996;3:31–6.

58. Magnusson Y, Wallukat G, Guillet JG, Hjalmarson A, Hoebeke J. Functional analysis of rabbit anti-peptide antibodies which mimic autoantibodies against the beta 1-adrenergic receptor in patients with idiopathic dilated cardiomyopathy. J Autoimmun. 1991;4(6):893–905.

59. Tate K, Magnusson Y, Viguier M, Lengagne R, Hjalmarson A, Guillet JG, Hoebeke J. Epitope analysis of T- and B-cell response against the human beta 1-adrenoceptor. Biochimie. 1994;76(2):159–64.

60. Wallukat G, Morwinski R, Magnusson Y, Hoebeke J, Wollenberger A. Autoantibodies against the beta 1-adrenergic receptor in myocarditis and dilated cardiomyopathy: localization of two epitopes. Z Kardiol. 1992;81(Suppl 4):79–83.

61. Stork S, Boivin V, Horf R, Hein L, Lohse MJ, Angermann CE, Jahns R. Stimulating autoantibodies directed against the cardiac beta1-adrenergic receptor predict increased mortality in idiopathic cardiomyopathy. Am Heart J. 2006;152(4):697–704. doi:10.1016/j. ahj.2006.05.004.

62. Jahns R, Boivin V, Hein L, Triebel S, Angermann CE, Ertl G, Lohse MJ. Direct evidence for a beta 1-adrenergic receptor-directed autoimmune attack as a cause of idiopathic dilated cardiomyopathy. J Clin Invest. 2004;113(10):1419–29. doi:10.1172/JCI20149.

63. Munch G, Boivin-Jahns V, Holthoff HP, Adler K, Lappo M, Truol S, Degen H, Steiger N, Lohse MJ, Jahns R, Ungerer M. Administration of the cyclic peptide COR-1 in humans (phase I study): ex vivo measurements of anti-beta1-adrenergic receptor antibody neutralization and of immune parameters. Eur J Heart Fail. 2012;14(11):1230–9. doi:10.1093/eurjhf/ hfs118.

64. Cohen-Sfady M, Nussbaum G, Pevsner-Fischer M, Mor F, Carmi P, Zanin-Zhorov A, Lider O, Cohen IR. Heat shock protein 60 activates B cells via the TLR4-MyD88 pathway. J Immunol. 2005;175(6):3594–602.

65. Coutinho A. Genetic control of B-cell responses. II. Identification of the spleen B-cell defect in C3H/HeJ mice. Scand J Immunol. 1976;5(1–2):129–40.

66. Peng SL. Signaling in B cells via Toll-like receptors. Curr Opin Immunol. 2005;17(3):230–6. doi:10.1016/j.coi.2005.03.003.

67. Teichmann LL, Schenten D, Medzhitov R, Kashgarian M, Shlomchik MJ. Signals via the adaptor MyD88 in B cells and DCs make distinct and synergistic contributions to immune activation and tissue damage in lupus. Immunity. 2013;38(3):528–40. doi:10.1016/j. immuni.2012.11.017.

68. Zouggari Y, Ait-Oufella H, Bonnin P, Simon T, Sage AP, Guerin C, Vilar J, Caligiuri G, Tsiantoulas D, Laurans L, Dumeau E, Kotti S, Bruneval P, Charo IF, Binder CJ, Danchin N, Tedgui A, Tedder TF, Silvestre JS, Mallat Z. B lymphocytes trigger monocyte mobilization and impair heart function after acute myocardial infarction. Nat Med. 2013;19(10):1273–80. doi:10.1038/nm.3284.

69. Iwata Y, Yoshizaki A, Komura K, Shimizu K, Ogawa F, Hara T, Muroi E, Bae S, Takenaka M, Yukami T, Hasegawa M, Fujimoto M, Tomita Y, Tedder TF, Sato S. CD19, a response regulator of B lymphocytes, regulates wound healing through hyaluronan-induced TLR4 signaling. Am J Pathol. 2009;175(2):649–60. doi:10.2353/ajpath.2009.080355.

70. Goodchild TT, Robinson KA, Pang W, Tondato F, Cui J, Arrington J, Godwin L, Ungs M, Carlesso N, Weich N, Poznansky MC, Chronos NA. Bone marrow-derived B cells preserve ventricular function after acute myocardial infarction. JACC Cardiovasc Interv. 2009;2(10):1005–16. doi:10.1016/j.jcin.2009.08.010.

71. Coutinho A. Innate immunity: from lymphocyte mitogens to Toll-like receptors and back. Curr Opin Immunol. 2003;15(6):599–602. doi:10.1016/j.coi.2003.09.020.

72. Jackson SW, Kolhatkar NS, Rawlings DJ. B cells take the front seat: dysregulated B cell signals orchestrate loss of tolerance and autoantibody production. Curr Opin Immunol. 2015;33:70–7. doi:10.1016/j.coi.2015.01.018.

73. Davis MM. T cell receptor gene diversity and selection. Annu Rev Biochem. 1990;59:475–96. doi:10.1146/annurev.bi.59.070190.002355.

74. Malissen B, Bongrand P. Early T cell activation: integrating biochemical, structural, and biophysical cues. Annu Rev Immunol. 2015;33:539–61. doi:10.1146/ annurev-immunol-032414-112158.

75. Rossjohn J, Gras S, Miles JJ, Turner SJ, Godfrey DI, McCluskey J. T cell antigen receptor recognition of antigen-presenting molecules. Annu Rev Immunol. 2015;33:169–200. doi:10.1146/annurev-immunol-032414-112334.
76. Rudolph MG, Stanfield RL, Wilson IA. How TCRs bind MHCs, peptides, and coreceptors. Annu Rev Immunol. 2006;24:419–66. doi:10.1146/annurev.immunol.23.021704.115658.
77. Komarowska I, Coe D, Wang G, Haas R, Mauro C, Kishore M, Cooper D, Nadkarni S, Fu H, Steinbruchel DA, Pitzalis C, Anderson G, Bucy P, Lombardi G, Breckenridge R, Marelli-Berg FM. Hepatocyte growth factor receptor c-Met instructs T cell cardiotropism and promotes T cell migration to the heart via autocrine chemokine release. Immunity. 2015;42(6):1087–99. doi:10.1016/j.immuni.2015.05.014.
78. Mosmann TR, Cherwinski H, Bond MW, Giedlin MA, Coffman RL. Two types of murine helper T cell clone. I. Definition according to profiles of lymphokine activities and secreted proteins. J Immunol. 1986;136(7):2348–57.
79. Zhu J, Paul WE. CD4 T cells: fates, functions, and faults. Blood. 2008;112(5):1557–69. doi:10.1182/blood-2008-05-078154.
80. Bennett CL, Christie J, Ramsdell F, Brunkow ME, Ferguson PJ, Whitesell L, Kelly TE, Saulsbury FT, Chance PF, Ochs HD. The immune dysregulation, polyendocrinopathy, enteropathy, X-linked syndrome (IPEX) is caused by mutations of FOXP3. Nat Genet. 2001;27(1):20–1. doi:10.1038/83713.
81. Liston A, Nutsch KM, Farr AG, Lund JM, Rasmussen JP, Koni PA, Rudensky AY. Differentiation of regulatory Foxp3+ T cells in the thymic cortex. Proc Natl Acad Sci U S A. 2008;105(33):11903–8. doi:10.1073/pnas.0801506105.
82. Sakaguchi S, Sakaguchi N, Asano M, Itoh M, Toda M. Immunologic self-tolerance maintained by activated T cells expressing IL-2 receptor alpha-chains (CD25). Breakdown of a single mechanism of self-tolerance causes various autoimmune diseases. J Immunol. 1995;155(3):1151–64.
83. Sakaguchi S, Yamaguchi T, Nomura T, Ono M. Regulatory T cells and immune tolerance. Cell. 2008;133(5):775–87. doi:10.1016/j.cell.2008.05.009.
84. Burzyn D, Kuswanto W, Kolodin D, Shadrach JL, Cerletti M, Jang Y, Sefik E, Tan TG, Wagers AJ, Benoist C, Mathis D. A special population of regulatory T cells potentiates muscle repair. Cell. 2013;155(6):1282–95. doi:10.1016/j.cell.2013.10.054.
85. Pacholczyk R, Ignatowicz H, Kraj P, Ignatowicz L. Origin and T cell receptor diversity of Foxp3+CD4+CD25+T cells. Immunity. 2006;25(2):249–59. doi:10.1016/j.immuni.2006.05.016.
86. Pacholczyk R, Kern J. The T-cell receptor repertoire of regulatory T cells. Immunology. 2008;125(4):450–8. doi:10.1111/j.1365-2567.2008.02992.x.
87. Arpaia N, Green JA, Moltedo B, Arvey A, Hemmers S, Yuan S, Treuting PM, Rudensky AY. A distinct function of regulatory T cells in tissue protection. Cell. 2015;162(5):1078–89. doi:10.1016/j.cell.2015.08.021.
88. Yang Z, Day YJ, Toufektsian MC, Xu Y, Ramos SI, Marshall MA, French BA, Linden J. Myocardial infarct-sparing effect of adenosine A2A receptor activation is due to its action on CD4+ T lymphocytes. Circulation. 2006;114(19):2056–64. doi:10.1161/CIRCULATIONAHA.106.649244.
89. Burzyn D, Benoist C, Mathis D. Regulatory T cells in nonlymphoid tissues. Nat Immunol. 2013;14(10):1007–13. doi:10.1038/ni.2683.
90. Schenkel JM, Masopust D. Tissue-resident memory T cells. Immunity. 2014;41(6):886–97. doi:10.1016/j.immuni.2014.12.007.
91. Ramos GC, van den Berg A, Nunes-Silva V, Weirather J, Peters L, Burkard M, Friedrich M, Pinnecker J, Abeßer M, Heinze KG, Schuh K, Beyersdorf N, Kerkau T, Demengeot J, Frantz S, and Hofmann U. Myocardial aging as a T-cell–mediated phenomenon PNAS. 2017;114(12):E2420–9. doi:10.1073/pnas.1621047114.
92. Hofmann U, Frantz S. Role of T-cells in myocardial infarction. Eur Heart J. 2015; doi:10.1093/eurheartj/ehv639.
93. Lu L, Li G, Rao J, Pu L, Yu Y, Wang X, Zhang F. In vitro induced CD4(+)CD25(+)Foxp3(+) Tregs attenuate hepatic ischemia-reperfusion injury. Int Immunopharmacol. 2009;9(5):549–52. doi:10.1016/j.intimp.2009.01.020.

94. Ke D, Fang J, Fan L, Chen Z, Chen L. Regulatory T cells contribute to rosuvastatin-induced cardioprotection against ischemia-reperfusion injury. Coron Artery Dis. 2013;24(4):334–41. doi:10.1097/MCA.0b013e3283608c12.

95. Mathes D, Weirather J, Nordbeck P, Arias-Loza AP, Burkard M, Pachel C, Kerkau T, Beyersdorf N, Frantz S, Hofmann U. CD4+ Foxp3+ T-cells contribute to myocardial ischemia-reperfusion injury. J Mol Cell Cardiol. 2016 Dec;101:99–105. doi: 10.1016/j.yjmcc.2016.10.007. Epub 2016 Oct 19.

96. Matsumoto K, Ogawa M, Suzuki J, Hirata Y, Nagai R, Isobe M. Regulatory T lymphocytes attenuate myocardial infarction-induced ventricular remodeling in mice. Int Heart J. 2011;52(6):382–7.

97. Saxena A, Bjorkbacka H, Strom A, Rattik S, Berg KE, Gomez MF, Fredrikson GN, Nilsson J, Hultgardh-Nilsson A. Mobilization of regulatory T cells in response to carotid injury does not influence subsequent neointima formation. PLoS One. 2012;7(12):e51556. doi:10.1371/journal.pone.0051556.

98. Saxena A, Dobaczewski M, Rai V, Haque Z, Chen W, Li N, Frangogiannis NG. Regulatory T cells are recruited in the infarcted mouse myocardium and may modulate fibroblast phenotype and function. Am J Physiol Heart Circ Physiol. 2014;307(8):H1233–42. doi:10.1152/ajpheart.00328.2014.

99. Sharir R, Semo J, Shimoni S, Ben-Mordechai T, Landa-Rouben N, Maysel-Auslender S, Shaish A, Entin-Meer M, Keren G, George J. Experimental myocardial infarction induces altered regulatory T cell hemostasis, and adoptive transfer attenuates subsequent remodeling. PLoS One. 2014;9(12):e113653. doi:10.1371/journal.pone.0113653.

100. Tang TT, Yuan J, Zhu ZF, Zhang WC, Xiao H, Xia N, Yan XX, Nie SF, Liu J, Zhou SF, Li JJ, Yao R, Liao MY, Tu X, Liao YH, Cheng X. Regulatory T cells ameliorate cardiac remodeling after myocardial infarction. Basic Res Cardiol. 2012;107(1):232. doi:10.1007/s00395-011-0232-6.

101. Hünig T. The rise and fall of the CD28 superagonist TGN1412 and its return as TAB08: a personal account. FEBS J. 2016;283(18):3325–34. doi: 10.1111/febs.13754. Epub 2016 Jun 6.

102. Wang YP, Xie Y, Ma H, Su SA, Wang YD, Wang JA, Xiang MX. Regulatory T lymphocytes in myocardial infarction: a promising new therapeutic target. Int J Cardiol. 2016;203:923–8. doi:10.1016/j.ijcard.2015.11.078.

103. Curato C, Slavic S, Dong J, Skorska A, Altarche-Xifro W, Miteva K, Kaschina E, Thiel A, Imboden H, Wang J, Steckelings U, Steinhoff G, Unger T, Li J. Identification of noncytotoxic and IL-10-producing CD8+AT2R+ T cell population in response to ischemic heart injury. J Immunol. 2010;185(10):6286–93. doi:10.4049/jimmunol.0903681.

104. Skorska A, von Haehling S, Ludwig M, Lux CA, Gaebel R, Kleiner G, Klopsch C, Dong J, Curato C, Altarche-Xifro W, Slavic S, Unger T, Steinhoff G, Li J, David R. The CD4(+) AT2R(+) T cell subpopulation improves post-infarction remodelling and restores cardiac function. J Cell Mol Med. 2015;19(8):1975–85. doi:10.1111/jcmm.12574.

105. Nindl V, Maier R, Ratering D, De Giuli R, Zust R, Thiel V, Scandella E, Di Padova F, Kopf M, Rudin M, Rulicke T, Ludewig B. Cooperation of Th1 and Th17 cells determines transition from autoimmune myocarditis to dilated cardiomyopathy. Eur J Immunol. 2012;42(9):2311–21. doi:10.1002/eji.201142209.

106. Eriksson U, Kurrer MO, Bingisser R, Eugster HP, Saremaslani P, Follath F, Marsch S, Widmer U. Lethal autoimmune myocarditis in interferon-gamma receptor-deficient mice: enhanced disease severity by impaired inducible nitric oxide synthase induction. Circulation. 2001;103(1):18–21.

107. Eriksson U, Kurrer MO, Sebald W, Brombacher F, Kopf M. Dual role of the IL-12/IFN-gamma axis in the development of autoimmune myocarditis: induction by IL-12 and protection by IFN-gamma. J Immunol. 2001;167(9):5464–9.

108. Moalem G, Leibowitz-Amit R, Yoles E, Mor F, Cohen IR, Schwartz M. Autoimmune T cells protect neurons from secondary degeneration after central nervous system axotomy. Nat Med. 1999;5(1):49–55. doi:10.1038/4734.

109. Schwartz M, Cohen I, Lazarov-Spiegler O, Moalem G, Yoles E. The remedy may lie in ourselves: prospects for immune cell therapy in central nervous system protection and repair. J Mol Med. 1999;77(10):713–7. doi:10.1007/s001099900047.

110. Schwartz M, Cohen IR. Autoimmunity can benefit self-maintenance. Immunol Today. 2000;21(6):265–8.

111. Christ T, Dobrev D, Wallukat G, Schuler S, Ravens U. Acute hemodynamic effects during immunoadsorption in patients with dilated cardiomyopathy positive for beta 1-adrenoceptor autoantibodies. Methods Find Exp Clin Pharmacol. 2001;23(3):141–4.

112. Dandel M, Wallukat G, Englert A, Lehmkuhl HB, Knosalla C, Hetzer R. Long-term benefits of immunoadsorption in beta(1)-adrenoceptor autoantibody-positive transplant candidates with dilated cardiomyopathy. Eur J Heart Fail. 2012;14(12):1374–88. doi:10.1093/eurjhf/hfs123.

113. Gullestad L, Aass H, Fjeld JG, Wikeby L, Andreassen AK, Ihlen H, Simonsen S, Kjekshus J, Nitter-Hauge S, Ueland T, Lien E, Froland SS, Aukrust P. Immunomodulating therapy with intravenous immunoglobulin in patients with chronic heart failure. Circulation. 2001;103(2):220–5.

114. Gullestad L, Orn S, Dickstein K, Eek C, Edvardsen T, Aakhus S, Askevold ET, Michelsen A, Bendz B, Skardal R, Smith HJ, Yndestad A, Ueland T, Aukrust P. Intravenous immunoglobulin does not reduce left ventricular remodeling in patients with myocardial dysfunction during hospitalization after acute myocardial infarction. Int J Cardiol. 2013;168(1):212–8. doi:10.1016/j.ijcard.2012.09.092.

115. Frenkel D, Pachori AS, Zhang L, Dembinsky-Vaknin A, Farfara D, Petrovic-Stojkovic S, Dzau VJ, Weiner HL. Nasal vaccination with troponin reduces troponin specific T-cell responses and improves heart function in myocardial ischemia-reperfusion injury. Int Immunol. 2009;21(7):817–29. doi:10.1093/intimm/dxp051.

116. Gonnella PA, Del Nido PJ, McGowan FX. Oral tolerization with cardiac myosin peptide (614-629) ameliorates experimental autoimmune myocarditis: role of STAT 6 genes in BALB/CJ mice. J Clin Immunol. 2009;29(4):434–43. doi:10.1007/s10875-009-9290-z.

117. Kaya Z, Dohmen KM, Wang Y, Schlichting J, Afanasyeva M, Leuschner F, Rose NR. Cutting edge: a critical role for IL-10 in induction of nasal tolerance in experimental autoimmune myocarditis. J Immunol. 2002;168(4):1552–6.

118. Ramos GC, Dalbo S, Leite DP, Goldfeder E, Carvalho CR, Vaz NM, Assreuy J. The autoimmune nature of post-infarct myocardial healing: oral tolerance to cardiac antigens as a novel strategy to improve cardiac healing. Autoimmunity. 2012;45(3):233–44. doi:10.3109/089169 34.2011.647134.

119. Wang Y, Afanasyeva M, Hill SL, Kaya Z, Rose NR. Nasal administration of cardiac myosin suppresses autoimmune myocarditis in mice. J Am Coll Cardiol. 2000;36(6):1992–9.

120. Eun HC, Jun-Ho L, Eun-Hye P, Hyo Eun P, Nam-Chul J, Tae-Hoon K, Yoon-Seok K, Eunmin K, Ki-Bae S, Cheongsoo P, Kwan-Soo H, Kwonyoon K, Jie-Young S, Han Geuk S, Dae-Seog L, Kiyuk C. Infarcted Myocardium-Primed Dendritic Cells Improve Remodeling and Cardiac Function After Myocardial Infarction by Modulating the Regulatory T Cell and Macrophage Polarization. Circulation. 2017;135:1444–1457. https://doi.org/10.1161/CIRCULATIONAHA.116.023106.

121. Tauber AI. Metchnikoff and the phagocytosis theory. Nat Rev Mol Cell Biol. 2003;4(11):897–901. doi:10.1038/nrm1244.

122. Porrello ER, Mahmoud AI, Simpson E, Hill JA, Richardson JA, Olson EN, Sadek HA. Transient regenerative potential of the neonatal mouse heart. Science. 2011;331(6020):1078–80. doi:10.1126/science.1200708.

123. Laflamme MA, Murry CE. Heart regeneration. Nature. 2011;473(7347):326–35. doi:10.1038/nature10147.

124. Metchnikoff E. Lectures on the comparative pathology of inflammation (trans: Starling FA, Starling EH.), Kegan Paul, Trench, Trübner & Co, Ltd. 1891.

125. Cohen IR. Activation of benign autoimmunity as both tumor and autoimmune disease immunotherapy: a comprehensive review. J Autoimmun. 2014;54:112–7. doi:10.1016/j.jaut.2014.05.002.

126. Ramos GC. Inflammation as an animal development phenomenon. Clin Dev Immunol. 2012;2012:983203. doi:10.1155/2012/983203.

127. Vaz NM, Carvalho CR. On the origin of immunopathology. J Theor Biol. 2015;375:61–70. doi:10.1016/j.jtbi.2014.06.006.

128. Kloner RA, Fishbein MC, Lew H, Maroko PR, Braunwald E. Mummification of the infarcted myocardium by high dose corticosteroids. Circulation. 1978;57(1):56–63.

129. Aurora AB, Porrello ER, Tan W, Mahmoud AI, Hill JA, Bassel-Duby R, Sadek HA, Olson EN. Macrophages are required for neonatal heart regeneration. J Clin Invest. 2014;124(3):1382–92. doi:10.1172/JCI72181.

130. Han C, Nie Y, Lian H, Liu R, He F, Huang H, Hu S. Acute inflammation stimulates a regenerative response in the neonatal mouse heart. Cell Res. 2015;25(10):1137–51. doi:10.1038/cr.2015.110.

131. Huang WC, Yang CC, Chen IH, Liu YM, Chang SJ, Chuang YJ. Treatment of glucocorticoids inhibited early immune responses and impaired cardiac repair in adult zebrafish. PLoS One. 2013;8(6):e66613. doi:10.1371/journal.pone.0066613.

Chapter 12
The Innate Immune Response in Myocardial Infarction, Repair, and Regeneration

Rebecca Gentek and Guillaume Hoeffel

12.1 Introduction

Accumulating evidence identifies the immune system as a key player in injury responses affecting practically all organs, including the heart. Not surprisingly, perhaps, the focus of regenerative medicine in recent years seems to have shifted from being stem cell oriented to investigating the role of "stromal cell types," including resident immune cells, and the innate immune system in particular [1]. The primary response to injuries in most adult mammalian organs is tissue repair by fibrotic scarring, which can cause differing degrees of functional impairment and is thus distinct from true regeneration.

The adult mammalian heart is non-regenerative: During ischemic heart disease, necrotic cardiomyocytes are replaced with noncontractile scars, ultimately inducing heart failure, the leading cause of death in developed countries [2, 3]. Although the distinction of repair and true regeneration is critical, especially for the heart, it is important to note that even non-regenerative repair processes are essential to ensure organ functionality. Similarly, although often considered "harmful" in an oversimplified manner, inflammation is an essential feature required for the initiation of successful healing, and even true regenerative responses to injury, and without an initial inflammatory phase, severe left ventricular dysfunction is the consequence of myocardial infarction.

Indeed, as suggested by Elie Metchnikoff, who also first described phagocytes, the immune system might have originally evolved to regulate developmental

R. Gentek • G. Hoeffel (✉)
Centre d'Immunologie de Marseille-Luminy (CIML),
Aix-Marseille Université, Centre National de la Recherche Scientifique (CNRS),
Institut National de la Santé et de la Recherche Médicale (INSERM),
Marseille 13288, France
e-mail: gentek@ciml.univ-mrs.fr; hoeffel@ciml.univ-mrs.fr

© Springer International Publishing AG 2017   251
S. Sattler, T. Kennedy-Lydon (eds.), *The Immunology of Cardiovascular Homeostasis and Pathology*, Advances in Experimental Medicine and Biology 1003, DOI 10.1007/978-3-319-57613-8_12

processes and tissue homeostasis [4], while inflammation could be regarded as an animal developmental process [5]. Metchnikoff focused on macrophages (MΦ) that indeed are involved in injury responses in virtually all organs, including the heart [6–8]. However, his concept might also apply to other members of the innate immune system, as discussed here.

Paradoxically, immune cells can mediate both *bona fide* regeneration and fibrotic scarring following injury, raising the question of what determines their exact function in the context of injury and repair or regeneration. Although classically considered non-regenerative, the mammalian heart retains the capacity to fully regenerate during embryonic development [9] and a short period of neonatal life [10–12]. Despite some initial controversies regarding the reproducibility and extent of "true" regeneration in such experimental models, the consensus now appears to be that indeed the neonatal mouse heart does regenerate following ligation of the left anterior descending coronary artery (LAD) and apical resection with minimal (residual) scar formation and full functional restoration as judged by left ventricular systolic function [10, 13, 14].

Innate Immune Players in Cardiovascular Repair and Regeneration Excitingly, neonatal heart regeneration has been shown to require MΦ, as demonstrated through systemic depletion using clodronate liposomes [7]. Other members of the innate immune system for which a role in cardiovascular repair and/or regeneration following myocardial infarction has been firmly established are monocytes and neutrophils as well as mast cells (MC).

In this chapter, the involvement of these cell types in myocardial repair and regeneration is summarized as far as known, with a particular focus on heart-resident populations such as MΦ and mast cells. Lineages recruited from the circulation will primarily be discussed insofar as they might contribute to the pool of resident innate cells and/or modulate their functional immunophenotype. We consider the role of the various lineages and their heterogeneity on the background of recent advances in our understanding of their fundamental biology, particularly their developmental dynamics. The data discussed here are largely derived from experimental animal studies, and, where applicable, we will pinpoint technical limitations of current approaches to studying innate immune lineages.

In addition to the subsets that have already been identified as key players, this chapter also explores the potential involvement of additional lineages, namely innate lymphoid cells, a recently identified family of lymphocytes with innate functions. Finally, emerging themes regarding the role of innate immunity in cardiovascular repair and regeneration are discussed, specifically the relevance of immune cell cross talk and the question as to what extent the specific functional outcome of the activation of the innate immune system is primarily defined by their developmental origin or their (micro)environment under non-homeostatic conditions such as acute myocardial infarction. We propose a model whereby immune cell functions are critically influenced by the balance between local adaptation and recruitment of additional mature or precursors cells.

The Sequential Events of the Innate Immune Response to Myocardial Infarction Following acute myocardial infarction, a dynamic, tightly orchestrated healing process is initiated which involves the innate immune system at multiple levels, and, importantly, relies on resident immune cells as well as additional populations recruited upon injury.

Strikingly, the overall mobilization of the immune system in tissues follows a consistent pattern, regardless of the specific cause of injury: Immediately following trauma, activated resident immune cells such as macrophages (MΦ), innate lymphoid cells (ILC), and mast cells (MC) coordinate the removal of damaged cells, the remodeling of the tissue stroma, and the recruitment of additional immune cells from the blood. While MΦ capture and phagocytose myocardial tissue debris, ILC can sustain MΦ activity through the production of IL-13 and IL-4 [15] promoting MΦ self-renewal and their anti-inflammatory phenotype. In damaged organs such as the ischemic heart, the release of TNFα, IL-1β by MΦ, and histamine by MC triggers vascular permeability and the transmigration of circulating innate cells [16, 17]. The quasi-immediate (minutes to hours) influx of neutrophils favories myocardial tissue debris elimination and reduces the expansion of the tissue lesion through the release of neutrophil extracellular traps (NETs) [18]. Subsequently, infiltrating monocytes differentiate locally to give rise either to scavenging MΦ or TNFα/iNOS-producing dendritic cells (TipDC, [19]), able to coordinate an adaptive immune response. This sequence of cellular events is crucial for tissue recovery. However, excessive activation and local expansion of MΦ can also be detrimental to the process of tissue healing and the initiation of a true regenerative program in particular.

12.2   Mononuclear Phagocytes: Monocytes and Macrophages (MΦ)

In recent years, MΦ have gained considerable scientific interest for fundamental immunology and cardiovascular biology owing to two seminal findings: [i] Unlike previously thought, embryonic MΦ can persist postnatally under homoeostatic conditions, and tissue-resident MΦ can maintain themselves *in situ* with minimal input from the circulation [20–28]. [ii] MΦ are required for *bona fide* heart regeneration in neonatal mice [7], identifying them as critical mediators of true regenerative programs and, hence, attractive therapeutic targets.

Recent Advances in Mononuclear Phagocyte System (MPS) Biology MΦ are long-lived myeloid cell members of the mononuclear phagocyte system (MPS) that are now known to derive from sequential waves of embryonic precursors [29]. MΦ reside in virtually all tissues, which they seed concomitantly with their development during embryonic or (early) postnatal life [30]. During organogenesis, they participate in tissue growth and remodeling, primarily through the clearance of senescent cells. Their absence leads to developmental abnormalities and, most notably, impairs the ability of tissues to regenerate, highlighting their importance in tissue homeostasis and healing after injury [31].

Until recently, the prevailing concept about the ontogeny of the MPS postulated that monocytes and MΦ derive from hematopoietic stem cells (HSC) through sequential commitment to MΦ and dendritic cell progenitors (MDP) [32]. MDP present in the bone marrow (BM) further differentiate through a newly described common monocyte precursor (cMoP) [33] that gives rise to the two main subsets of circulating monocytes, which can be distinguished by differential expression of Ly6C [34]. Ly6C$^+$ monocytes patrol the body through the blood circulation and are actively and rapidly recruited to the heart after MI. They subsequently differentiate in Ly6C^{low} monocytes through the NR4A1-dependent transcriptional program [35] and finally mature into MΦ at the site of injury.

This vision of the MPS has changed drastically in recent years, causing immunologists to revise the facultative monocytic origin of tissue-resident MΦ originally proposed and put forward by Van Furth [36]. The use of parabiotic mice and genetic fate-mapping models revealed that resident MΦ receive minimal input from HSC-derived circulating cells under homeostatic conditions, but rather, originate from embryonic precursors initially emerging in the yolk sac [20–27], seeding the fetal liver and eventually giving rise to fetal monocytes [23, 28]. These fetal monocytes circulate throughout the embryo and, with the notable exception of the brain [28], constantly infiltrate peripheral tissues including the heart [37], where they differentiate into resident MΦ. This continues to be the major developmental pathway until (at least) the onset of definitive hematopoiesis in the BM after birth. More recent work has further refined our understanding of MΦ biology, demonstrating that the capacity to self-maintain is not restricted to embryonic MΦ [38]. Extreme cases such as microglia exclusively depend on primitive yolk sac macrophages [20, 26, 39], while dermal and intestinal MΦ [40–42] continually recruit HSC-derived adult monocytes after birth. The majority of tissue-resident MΦ populations, however, appears to be of mixed origin. This is also the case for the highly heterogeneous MΦ population of the heart [37, 43]. Together, these observations support the concept of layered immunity, whereby each tissue-resident MΦ population originates from the sequential seeding of multiple waves of precursors over the lifespan of an animal [29]. As distinction of "embryonic" versus "adult" MΦ solely based on surface marker phenotype is not possible, the tissue-specific functions of each of these waves remain to be investigated through the use of refined fate-mapping systems. This will be key in uncovering the exact mechanisms by which MΦ affect cardiac healing and regeneration after MI and the question whether their developmental origin influences these functions.

12.2.1   The MPS in Myocardial Infarction, Repair and Regeneration

Cardiac MΦ   In the heart, resident MΦ are localized in the interstitial space from where they constantly sample the environment by phagocytosis and the expression of a large panel of pattern recognition receptors (PRR, for review [44]). In doing so, cardiac MΦ can identify and process pathogen- and danger-associated molecular patterns (PAMPS and DAMPS, respectively) released, for example, by dying or injured myocardial cells after MI. As these mechanisms rely on close cellular interactions, heart-resident MΦ limit the spread of inflammatory molecules to neighboring myocardial cells in proximity to the ischemic site and, thus, maintain local homeostasis. The adult murine heart is inhabited by relatively abundant, phenotypically, and developmentally heterogeneous MΦ [45, 46]. Based on their relative expression of MHCII and CCR2, three subsets have been described [37]. The CCR2⁻ cardiac MΦ can be further separated into MHCII⁺ and MHCII⁻ populations, which mainly derive from embryonic precursors [37, 43]. In steady-state mice, these resident cardiac MΦ have been proposed to largely maintain themselves through local self-renewal [37]; however, partial dilution of the resident embryonic-derived MΦ by bone marrow-derived MΦ is observed over time [43]. While the CCR2⁺ MΦ population has been considered part of the resident macrophage pool, they are likely more related to circulating [47] monocytes. These are functionally distinct from true resident cardiac MΦ in that they could provide more efficient protection against invading pathogens but could also be detrimental for tissue integrity under inappropriate activation situations. This emerging ontogenic disparity raises the question to what extent the cellular identity and function of MΦ is influenced by their origin. Albeit seemingly of academic nature, this question has significant direct implications for the role of MΦ in cardiovascular repair and regeneration: According to the current consensus, which is largely based on state-of-the-art genomics and epigenomics approaches [48], MΦ identity appears to be primarily shaped by the microenvironment and not their developmental origin [49, 50]. However, functional differences might only be apparent under non-homeostatic conditions. Indeed, monocyte-derived cells recruited during acute injury differ substantially from resident MΦ in that they remain more pro-inflammatory and pro-fibrotic [51]. Hence, in the context of myocardial infarction, it is tempting to speculate that the balance between self-maintenance of fully locally adapted cells and recruitment of circulating progenitors critically influences the regenerative potential of heart-resident MΦ. Seemingly in agreement with this hypothesis, the cardiac MΦ population changes over time, which appears to be at least partially due to a decline in the local self-renewal capacity and compensation by increased monocyte recruitment [43]. Strikingly, these changes coincide with loss of the regenerative potential in postnatal life, suggesting a causal link. Accordingly, it has been proposed that the capacity of cardiac MΦ to self-renew and/or their balance with recruitment from circulating progenitors might represent a critical determining factor for cardiac regeneration as opposed to tissue repair.

Interestingly, embryonic cardiac MΦ have been ascribed a critical role in coronary plexus remodeling [52] and thereby a developmental function, which is often regarded as the physiological counterpart to regenerative programs. Using a combination of a novel inducible cardiomyocyte ablation model and genetic lineage tracing, a recent study pioneered in addressing the question whether cardiac MΦ origin matters in the context of heart injury and repair [8]. This work relied on Rosa26-DTR mice crossed to a line in which Cre is expressed under control of the myosin light chain 2v (Mlc2v^{Cre}: Rosa26-DTR). In the resulting compound mice, cardiomyocytes are depleted upon administration of diphtheria toxin. Unlike adult mice, neonatal mice showed minimal mortality upon cardiomyocyte depletion. In neonatal, but not adult mice, embryo-derived MΦ supported healing through promoting angiogenesis and cardiomyocyte proliferation. Although some embryonic MΦ were found to persist in adult hearts, confirming earlier work [37], pro-inflammatory monocytes instead dominated the response to injury in the adult, resulting in impaired cardiac healing, a situation which, in turn, was improved when monocyte recruitment was dampened using CCR2-deficient mice. While cardiomyocyte ablation in this model [8] is rather strong and these results do not formally prove a strict dependence on either origin or environmental imprinting, they are in line with a model in which the fine-tuned balance between local adaptation and self-maintenance of resident MΦ, including those of embryonic origin, and recruitment of cells from additional sources (see below) determines the outcome of the regenerative or reparative program initiated and orchestrated by tissue-resident MΦ following sterile injury (see Fig. 12.1).

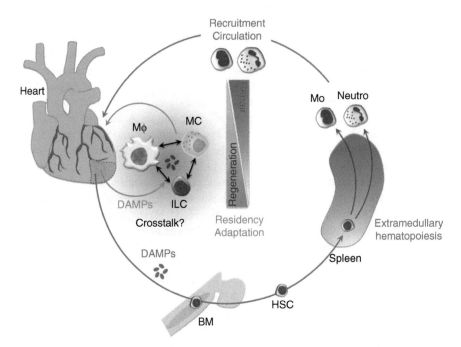

Fig. 12.1 The innate immune system in myocardial repair and regeneration following myocardial infarction. Scheme depicting the network of resident and circulating innate immune cells implicated in the response to myocardial infarction. Local interactions between resident macrophages, innate lymphoid cells and mast cells orchestrate cardiac tissue homeostasis at the site of injury. If the local immune response does not contain tissue injury expansion, excessive DAMPs and inflammatory signals from activated immune cells can trigger extramedullary hematopoiesis in the spleen. The newly generated monocytes and neutrophils then reach the site of injury and participate in controlling tissue damage. This finely tuned balance between local adaptation and expansion of resident and recruited cells determines the outcome of cardiac tissue regeneration or repair (scar formation). *BM* bone marrow, *HSC* hematopoietic stem cells, *Mo* monocytes, *Neutro* neutrophils, *MC* mast cells, *ILC* innate lymphoid cells, *MΦ* macrophages, *DAMPs* danger-associated molecular patterns

Extramedullary ("Emergency") Hematopoiesis Complementing local processes, tissue damage is sensed and the healing response coordinated also at the systemic level. As outlined above, this involves mechanisms of selective immune cell recruitment from circulating progenitors derived from the BM. In addition, recruitment of myeloid cells, like granulocytes and monocytes, can also occur from extramedullary "reservoirs" such as the spleen in a process referred to as "emergency hematopoiesis" [53]. Excessive amounts of DAMPs released from the injured tissue can reach the hematopoietic stem cell niche in the BM. Recent reports suggest that committed progenitors and HSCs are mobilized from the BM to seed the spleen in response to external threat or repetitive exposure to stress through the β3-adrenergic receptor [54]. Emergency hematopoiesis can be initiated by circulating pathogen-derived factors [55], but other pro-inflammatory factors derived from injured tissues such as DAMPs and pro-inflammatory cytokines can also be triggers. Additional endogenous signals, such as those derived from the nervous system, start to be explored in this context. For example, the perception of stress or pain itself is suspected to contribute to cardiac conditions through induction of extramedullary hematopoiesis [56]. To better control the number of infiltrating monocytes and MΦ, splenic hematopoiesis could be stimulated or regulated after MI [57], for example through activation or inhibition of the sympathetic nervous system via adrenoreceptor agonists or antagonists to promote or reduce the mobilization to the splenic monocyte reservoir, respectively [56]. Thus, this strategy might be relevant in regulating inflammatory monopoiesis, splenic release, and influx to the myocardium. This mechanism generally results in the generation of myeloid cells more adapted against invaders but also seems to have an overall protective role after MI, as splenectomy impairs the cardiac healing process [57]. Moreover, approaches to deplete monocytes and MΦ highlighted their importance in local collagen production, which is necessary for tissue repair and remodeling after MI. Other studies using CCR2 knockout mice, however, have also shown that Ly6C$^+$ monocyte recruitment promotes cardiac tissue fibrosis, local inflammation, and scar formation [51]. Hence, excessive inflammatory monocyte recruitment seems to increase cardiac pathology and further promote myocardial fragility. This discrepancy in monocyte functions could be explained by the existence of discrete monocytic subsets within the circulating monocyte pool, which is only being fully appreciated in more recent times [58].

12.3   Neutrophils

Neutrophil Biology Neutrophils are polymorphonuclear myeloid cells specialized in bacterial killing through multiple intra- and extracellular means. They are equipped with three types of granules [59]. These are azurophilic (primary) granules, which contain myeloperoxidase (MPO); specific (secondary) granules containing lactoferrin; and gelatinase (tertiary) granules that contain matrix metalloproteinase 9 (MMP9; also known as gelatinase B). Neutrophils can phagocytose invading pathogens very efficiently and kill them through the production of reactive oxygen species (ROS) generated in an NADPH-oxygenase-dependent manner. They also release antibacterial proteins (cathepsins, defensins, lactoferrin, and lysozyme) [60]. Highly activated neutrophils can also eliminate extracellular pathogens by releasing NETs. NETs are composed of a core DNA element to which histones, proteins, and enzymes from their granules are attached. Neutrophils are extremely motile and are the first leukocytes mobilized regardless of the cause of the injury [61]. This arsenal of biological "weapons" makes them true "killing machines" that prevent pathogen dissemination. Beyond these well-known functions, more recent reports also suggest functional plasticity within neutrophils. For example, neutrophils activated upon *Trypanosoma cruzi* infection produce IL-10, thereby inhibiting T-cell proliferation and interferon-γ (IFNγ) production [62]. Another report suggests that specific subsets of neutrophils respond to specific signals: CXCR4^{low} pro-inflammatory neutrophils respond to CXCL2 to reach the site of injury, whereas CXCR4^{high} MMP9^{high} pro-angiogenic neutrophils respond to vascular endothelial growth factor A (VEGFA) [63]. Such pathways could be targeted to control the recruitment of specific neutrophil subsets following MI.

Role of Neutrophils in Myocardial Repair Following Infarction Neutrophils attracted to the myocardium after MI release large amounts of reactive oxygen species (ROS), a phenomenon known as respiratory burst [64]. These can directly react with myocardial membrane lipids, proteins, and DNA, causing cell injury in the early phase of MI [65]. However, antioxidant treatment 7 days post-MI reduces microvascular density, suggesting that ROS production can also promote angiogenesis and thus be beneficial for cardiac tissue repair [66]. Granule components of neutrophils such as MPO, known as a diagnostic plasma marker of MI patients, are also harmful as they are associated with increased long-term mortality in acute MI patients [67] and predict adverse long-term prognosis and heart failure after MI. Furthermore, the generation of NETs can also be detrimental during the recovery phase after MI. Experimental cleaving and clearance of NETs' chromatin through DNase administration has cardioprotective effects, resulting in subsequent improvement of cardiac contractile function in ischemia/reperfusion models [68]. Therefore, inhibition of NET formation or its degradation could be a new therapeutic strategy to reduce ischemic cardiac injury. In the opposite situation, phagocytosis of apoptotic neutrophils leads MΦ to produce anti-inflammatory cytokines such as transforming growth factor beta (TGF-β) and IL-10, as well as lipoxins and resolvins [69]. Thus, the clearance of apoptotic neutrophils appears to reprogram MΦ towards an anti-inflammatory phenotype crucial for the resolution of inflammation after MI.

12.4   Mast Cells (MC)

MC Biology Best known as effector cells mediating anaphylactic reactions in allergy, mast cells (MC) are characterized by cytosolic secretory granules equipped with effector molecules that can be released instantly upon MC activation. These effectors are either preformed or synthesized *de novo*. They encompass chemokines and cytokines, proteases, heparin, histamine and various other classes of molecules, including growth factors, fatty acid metabolites, as well as vaso- and neuroactive substances.

As is the case for their effectors, the stimuli activating MC range widely. MC express pattern recognition receptors (PRRs) that respond to pathogen- and damage-associated molecular patterns (PAMPs and DAMPs, respectively), both of which are released by the damaged, infarcted myocardium. MC also express ST2, the receptor for IL-33, an IL-1 family member that functions as a so-called alarmin in that it is constitutively expressed and intracellularly stored primarily by epithelial cells, which release it upon damage [70]. Thus, MC are rapid responders providing a "first line of defense" to pathogens as well as tissue damage. MC have long been known to be capable of re-granulating [71, 72], (Kobayasi 1969), [73]), and the exact composition of MC mediators released is defined by the nature of the activating stimulus. Perhaps counterintuitively, therefore, MC degranulation appears to be a specific process.

Similar to MΦ, MC are long-lived [73, 74] tissue-resident innate immune cells of the myeloid lineage. They originate from BM-derived progenitors downstream of HSC and commonly thought to be contained within the common granulocyte-monocyte progenitor (GMP) population. Using state-of-the-art single-cell RNA sequencing, a recent study resolved a long-standing controversy and found that the bipotent progenitors for mast cells and basophil and eosinophil progenitors segregate from those for monocytes and neutrophils earlier than previously thought [75]. Precursors with restricted MC potential are also transiently present in the fetal circulation during late gestation [76]; however, their relevance for and relation to adult MC development are currently unknown.

MC reside in a variety of organs, but, with the exception of the skin, their abundance in unchallenged conditions is rather low. In contrast, MC numbers are known to increase sometimes drastically in pathology both in animal models [71, 77, 78] and humans [79–82]. Paralleling the situation for MΦ, three main, non-mutually exclusive mechanisms can be envisioned by which MC increase in an organ affected by disease: While thought to be uncommon at steady state, local proliferation of mature MC could contribute to (rapid) local increases in MC numbers. Similarly, circulating MC progenitors continuously home to peripheral tissues at low frequency, which could be enhanced, for example, in response to sterile injury. Alternatively, or in addition, precursors already present in the affected tissue could divide and mature locally. In this context, it is noteworthy that indeed MC progenitors have been identified in various peripheral organs including the skin, gut, white adipose tissue (WAT), and lung [83–86].

As with MΦ and recruited monocytes, it is tempting to speculate that the balance between freshly recruited MC progenitors and their locally adapted resident or resident precursor-derived counterpart influences the functional phenotype of the composite resident population. This would be particularly relevant for the transition from the early inflammatory to the anti-inflammatory, reparative phase after myocardial infarction, a possibility that will be further explored below.

Support for the notion that the (micro)environment determines MC phenotypes comes from data collected by the Immunological Genome Consortium, which recently determined the core transcriptomic signature of tissue-resident MC through genome-wide expression [87]. In addition to the shared core signature defining MC lineage identity, MC populations also express genes dependent on the organ they reside in, reminiscent of what the consortium had previously shown for MΦ using the same approach [88].

Cardiac MC and Their Functions in Myocardial Remodeling After Infarction The adult mammalian heart contains low numbers of mature c-Kit$^+$ FcεR1$^+$ MC [77, 89, 90]. In stark contrast to MΦ (see above and chapter "The Role of Cardiac Tissue Macrophages in Homeostasis and Disease"), very little is known about this population in the resting state.

Pathophysiologically, MC have been initially implicated in cardiovascular disease owing to the seminal observation that they are found (more) abundantly in atherosclerotic lesions of human patients [91], followed by the finding that they can directly convert MΦ into plaque-forming foam cells through modulating their lipoprotein metabolism [92, 93]. Thus, MC are generally thought to be pro-atherogenic both during initiation, but also progression of atherosclerosis. Indeed, clinically, the numbers of mature MC in atherosclerotic lesions correlate with disease stage and the microvessel density within the plaques [94].

Our knowledge about the involvement of MC in the immediate response to and remodeling following myocardial infarction is comparably sparse, although MI can, in its extremity, even represent a cardiovascular manifestation of anaphylaxis, and, reversely, cardiovascular disease increases the risk of severe and especially of fatal allergic complications [95], as does obesity [96]. Evidence for an involvement of MC in human MI largely derived from traditional approaches like the assessment of circulating levels of MC mediators and activators such as tryptase and IgE, respectively. Similarly, classical immunohistochemistry is used to detect MC *in situ* in pathological samples, often by means of their metachromatic granules.

Together, experimental and clinical data have identified multiple roles for MC in myocardial healing after acute infarction. By means of their activating receptors, MC rapidly sense cardiac damage and release histamine and TNF-α, thereby participating in the initiation of sterile inflammation [97]. As outlined above, this inflammatory response is further enhanced through activation of resident MΦ and infiltrating neutrophils. MC effectors, particularly pro-inflammatory cytokines, also directly partake in the recruitment of immune cells, such as T cells and monocytes, as reduced numbers of inflammatory monocytes and MΦ are found in mice treated with MC stabilizers or MC-deficient mice [98]. Finally, accumulating evidence suggests MC might be involved in the reparative phase, primarily through their effects on ECM remodeling [90, 99]. Thus, MC appear to be involved throughout the distinct stages of myocardial healing. Unlike their disease-promoting role in atherosclerosis, however, they appear to have both detrimental and beneficial effects in the context of MI. For example, MC can promote fibrosis through stimulation of collagen synthesis, while collagen degradation through MC-mediated activation of matrix metalloproteinases (MMP) has also been reported [100].

Some of this controversy might be attributable to the widespread use of c-Kit mutant mice as MC-deficient mouse models. In addition to its role in MC development, proliferation, and survival, signaling of stem cell factor (SCF) through its receptor c-Kit has many nonredundant functions in other cell types both within and outside the hematopoietic system [101]. Therefore, data solely derived from c-Kit mutant mice need to be interpreted with caution. In the light of these issues, several teams have recently developed novel genetic tools to study MC function more specifically [101]. Using one such mouse model, the so-called Cre-Master mice, in which MC are selectively depleted owing to Cre-induced genotoxicity when expressed under control of the MC protease carboxypeptidase A3 (Cpa3) [102], a recent study revealed a somewhat unexpected function for MC in the repair phase following acute myocardial infarction [77]. In these mice, MC deficiency results in calcium desensitization of the cardiac myofilaments in a mechanism dependent on MC tryptase, causing impaired contractility [77].

As discussed above, cardiac MC significantly increase in numbers in various diseases and disease models, yet the mechanisms responsible for this increase have barely been deciphered. Interestingly, these might differ depending on the conditions: In a model for chronic volume overload, for instance, MC numbers increase within 12 hours, which has been attributed to the fast maturation of immature resident cells or local precursors in the absence of (increased) proliferation [100, 103]. Contrary to this rapid increase from a pool of immature, resident cells, MC numbers show a marked increase and peak only 7 days after myocardial infarction, succeeding an increase in local progenitors after 3 days [77]. Interestingly, not only do these data suggest a different mechanism underlying the increase in MC numbers following MI, namely, recruitment of a progenitor, the study also convincingly demonstrated that these progenitors do not originate from the BM, but instead, derive from the WAT [77].

As summarized here, MC are involved in various stages of the cardiac remodeling process following acute infarction. Taking into account the diversity of the reported functions and the controversy of some findings, however, much remains to be learned about their roles in acute myocardial infarction and return to homeostasis. The advent of alternative, c-Kit-independent MC mouse models [101] will allow a better dissection of their diverse functions at distinct stages of cardiac remodeling. Such models allow for the identification of previously unknown functions, as illustrated by the example of the modulation of myofilament contractility by MC [77]. Such models will also enable addressing some as of yet unresolved questions, for instance, whether MC are also required for the *bona fide* regenerative capacity of newborn mouse hearts, a possibility that seems likely considering the need for removal of the initially formed fibrotic scar and the equipment of MC with potent mediators of ECM remodeling.

12.5   Innate Lymphoid Cells (ILC)

ILC Biology   Innate lymphoid cells (ILC) are a recently described family of tissue-resident immune cells that derive from the common lymphoid progenitor in an IL-7-dependent manner and, hence, developmentally belong to the lymphoid lineage [104]. Unlike classical T- and B-lymphocytes, however, ILC display characteristics of innate immune cells as they lack rearranged antigen receptors and, instead, readily produce cytokines in response to activation. In doing so, ILC contribute to the "first line of defense" against pathogens but also partake in the rapid response to non-immunological challenges such as tissue damage, functions classically assigned to the myeloid lineage. Indeed, ILC are now well recognized for their involvement in tissue homeostasis as they mediate organogenesis [105–107] as well as repair and regeneration following injury [108–113].

The different members of the ILC family can be distinguished according to their upstream activators and corresponding surface receptors, the signature cytokines they produce, as well as the transcriptomic circuits required for their development and lineage specification. As these features mirror the different T helper cell lineages, ILC are commonly regarded as their innate counterparts. Paying tribute to this striking resemblance, three main ILC lineages are now distinguished: Group 1 ILC produce IFNγ and TNF and depend on the transcription factor T-bet; group 2 ILC require RORα and GATA3 expression and produce the type 2 cytokines IL-4, IL-5, and IL-13, while group 3 ILC resemble Th17 cells in that they depend on the transcription factor RORγt and secrete IL-17A and/or IL-22 [15]. Adding further complexity to this classification, the ILC family also encompasses conventional natural killer (NK) cells and the prototypical ILC, lymphoid tissue inducer (LTi) cells [105], that are now classed as group 1 and 3 ILC, respectively. Taking their broad functions into account, a refined nomenclature has been put forward that further distinguishes "helper-like" ILC (members of ILC1, ILC2, ILC3) from "killer-like" ILC (NK cells, some ILC1) [114].

Not unlike myeloid cells, ILC display remarkable phenotypic plasticity in response to environmental stimuli. While much of the current knowledge about ILC is derived from mouse studies, many aspects of their biology have been explored and confirmed in human (recently reviewed in [115, 116]). Moreover, ILC have been directly implicated in a variety of human pathologies, ranging from infectious diseases [117] to autoimmunity such as allergy, asthma, and inflammatory bowel disease [115] to the development of graft-versus-host disease following hematopoietic stem cell transplantation [118, 119]. Not surprisingly, therefore, ILC have been in the focus of immunological research ever since their recent identification.

Developmentally, fetal liver and adult bone marrow progenitors [120–123] have been identified for ILC. Strikingly, in naïve mice, helper-like ILC resident in non-lymphoid organs are relatively long-lived and self-maintain through local proliferation largely independently from hematopoietic input [124]. Thus, ILC development and maintenance mechanisms appear in many ways reminiscent of what has recently become known for MΦ (see above and chapter "The Role of Cardiac Tissue Macrophages in Homeostasis and Disease"). Although it is currently unclear which exact hematopoietic stage(s) ILC originate from in the embryo and whether embryonic ILC persist postnatally, it is tempting to speculate that more similarities exist between the different arms of the innate immune system, which, as outlined above and discussed in more detail below, might have direct functional implications for their roles in heart repair and *bona fide* regeneration.

Thus, our fundamental understanding of ILC biology and their involvement in pathophysiology has grown exponentially, yet, comparably, little is known about the involvement of ILC in cardiovascular disease. Of note, however, several recent studies identified critical roles for ILC, and group 2 ILC in particular, in adipose tissue function and metabolic diseases such as diabetes, obesity, and atherosclerosis [125–128], all of which are inherently linked with (the risk for) myocardial infarction.

Under homeostatic conditions, murine and human ILC appear to be enriched at border surfaces such as the skin and mucosal epithelia of the lung and gastrointestinal systems, while their numbers in other organs are comparably low in the adult, circumstances which have likely contributed to their late discovery [104]. Interestingly, ILC seem to be generally more abundant during embryonic and early postnatal life [129], further underlining their (potential) involvement in developmental processes that, in turn, are often regarded as the developmental "blueprints" to regeneration. Such developmental functions have been formally demonstrated, for example for LTi cells, which are required for the establishment of lymph nodes [105].

Cardiac ILC NK cells, founding members of the ILC family, rapidly appear in the myocardium upon infarction, along with adaptive T, B cells and monocytes [130]. An early study reported reduced function of circulating NK cells following myocardial infarction in patients [131]. Mechanistically, NK cells and monocytes are known to engage in reciprocal functional modulation through interferon-γ (IFNγ) and IL-12 and IL-18, respectively [132]. Although this appears to be important in the acute inflammatory phase, the question whether NK cells can integrate in the pool of resident immune cells as well as their exact contribution to cardiac remodeling following infarction remains largely enigmatic.

Until recently, NK cells were the only ILC family members whose presence was documented in the murine heart. This changed with a seminal study that identified tissue-resident cardiac ILC2, notably in the resting heart of naïve adult IL-5 reporter mice [133]. Numbers of cardiac ILC2 are low at steady state. However, it can be envisioned that these increase in response to myocardial infarction. As is the case for other innate immune cells such as MC, low abundance at steady state does not preclude critical functions following an insult such as myocardial infarction. Moreover, not only has a resident cardiac ILC2 population been identified; their upstream-activating cytokines IL-25 and IL-33 have been shown to be contributing factors to atherosclerosis [134, 135], and critically, IL-13, a signature cytokine produced by ILC2, might be cardioprotective following MI [136].

(Potential) Involvement of ILC in Myocardial Infarction, Repair, and Regeneration ILC are increasingly recognized for their critical functions in tissue remodeling in various infectious but also chronic and acute inflammatory conditions, including sterile injuries [108, 137, 138]. Regeneration of the gastrointestinal tract, for instance, depends on ILC, which, intriguingly, appear to directly act on intestinal stem cells [113, 139].

As prototypical type 2 immune cells, ILC2 express receptors that respond to epithelial-derived cytokines known to be involved in fibrosis in both animal models and human disease, namely, IL-25, IL-33, and TSLP, some of which are regarded as "emergency" signals or so-called alarmins. Therefore, ILC, and (cardiac) ILC2 especially, represent prime candidates for partaking in the regenerative and reparative response following myocardial infarction: Unlike their adaptive counterparts, they are equipped with cytokines to readily respond to tissue damage, many of which are produced constitutively and secreted upon activation, the virtue by which cardiac ILC2 have been identified in the first place [133].

Although formal proof of their involvement in cardiac remodeling following acute infarction is currently lacking, several lines of evidence support this notion: Elevated levels of circulating IL-13, a signature cytokine produced by ILC2, have been found in patients suffering from chronic heart failure, where they were found to inversely correlative with left ventricular ejection fraction [140]. Moreover, IL-13 might be a critical parameter also for acute infarction, as its genetic deficiency worsened the outcome following MI in a rodent model [136]. While this effect has been attributed to Th2 cells, these data were obtained from a non-conditional knockout for IL-13 and, hence, would be consistent with an involvement of ILC [2]. Not only do ILC2 produce IL-13 themselves in both mice and humans [141, 142], they can also initiate and further potentiate Th2 responses [143]. Mechanistically, IL-13 deficiency caused an increase in overall leukocytes, especially myeloid cells, which displayed a more pro-inflammatory and pro-fibrotic phenotype. This suggests that type 2 immune cells phenotypically modulate recruited monocytes and resident MΦ by means of IL-13 secretion in response to MI. Such modulatory cross talk is emerging as a cardinal feature of immune cell networks, including ILC (see Fig. 12.1).

Indeed, ILC are known to engage in extensive cross talk, particularly with myeloid lineages, resulting in reciprocal modulation of immune cell phenotype and activation status. ILC2, for example, intimately interact with MC in the dermis and modulate their IgE-dependent cytokine release through IL-13 [144]. Notably, evidence for functional ILC-MΦ cross talk has also been obtained in the context of injury, as systemically administered IL-33 improves skin wound healing by promoting alternative MΦ activation [111], whereas deletion of the IL-33 receptor ST2 favors inflammatory MΦ and results in impaired healing [145]. Conversely, ILC function is also subject to modulation by other lineages, as alveolar MΦ contribute to airway hyperreactivity by potentiating IL-13 secretion of ILC2 [146], while intestinal MΦ regulate IL-22 expression by ILC [147–149]. Thus, ILC cross talk with other (innate) immune cells, such as MΦ and MC, occurs in various organs both at steady state and following infection or injury, suggesting it represents a more general mechanism that might also apply to the heart upon acute infarction.

In conclusion, studying the role of ILC in the context of heart repair and regeneration bears great potential. Unfortunately, however, it faces technical challenges. These are largely attributable to the inherent limitation of functional studies using human material and the paucity of specific mouse models. Common ILC-deficient mouse models such as Id2$^{-/-}$ and Rag2$^{-/-}$ Il2rg$^{-/-}$ mice can be difficult to interpret: Id2$^{-/-}$ mice appear grossly normal at birth, but display gradual growth retardation [150]. Another commonly used model, Rag2$^{-/-}$ Il2rg$^{-/-}$ mice, additionally lack adaptive lymphocytes, which also play critical roles in the response to MI [136, 151, 152] (see chapter "Lymphocytes"). Thus, better distinction of ILC from T cells will be critical. A suitable approach is to compare mice in which expression of a floxed diphtheria toxin receptor (DTR) transgene affects either both ILC and T cells, or T cells only [153]. Subjecting such mice to microsurgical models of myocardial infarction would allow researchers to directly and specifically assess the role of and requirement for ILC2 in cardiac repair (adult mice) and regeneration (neonatal mice). Supplemented with clinical data, such studies will likely yield critical insight regarding the involvement of ILC in myocardial infarction and, ultimately, repair and regeneration.

References

1. Forbes SJ, Rosenthal N. Preparing the ground for tissue regeneration: from mechanism to therapy. Nat Med. 2014;20(8):857–69.
2. Moran AE, Forouzanfar MH, Roth GA, Mensah GA, Ezzati M, Flaxman A, et al. The global burden of ischemic heart disease in 1990 and 2010: the global burden of disease 2010 study. Circulation. 2014;129(14):1493–501.
3. Nowbar AN, Howard JP, Finegold JA, Asaria P, Francis DP. 2014 global geographic analysis of mortality from ischaemic heart disease by country, age and income: statistics from World Health Organisation and United Nations. Int J Cardiol. 2014;174(2):293–8.
4. Tauber AI. Metchnikoff and the phagocytosis theory. Nat Rev Mol Cell Biol. 2003;4(11):897–901.
5. Ramos GC. Inflammation as an animal development phenomenon. Clin Dev Immunol. 2012;2012:983203.
6. Leor J, Rozen L, Zuloff-Shani A, Feinberg MS, Amsalem Y, Barbash IM, et al. Ex vivo activated human macrophages improve healing, remodeling, and function of the infarcted heart. Circulation. 2006;114(1 Suppl):I94–100.
7. Aurora AB, Porrello ER, Tan W, Mahmoud AI, Hill JA, Bassel-Duby R, et al. Macrophages are required for neonatal heart regeneration. J Clin Invest. 2014;124(3):1382–92.
8. Lavine KJ, Epelman S, Uchida K, Weber KJ, Nichols CG, Schilling JD, et al. Distinct macrophage lineages contribute to disparate patterns of cardiac recovery and remodeling in the neonatal and adult heart. Proc Natl Acad Sci U S A. 2014;111(45):16029–34.
9. Drenckhahn JD, Schwarz QP, Gray S, Laskowski A, Kiriazis H, Ming Z, et al. Compensatory growth of healthy cardiac cells in the presence of diseased cells restores tissue homeostasis during heart development. Dev Cell. 2008;15(4):521–33.
10. Porrello ER, Mahmoud AI, Simpson E, Hill JA, Richardson JA, Olson EN, et al. Transient regenerative potential of the neonatal mouse heart. Science. 2011;331(6020):1078–80.
11. Haubner BJ, Adamowicz-Brice M, Khadayate S, Tiefenthaler V, Metzler B, Aitman T, et al. Complete cardiac regeneration in a mouse model of myocardial infarction. Aging. 2012;4(12):966–77.
12. Robledo M. Myocardial regeneration in young rats. Am J Pathol. 1956;32(6):1215–39.
13. Konfino T, Landa N, Ben-Mordechai T, Leor J. The type of injury dictates the mode of repair in neonatal and adult heart. J Am Heart Assoc. 2015;4(1):e001320.
14. Darehzereshki A, Rubin N, Gamba L, Kim J, Fraser J, Huang Y, et al. Differential regenerative capacity of neonatal mouse hearts after cryoinjury. Dev Biol. 2015;399(1):91–9.
15. Spits H, Artis D, Colonna M, Diefenbach A, Di Santo JP, Eberl G, et al. Innate lymphoid cells--a proposal for uniform nomenclature. Nat Rev Immunol. 2013;13(2):145–9.
16. Ley K, Laudanna C, Cybulsky MI, Nourshargh S. Getting to the site of inflammation: the leukocyte adhesion cascade updated. Nat Rev Immunol. 2007;7(9):678–89.
17. Ajuebor MN, Das AM, Virag L, Flower RJ, Szabo C, Perretti M. Role of resident peritoneal macrophages and mast cells in chemokine production and neutrophil migration in acute inflammation: evidence for an inhibitory loop involving endogenous IL-10. J Immunol. 1999;162(3):1685–91.

18. Brinkmann V, Reichard U, Goosmann C, Fauler B, Uhlemann Y, Weiss DS, et al. Neutrophil extracellular traps kill bacteria. Science. 2004;303(5663):1532–5.

19. Serbina NV, Salazar-Mather TP, Biron CA, Kuziel WA, Pamer EG. TNF/iNOS-producing dendritic cells mediate innate immune defense against bacterial infection. Immunity. 2003;19(1):59–70.

20. Ginhoux F, Greter M, Leboeuf M, Nandi S, See P, Gokhan S, et al. Fate mapping analysis reveals that adult microglia derive from primitive macrophages. Science. 2010;330(6005):841–5.

21. Jenkins SJ, Ruckerl D, Cook PC, Jones LH, Finkelman FD, van Rooijen N, et al. Local macrophage proliferation, rather than recruitment from the blood, is a signature of TH2 inflammation. Science. 2011;332(6035):1284–8.

22. Schulz C, Gomez Perdiguero E, Chorro L, Szabo-Rogers H, Cagnard N, Kierdorf K, et al. A lineage of myeloid cells independent of Myb and hematopoietic stem cells. Science. 2012;336(6077):86–90.

23. Hoeffel G, Wang Y, Greter M, See P, Teo P, Malleret B, et al. Adult Langerhans cells derive predominantly from embryonic fetal liver monocytes with a minor contribution of yolk sac-derived macrophages. J Exp Med. 2012;209(6):1167–81.

24. Yona S, Kim KW, Wolf Y, Mildner A, Varol D, Breker M, et al. Fate mapping reveals origins and dynamics of monocytes and tissue macrophages under homeostasis. Immunity. 2013;38(1):79–91.

25. Hashimoto D, Chow A, Noizat C, Teo P, Beasley MB, Leboeuf M, et al. Tissue-resident macrophages self-maintain locally throughout adult life with minimal contribution from circulating monocytes. Immunity. 2013;38(4):792–804.

26. Kierdorf K, Erny D, Goldmann T, Sander V, Schulz C, Perdiguero EG, et al. Microglia emerge from erythromyeloid precursors via Pu.1- and Irf8-dependent pathways. Nat Neurosci. 2013;16(3):273–80.

27. Gomez Perdiguero E, Klapproth K, Schulz C, Busch K, Azzoni E, Crozet L, et al. Tissue-resident macrophages originate from yolk-sac-derived erythro-myeloid progenitors. Nature. 2015;518(7540):547–51.

28. Hoeffel G, Chen J, Lavin Y, Low D, Almeida FF, See P, et al. C-myb(+) erythro-myeloid progenitor-derived fetal monocytes give rise to adult tissue-resident macrophages. Immunity. 2015;42(4):665–78.

29. Hoeffel G, Ginhoux F. Ontogeny of tissue-resident macrophages. Front Immunol. 2015;6:486.

30. Mass E, Ballesteros I, Farlik M, Halbritter F, Gunther P, Crozet L, et al. Specification of tissue-resident macrophages during organogenesis. Science. 2016;353(6304):aaf4238.

31. McKercher SR, Torbett BE, Anderson KL, Henkel GW, Vestal DJ, Baribault H, et al. Targeted disruption of the PU.1 gene results in multiple hematopoietic abnormalities. EMBO J. 1996;15(20):5647–58.

32. Auffray C, Fogg DK, Narni-Mancinelli E, Senechal B, Trouillet C, Saederup N, et al. CX3CR1+ CD115+ CD135+ common macrophage/DC precursors and the role of CX3CR1 in their response to inflammation. J Exp Med. 2009;206(3):595–606.

33. Hettinger J, Richards DM, Hansson J, Barra MM, Joschko AC, Krijgsveld J, et al. Origin of monocytes and macrophages in a committed progenitor. Nat Immunol. 2013;14(8):821–30.

34. Geissmann F, Jung S, Littman DR. Blood monocytes consist of two principal subsets with distinct migratory properties. Immunity. 2003;19(1):71–82.

35. Hanna RN, Carlin LM, Hubbeling HG, Nackiewicz D, Green AM, Punt JA, et al. The transcription factor NR4A1 (Nur77) controls bone marrow differentiation and the survival of Ly6C- monocytes. Nat Immunol. 2011;12(8):778–85.

36. van Furth R, Cohn ZA. The origin and kinetics of mononuclear phagocytes. J Exp Med. 1968;128(3):415–35.

37. Epelman S, Lavine KJ, Beaudin AE, Sojka DK, Carrero JA, Calderon B, et al. Embryonic and adult-derived resident cardiac macrophages are maintained through distinct mechanisms at steady state and during inflammation. Immunity. 2014;40(1):91–104.

38. van de Laar L, Saelens W, De Prijck S, Martens L, Scott CL, Van Isterdael G, et al. Yolk sac macrophages, fetal liver, and adult monocytes can colonize an empty niche and develop into functional tissue-resident macrophages. Immunity. 2016;44(4):755–68.

39. Ajami B, Bennett JL, Krieger C, Tetzlaff W, Rossi FM. Local self-renewal can sustain CNS microglia maintenance and function throughout adult life. Nat Neurosci. 2007;10(12):1538–43.
40. Bain CC, Bravo-Blas A, Scott CL, Gomez Perdiguero E, Geissmann F, Henri S, et al. Constant replenishment from circulating monocytes maintains the macrophage pool in the intestine of adult mice. Nat Immunol. 2014;15(10):929–37.
41. Zigmond E, Varol C, Farache J, Elmaliah E, Satpathy AT, Friedlander G, et al. Ly6C hi monocytes in the inflamed colon give rise to proinflammatory effector cells and migratory antigen-presenting cells. Immunity. 2012;37(6):1076–90.
42. Tamoutounour S, Guilliams M, Montanana Sanchis F, Liu H, Terhorst D, Malosse C, et al. Origins and functional specialization of macrophages and of conventional and monocyte-derived dendritic cells in mouse skin. Immunity. 2013;39(5):925–38.
43. Molawi K, Wolf Y, Kandalla PK, Favret J, Hagemeyer N, Frenzel K, et al. Progressive replacement of embryo-derived cardiac macrophages with age. J Exp Med. 2014;211(11):2151–8.
44. Underhill DM, Goodridge HS. Information processing during phagocytosis. Nat Rev Immunol. 2012;12(7):492–502.
45. Pinto AR, Paolicelli R, Salimova E, Gospocic J, Slonimsky E, Bilbao-Cortes D, et al. An abundant tissue macrophage population in the adult murine heart with a distinct alternatively-activated macrophage profile. PLoS One. 2012;7(5):e36814.
46. Pinto AR, Godwin JW, Chandran A, Hersey L, Ilinykh A, Debuque R, et al. Age-related changes in tissue macrophages precede cardiac functional impairment. Aging. 2014;6(5):399–413.
47. Rea D, Francis A, Hanby AM, Speirs V, Rakha E, Shaaban A, et al. Inflammatory breast cancer: time to standardise diagnosis assessment and management, and for the joining of forces to facilitate effective research. Br J Cancer. 2015;112(9):1613–5.
48. Alvarez-Errico D, Vento-Tormo R, Sieweke M, Ballestar E. Epigenetic control of myeloid cell differentiation, identity and function. Nat Rev Immunol. 2015;15(1):7–17.
49. Lavin Y, Winter D, Blecher-Gonen R, David E, Keren-Shaul H, Merad M, et al. Tissue-resident macrophage enhancer landscapes are shaped by the local microenvironment. Cell. 2014;159(6):1312–26.
50. Gosselin D, Link VM, Romanoski CE, Fonseca GJ, Eichenfield DZ, Spann NJ, et al. Environment drives selection and function of enhancers controlling tissue-specific macrophage identities. Cell. 2014;159(6):1327–40.
51. Majmudar MD, Keliher EJ, Heidt T, Leuschner F, Truelove J, Sena BF, et al. Monocyte-directed RNAi targeting CCR2 improves infarct healing in atherosclerosis-prone mice. Circulation. 2013;127(20):2038–46.
52. Leid J, Carrelha J, Boukarabila H, Epelman S, Jacobsen SE, Lavine KJ. Primitive embryonic macrophages are required for coronary development and maturation. Circ Res. 2016;118(10):1498–511.
53. Swirski FK, Nahrendorf M, Etzrodt M, Wildgruber M, Cortez-Retamozo V, Panizzi P, et al. Identification of splenic reservoir monocytes and their deployment to inflammatory sites. Science. 2009;325(5940):612–6.
54. Heidt T, Sager HB, Courties G, Dutta P, Iwamoto Y, Zaltsman A, et al. Chronic variable stress activates hematopoietic stem cells. Nat Med. 2014;20(7):754–8.
55. Khosravi A, Yanez A, Price JG, Chow A, Merad M, Goodridge HS, et al. Gut microbiota promote hematopoiesis to control bacterial infection. Cell Host Microbe. 2014;15(3):374–81.
56. Dutta P, Courties G, Wei Y, Leuschner F, Gorbatov R, Robbins CS, et al. Myocardial infarction accelerates atherosclerosis. Nature. 2012;487(7407):325–9.
57. Leuschner F, Rauch PJ, Ueno T, Gorbatov R, Marinelli B, Lee WW, et al. Rapid monocyte kinetics in acute myocardial infarction are sustained by extramedullary monocytopoiesis. J Exp Med. 2012;209(1):123–37.
58. Menezes S, Melandri D, Anselmi G, Perchet T, Loschko J, Dubrot J, et al. The heterogeneity of Ly6Chi monocytes controls their differentiation into iNOS+ macrophages or monocyte-derived dendritic cells. Immunity. 2016;45(6):1205–18.
59. Hager M, Cowland JB, Borregaard N. Neutrophil granules in health and disease. J Intern Med. 2010;268(1):25–34.

60. Borregaard N. Neutrophils, from marrow to microbes. Immunity. 2010;33(5):657–70.
61. Lammermann T, Afonso PV, Angermann BR, Wang JM, Kastenmuller W, Parent CA, et al. Neutrophil swarms require LTB4 and integrins at sites of cell death in vivo. Nature. 2013;498(7454):371–5.
62. Tosello Boari J, Amezcua Vesely MC, Bermejo DA, Ramello MC, Montes CL, Cejas H, et al. IL-17RA signaling reduces inflammation and mortality during Trypanosoma cruzi infection by recruiting suppressive IL-10-producing neutrophils. PLoS Pathog. 2012;8(4):e1002658.
63. Christoffersson G, Vagesjo E, Vandooren J, Liden M, Massena S, Reinert RB, et al. VEGF-A recruits a proangiogenic MMP-9-delivering neutrophil subset that induces angiogenesis in transplanted hypoxic tissue. Blood. 2012;120(23):4653–62.
64. Ciz M, Denev P, Kratchanova M, Vasicek O, Ambrozova G, Lojek A. Flavonoids inhibit the respiratory burst of neutrophils in mammals. Oxidative Med Cell Longev. 2012;2012:1–6. 181295.
65. Amulic B, Cazalet C, Hayes GL, Metzler KD, Zychlinsky A. Neutrophil function: from mechanisms to disease. Annu Rev Immunol. 2012;30:459–89.
66. Zhao W, Zhao T, Chen Y, Ahokas RA, Sun Y. Reactive oxygen species promote angiogenesis in the infarcted rat heart. Int J Exp Pathol. 2009;90(6):621–9.
67. Mocatta TJ, Pilbrow AP, Cameron VA, Senthilmohan R, Frampton CM, Richards AM, et al. Plasma concentrations of myeloperoxidase predict mortality after myocardial infarction. J Am Coll Cardiol. 2007;49(20):1993–2000.
68. Savchenko AS, Borissoff JI, Martinod K, De Meyer SF, Gallant M, Erpenbeck L, et al. VWF-mediated leukocyte recruitment with chromatin decondensation by PAD4 increases myocardial ischemia/reperfusion injury in mice. Blood. 2014;123(1):141–8.
69. Soehnlein O, Lindbom L. Phagocyte partnership during the onset and resolution of inflammation. Nat Rev Immunol. 2010;10(6):427–39.
70. Martin NT, Martin MU. Interleukin 33 is a guardian of barriers and a local alarmin. Nat Immunol. 2016;17(2):122–31.
71. Dahlin JS, Feinstein R, Cui Y, Heyman B, Hallgren J. CD11c+ cells are required for antigen-induced increase of mast cells in the lung. J Immunol. 2012;189(8):3869–77.
72. Walker BE. Mast cell turn-over in adult mice. Nature. 1961;192:980–1.
73. Padawer J. Mast cells: extended lifespan and lack of granule turnover under normal in vivo conditions. Exp Mol Pathol. 1974;20(2):269–80.
74. Dahlin JS, Hallgren J. Mast cell progenitors: origin, development and migration to tissues. Mol Immunol. 2015;63(1):9–17.
75. Drissen R, Buza-Vidas N, Woll P, Thongjuea S, Gambardella A, Giustacchini A, et al. Distinct myeloid progenitor-differentiation pathways identified through single-cell RNA sequencing. Nat Immunol. 2016;17(6):666–76.
76. Rodewald HR, Dessing M, Dvorak AM, Galli SJ. Identification of a committed precursor for the mast cell lineage. Science. 1996;271(5250):818–22.
77. Ngkelo A, Richart A, Kirk JA, Bonnin P, Vilar J, Lemitre M, et al. Mast cells regulate myofilament calcium sensitization and heart function after myocardial infarction. J Exp Med. 2016;213(7):1353–74.
78. Hallgren J, Jones TG, Abonia JP, Xing W, Humbles A, Austen KF, et al. Pulmonary CXCR2 regulates VCAM-1 and antigen-induced recruitment of mast cell progenitors. Proc Natl Acad Sci U S A. 2007;104(51):20478–83.
79. Patella V, Marino I, Arbustini E, Lamparter-Schummert B, Verga L, Adt M, et al. Stem cell factor in mast cells and increased mast cell density in idiopathic and ischemic cardiomyopathy. Circulation. 1998;97(10):971–8.
80. Terada T, Matsunaga Y. Increased mast cells in hepatocellular carcinoma and intrahepatic cholangiocarcinoma. J Hepatol. 2000;33(6):961–6.
81. Molin D, Edstrom A, Glimelius I, Glimelius B, Nilsson G, Sundstrom C, et al. Mast cell infiltration correlates with poor prognosis in Hodgkin's lymphoma. Br J Haematol. 2002;119(1):122–4.
82. Sugamata M, Ihara T, Uchiide I. Increase of activated mast cells in human endometriosis. Am J Reprod Immunol. 2005;53(3):120–5.

83. Abonia JP, Hallgren J, Jones T, Shi T, Xu Y, Koni P, et al. Alpha-4 integrins and VCAM-1, but not MAdCAM-1, are essential for recruitment of mast cell progenitors to the inflamed lung. Blood. 2006;108(5):1588–94.

84. Poglio S, De Toni-Costes F, Arnaud E, Laharrague P, Espinosa E, Casteilla L, et al. Adipose tissue as a dedicated reservoir of functional mast cell progenitors. Stem Cells. 2010;28(11):2065–72.

85. Gurish MF, Tao H, Abonia JP, Arya A, Friend DS, Parker CM, et al. Intestinal mast cell progenitors require CD49dbeta7 (alpha4beta7 integrin) for tissue-specific homing. J Exp Med. 2001;194(9):1243–52.

86. Dahlin JS, Ivarsson MA, Heyman B, Hallgren J. IgE immune complexes stimulate an increase in lung mast cell progenitors in a mouse model of allergic airway inflammation. PLoS One. 2011;6(5):e20261.

87. Dwyer DF, Barrett NA, Austen KF, Immunological Genome Project Consortium. Expression profiling of constitutive mast cells reveals a unique identity within the immune system. Nat Immunol. 2016;17(7):878–87.

88. Gautier EL, Shay T, Miller J, Greter M, Jakubzick C, Ivanov S, et al. Gene-expression profiles and transcriptional regulatory pathways that underlie the identity and diversity of mouse tissue macrophages. Nat Immunol. 2012;13(11):1118–28.

89. Patella V, de Crescenzo G, Lamparter-Schummert B, De Rosa G, Adt M, Marone G. Increased cardiac mast cell density and mediator release in patients with dilated cardiomyopathy. Inflamm Res. 1997;46(Suppl 1):31–2.

90. Levick SP, McLarty JL, Murray DB, Freeman RM, Carver WE, Brower GL. Cardiac mast cells mediate left ventricular fibrosis in the hypertensive rat heart. Hypertension. 2009;53(6):1041–7.

91. Cairns A, Constantinides P. Mast cells in human atherosclerosis. Science. 1954;120(3105):31–2.

92. Kokkonen JO, Kovanen PT. Low density lipoprotein degradation by rat mast cells. Demonstration of extracellular proteolysis caused by mast cell granules. J Biol Chem. 1985;260(27):14756–63.

93. Kokkonen JO, Kovanen PT. Stimulation of mast cells leads to cholesterol accumulation in macrophages in vitro by a mast cell granule-mediated uptake of low density lipoprotein. Proc Natl Acad Sci U S A. 1987;84(8):2287–91.

94. Willems S, Vink A, Bot I, Quax PH, de Borst GJ, de Vries JP, et al. Mast cells in human carotid atherosclerotic plaques are associated with intraplaque microvessel density and the occurrence of future cardiovascular events. Eur Heart J. 2013;34(48):3699–706.

95. Sinkiewicz W, Sobanski P, Bartuzi Z. Allergic myocardial infarction. Cardiol J. 2008;15(3):220–5.

96. Shore SA. Obesity and asthma: possible mechanisms. J Allergy Clin Immunol. 2008;121(5):1087–93. quiz 94-5.

97. Frangogiannis NG, Lindsey ML, Michael LH, Youker KA, Bressler RB, Mendoza LH, et al. Resident cardiac mast cells degranulate and release preformed TNF-alpha, initiating the cytokine cascade in experimental canine myocardial ischemia/reperfusion. Circulation. 1998;98(7):699–710.

98. Bot I, van Berkel TJ, Biessen EA. Mast cells: pivotal players in cardiovascular diseases. Curr Cardiol Rev. 2008;4(3):170–8.

99. Hara M, Ono K, Hwang MW, Iwasaki A, Okada M, Nakatani K, et al. Evidence for a role of mast cells in the evolution to congestive heart failure. J Exp Med. 2002;195(3):375–81.

100. Janicki JS, Brower GL, Levick SP. The emerging prominence of the cardiac mast cell as a potent mediator of adverse myocardial remodeling. Methods Mol Biol. 2015;1220:121–39.

101. Reber LL, Marichal T, Galli SJ. New models for analyzing mast cell functions in vivo. Trends Immunol. 2012;33(12):613–25.

102. Feyerabend TB, Weiser A, Tietz A, Stassen M, Harris N, Kopf M, et al. Cre-mediated cell ablation contests mast cell contribution in models of antibody- and T cell-mediated autoimmunity. Immunity. 2011;35(5):832–44.

103. Forman MF, Brower GL, Janicki JS. Rat cardiac mast cell maturation and differentiation following acute ventricular volume overload. Inflamm Res. 2006;55(10):408–15.

104. Walker JA, Barlow JL, McKenzie AN. Innate lymphoid cells--how did we miss them? Nat Rev Immunol. 2013;13(2):75–87.
105. Mebius RE, Rennert P, Weissman IL. Developing lymph nodes collect CD4+CD3- LTbeta+ cells that can differentiate to APC, NK cells, and follicular cells but not T or B cells. Immunity. 1997;7(4):493–504.
106. Eberl G, Marmon S, Sunshine MJ, Rennert PD, Choi Y, Littman DR. An essential function for the nuclear receptor RORgamma(t) in the generation of fetal lymphoid tissue inducer cells. Nat Immunol. 2004;5(1):64–73.
107. Kruglov AA, Grivennikov SI, Kuprash DV, Winsauer C, Prepens S, Seleznik GM, et al. Nonredundant function of soluble LTalpha3 produced by innate lymphoid cells in intestinal homeostasis. Science. 2013;342(6163):1243–6.
108. Monticelli LA, Sonnenberg GF, Abt MC, Alenghat T, Ziegler CG, Doering TA, et al. Innate lymphoid cells promote lung-tissue homeostasis after infection with influenza virus. Nat Immunol. 2011;12(11):1045–54.
109. Scandella E, Bolinger B, Lattmann E, Miller S, Favre S, Littman DR, et al. Restoration of lymphoid organ integrity through the interaction of lymphoid tissue-inducer cells with stroma of the T cell zone. Nat Immunol. 2008;9(6):667–75.
110. Sawa S, Lochner M, Satoh-Takayama N, Dulauroy S, Berard M, Kleinschek M, et al. RORgammat+ innate lymphoid cells regulate intestinal homeostasis by integrating negative signals from the symbiotic microbiota. Nat Immunol. 2011;12(4):320–6.
111. Rak GD, Osborne LC, Siracusa MC, Kim BS, Wang K, Bayat A, et al. IL-33-dependent group 2 innate lymphoid cells promote cutaneous wound healing. J Invest Dermatol. 2016;136(2):487–96.
112. Dudakov JA, Hanash AM, Jenq RR, Young LF, Ghosh A, Singer NV, et al. Interleukin-22 drives endogenous thymic regeneration in mice. Science. 2012;336(6077):91–5.
113. Lindemans CA, Calafiore M, Mertelsmann AM, O'Connor MH, Dudakov JA, Jenq RR, et al. Interleukin-22 promotes intestinal-stem-cell-mediated epithelial regeneration. Nature. 2015;528(7583):560–4.
114. Diefenbach A, Colonna M, Koyasu S. Development, differentiation, and diversity of innate lymphoid cells. Immunity. 2014;41(3):354–65.
115. Mjosberg J, Spits H. Type 2 innate lymphoid cells-new members of the "type 2 franchise" that mediate allergic airway inflammation. Eur J Immunol. 2012;42(5):1093–6.
116. Hazenberg MD, Spits H. Human innate lymphoid cells. Blood. 2014;124(5):700–9.
117. Kloverpris HN, Kazer SW, Mjosberg J, Mabuka JM, Wellmann A, Ndhlovu Z, et al. Innate lymphoid cells are depleted irreversibly during acute HIV-1 infection in the absence of viral suppression. Immunity. 2016;44(2):391–405.
118. Munneke JM, Bjorklund AT, Mjosberg JM, Garming-Legert K, Bernink JH, Blom B, et al. Activated innate lymphoid cells are associated with a reduced susceptibility to graft-versus-host disease. Blood. 2014;124(5):812–21.
119. Karrich JJ, Cupedo T. Group 3 innate lymphoid cells in tissue damage and graft-versus-host disease pathogenesis. Curr Opin Hematol. 2016;23(4):410–5.
120. Constantinides MG, McDonald BD, Verhoef PA, Bendelac A. A committed precursor to innate lymphoid cells. Nature. 2014;508(7496):397–401.
121. Klose CS, Flach M, Mohle L, Rogell L, Hoyler T, Ebert K, et al. Differentiation of type 1 ILCs from a common progenitor to all helper-like innate lymphoid cell lineages. Cell. 2014;157(2):340–56.
122. Xu W, Domingues RG, Fonseca-Pereira D, Ferreira M, Ribeiro H, Lopez-Lastra S, et al. NFIL3 orchestrates the emergence of common helper innate lymphoid cell precursors. Cell Rep. 2015;10(12):2043–54.
123. Yu Y, Tsang JC, Wang C, Clare S, Wang J, Chen X, et al. Single-cell RNA-seq identifies a PD-1hi ILC progenitor and defines its development pathway. Nature. 2016;539(7627):102–6.
124. Gasteiger G, Fan X, Dikiy S, Lee SY, Rudensky AY. Tissue residency of innate lymphoid cells in lymphoid and nonlymphoid organs. Science. 2015;350(6263):981–5.

125. O'Sullivan TE, Rapp M, Fan X, Weizman OE, Bhardwaj P, Adams NM, et al. Adipose-resident group 1 innate lymphoid cells promote obesity-associated insulin resistance. Immunity. 2016;45(2):428–41.

126. Stanya KJ, Jacobi D, Liu S, Bhargava P, Dai L, Gangl MR, et al. Direct control of hepatic glucose production by interleukin-13 in mice. J Clin Invest. 2013;123(1):261–71.

127. Brestoff JR, Kim BS, Saenz SA, Stine RR, Monticelli LA, Sonnenberg GF, et al. Group 2 innate lymphoid cells promote beiging of white adipose tissue and limit obesity. Nature. 2015;519(7542):242–6.

128. Lee MW, Odegaard JI, Mukundan L, Qiu Y, Molofsky AB, Nussbaum JC, et al. Activated type 2 innate lymphoid cells regulate beige fat biogenesis. Cell. 2015;160(1–2):74–87.

129. Vivier E, van de Pavert SA, Cooper MD, Belz GT. The evolution of innate lymphoid cells. Nat Immunol. 2016;17(7):790–4.

130. Yan X, Anzai A, Katsumata Y, Matsuhashi T, Ito K, Endo J, et al. Temporal dynamics of cardiac immune cell accumulation following acute myocardial infarction. J Mol Cell Cardiol. 2013;62:24–35.

131. Klarlund K, Pedersen BK, Theander TG, Andersen V. Depressed natural killer cell activity in acute myocardial infarction. Clin Exp Immunol. 1987;70(1):209–16.

132. Atochina O, Harn D. LNFPIII/LeX-stimulated macrophages activate natural killer cells via CD40-CD40L interaction. Clin Diagn Lab Immunol. 2005;12(9):1041–9.

133. Nussbaum JC, Van Dyken SJ, von Moltke J, Cheng LE, Mohapatra A, Molofsky AB, et al. Type 2 innate lymphoid cells control eosinophil homeostasis. Nature. 2013;502(7470):245–8.

134. Miller AM, Xu D, Asquith DL, Denby L, Li Y, Sattar N, et al. IL-33 reduces the development of atherosclerosis. J Exp Med. 2008;205(2):339–46.

135. Mantani PT, Duner P, Bengtsson E, Alm R, Ljungcrantz I, Soderberg I, et al. IL-25 inhibits atherosclerosis development in apolipoprotein E deficient mice. PLoS One. 2015;10(1):e0117255.

136. Hofmann U, Knorr S, Vogel B, Weirather J, Frey A, Ertl G, et al. Interleukin-13 deficiency aggravates healing and remodeling in male mice after experimental myocardial infarction. Circ Heart Fail. 2014;7(5):822–30.

137. Sonnenberg GF, Artis D. Innate lymphoid cells in the initiation, regulation and resolution of inflammation. Nat Med. 2015;21(7):698–708.

138. Li Z, Hodgkinson T, Gothard EJ, Boroumand S, Lamb R, Cummins I, et al. Epidermal Notch1 recruits RORgamma(+) group 3 innate lymphoid cells to orchestrate normal skin repair. Nat Commun. 2016;7:11394.

139. Aparicio-Domingo P, Romera-Hernandez M, Karrich JJ, Cornelissen F, Papazian N, Lindenbergh-Kortleve DJ, et al. Type 3 innate lymphoid cells maintain intestinal epithelial stem cells after tissue damage. J Exp Med. 2015;212(11):1783–91.

140. Nishimura Y, Inoue T, Nitto T, Morooka T, Node K. Increased interleukin-13 levels in patients with chronic heart failure. Int J Cardiol. 2009;131(3):421–3.

141. Mjosberg JM, Trifari S, Crellin NK, Peters CP, van Drunen CM, Piet B, et al. Human IL-25- and IL-33-responsive type 2 innate lymphoid cells are defined by expression of CRTH2 and CD161. Nat Immunol. 2011;12(11):1055–62.

142. Klein Wolterink RG, Kleinjan A, van Nimwegen M, Bergen I, de Bruijn M, Levani Y, et al. Pulmonary innate lymphoid cells are major producers of IL-5 and IL-13 in murine models of allergic asthma. Eur J Immunol. 2012;42(5):1106–16.

143. Neill DR, Wong SH, Bellosi A, Flynn RJ, Daly M, Langford TK, et al. Nuocytes represent a new innate effector leukocyte that mediates type-2 immunity. Nature. 2010;464(7293):1367–70.

144. Roediger B, Kyle R, Yip KH, Sumaria N, Guy TV, Kim BS, et al. Cutaneous immunosurveillance and regulation of inflammation by group 2 innate lymphoid cells. Nat Immunol. 2013;14(6):564–73.

145. Lee JS, Seppanen E, Patel J, Rodero MP, Khosrotehrani K. ST2 receptor invalidation maintains wound inflammation, delays healing and increases fibrosis. Exp Dermatol. 2016;25(1):71–4.

146. Chang YJ, Kim HY, Albacker LA, Baumgarth N, McKenzie AN, Smith DE, et al. Innate lymphoid cells mediate influenza-induced airway hyper-reactivity independently of adaptive immunity. Nat Immunol. 2011;12(7):631–8.

147. Mizuno S, Mikami Y, Kamada N, Handa T, Hayashi A, Sato T, et al. Cross-talk between RORgammat+ innate lymphoid cells and intestinal macrophages induces mucosal IL-22 production in Crohn's disease. Inflamm Bowel Dis. 2014;20(8):1426–34.

148. Manta C, Heupel E, Radulovic K, Rossini V, Garbi N, Riedel CU, et al. CX(3)CR1(+) macrophages support IL-22 production by innate lymphoid cells during infection with Citrobacter rodentium. Mucosal Immunol. 2013;6(1):177–88.

149. Longman RS, Diehl GE, Victorio DA, Huh JR, Galan C, Miraldi ER, et al. CX(3)CR1(+) mononuclear phagocytes support colitis-associated innate lymphoid cell production of IL-22. J Exp Med. 2014;211(8):1571–83.

150. Yokota Y, Mansouri A, Mori S, Sugawara S, Adachi S, Nishikawa S, et al. Development of peripheral lymphoid organs and natural killer cells depends on the helix-loop-helix inhibitor Id2. Nature. 1999;397(6721):702–6.

151. Hofmann U, Beyersdorf N, Weirather J, Podolskaya A, Bauersachs J, Ertl G, et al. Activation of CD4+ T lymphocytes improves wound healing and survival after experimental myocardial infarction in mice. Circulation. 2012;125(13):1652–63.

152. Weirather J, Hofmann UD, Beyersdorf N, Ramos GC, Vogel B, Frey A, et al. Foxp3+ CD4+ T cells improve healing after myocardial infarction by modulating monocyte/macrophage differentiation. Circ Res. 2014;115(1):55–67.

153. Oliphant CJ, Hwang YY, Walker JA, Salimi M, Wong SH, Brewer JM, et al. MHCII-mediated dialog between group 2 innate lymphoid cells and CD4(+) T cells potentiates type 2 immunity and promotes parasitic helminth expulsion. Immunity. 2014;41(2):283–95.

Index

© Springer International Publishing AG 2017
S. Sattler, T. Kennedy-Lydon (eds.), *The Immunology of Cardiovascular Homeostasis and Pathology*, Advances in Experimental Medicine and Biology 1003, DOI 10.1007/978-3-319-57613-8

CPI Antony Rowe
Chippenham, UK
2017-07-11 21:36